EMERGING INFECTIONS

Microbial Threats to Health in the United States

Joshua Lederberg, Robert E. Shope,
and Stanley C. Oaks, Jr., *Editors*

Committee on Emerging Microbial Threats to Health
Division of Health Sciences Policy
Division of International Health

INSTITUTE OF MEDICINE

NATIONAL ACADEMY PRESS
Washington, D.C. 1992

NATIONAL ACADEMY PRESS • 2101 Constitution Avenue, N.W. • Washington, D.C. 20418

NOTICE: The project that is the subject of this report was approved by the Governing Board of the National Research Council, whose members are drawn from the councils of the National Academy of Sciences, the National Academy of Engineering, and the Institute of Medicine. The members of the committee responsible for the report were chosen for their special competences and with regard for appropriate balance.

This report has been reviewed by a group other than the authors according to procedures approved by a Report Review Committee consisting of members of the National Academy of Sciences, the National Academy of Engineering, and the Institute of Medicine.

The Institute of Medicine was chartered in 1970 by the National Academy of Sciences to enlist distinguished members of the appropriate professions in the examination of policy matters pertaining to the health of the public. In this, the Institute acts under both the Academy's 1863 congressional charter responsibility to be an adviser to the federal government and its own initiative in identifying issues of medical care, research, and education. Dr. Kenneth I. Shine is president of the Institute of Medicine.

Funding for this study was provided by the Centers for Disease Control, the Fogarty International Center, Lederle-Praxis Laboratories, the Lucille P. Markey Charitable Trust, the National Institute of Allergy and Infectious Diseases of the National Institutes of Health, the Rockefeller Foundation, and the U.S. Army Medical Research and Development Command.

Library of Congress Cataloging-in-Publication Data

Emerging infections : Microbial threats to health in the United States
  / Joshua Lederberg, Robert E. Shope, and Stanley C. Oaks, Jr.,
  editors.
            p.   cm.   Sixth Printing, June 1997
        Includes bibliographical references and index.
        ISBN 0-309-04741-2
        1. Communicable diseases—United States. I. Lederberg, Joshua.
    II. Shope, Robert E. III. Oaks, S. C.
    RA643.5.E43 1992
    614.4'273—dc20   92-26480
                                                             CIP

Printed in the United States of America

The serpent has been a symbol of long life, healing, and knowledge among almost all cultures and religions since the beginning of recorded history. The image adopted as a logotype by the Institute of Medicine is based on a relief carving from ancient Greece, now held by the Staatlichemuseen in Berlin.

COVER: The background for the cover of this report is a photograph of batik designed and printed specifically for the Malaysian Society of Parasitology and Tropical Medicine. The print contains drawings of various parasites and insects; it is used with the kind permission of the Society.

COMMITTEE ON EMERGING MICROBIAL THREATS TO HEALTH

JOSHUA LEDERBERG (*Co-chair*),[*] University Professor and Sackler Foundation Scholar, Rockefeller University, New York, New York

ROBERT E. SHOPE (*Co-chair*), Professor of Epidemiology and Director, Yale Arbovirus Research Unit, Yale University School of Medicine, New Haven, Connecticut

BARRY R. BLOOM,[*] Weinstock Professor and Chairman, Department of Microbiology and Immunology, and Investigator, Howard Hughes Medical Institute, Albert Einstein College of Medicine, Yeshiva University, Bronx, New York

ROBERT L. BUCHANAN, Research Leader, Microbial Food Safety Research Unit, Agricultural Research Service, Eastern Regional Research Center, U.S. Department of Agriculture, Philadelphia, Pennsylvania

JOHN R. DAVID,[†] Richard Pearson Strong Professor and Chairman, Department of Tropical Public Health, Harvard School of Public Health, and Professor of Medicine, Harvard Medical School, Boston, Massachusetts

CIRO A. DE QUADROS, Regional Advisor, Expanded Programme on Immunization, Pan American Health Organization, Washington, D.C.

PATRICIA N. FULTZ, Associate Professor, Department of Microbiology, University of Alabama, Birmingham

JOHN J. HOLLAND, Professor, Department of Biology and Institute for Molecular Biology, University of California, San Diego, La Jolla, California

DEAN T. JAMISON, Professor, Department of Community Health Sciences and Department of Education, University of California, Los Angeles

EDWIN D. KILBOURNE,[§] Distinguished Service Professor, Department of Microbiology, Mount Sinai School of Medicine, New York, New York

ADEL A. F. MAHMOUD,[†] John H. Hord Professor of Medicine and Chairman, Department of Medicine, Case Western Reserve University, University Hospitals of Cleveland, Cleveland, Ohio

GERALD L. MANDELL, Professor of Medicine, Owen R. Cheatham Professor of Sciences, and Head, Division of Infectious Diseases, Department of Internal Medicine, University of Virginia, Charlottesville

STEPHEN S. MORSE, Assistant Professor, Rockefeller University, New York, New York

JUNE E. OSBORN,[†] Dean and Professor of Epidemiology, School of Public Health, and Professor of Pediatrics and Communicable Disease, Medical School, University of Michigan, Ann Arbor

WILLIAM C. REEVES, Professor Emeritus of Epidemiology, School of Public Health, University of California, Berkeley

iii

PHILIP K. RUSSELL, Professor of International Health, School of Hygiene and Public Health, Johns Hopkins University, Baltimore, Maryland

ALEXIS SHELOKOV, Director of Medical Affairs, the Salk Institute-Government Services Division, San Antonio, Texas

P. FREDERICK SPARLING, Chairman, Department of Medicine, University of North Carolina School of Medicine, Chapel Hill

ANDREW SPIELMAN, Professor of Tropical Public Health, Department of Tropical Public Health, Harvard School of Public Health, Boston, Massachusetts

PROJECT STAFF

RUTH ELLEN BULGER, Director, Division of Health Sciences Policy
POLLY F. HARRISON, Director, Division of International Health
STANLEY C. OAKS, JR., Study Director
ELIZABETH E. MEYER, Research Associate
NANCY DIENER, Budget Analyst
GREG W. PEARSON, Consultant Writer/Editor

---

*Member, Institute of Medicine and National Academy of Sciences
†Member, Institute of Medicine
§Member, National Academy of Sciences

iv

Preface

As the human immunodeficiency virus (HIV) disease pandemic surely should have taught us, in the context of infectious diseases, there is nowhere in the world from which we are remote and no one from whom we are disconnected. Consequently, some infectious diseases that now affect people in other parts of the world represent potential threats to the United States because of global interdependence, modern transportation, trade, and changing social and cultural patterns.

The United States currently expends 14 percent of its gross national product on health; the vast majority of the money is spent on curative medicine to treat people who are already ill. The major premise of this report is that anticipation and prevention of infectious diseases are possible, necessary, and ultimately cost-effective.

In the battle against infectious disease, drugs, vaccines, and pesticides are important weapons. Because of the evolutionary potential of many microbes, however, the use of these weapons may inadvertently contribute to the selection of certain mutations, adaptations, and migrations that enable pathogens to proliferate or nonpathogens to acquire virulence. In those circumstances in which humankind has been successful in the battle against specific diseases, complacency (i.e., the assumption that we have conquered a disease and can thus shift our concern to other pressing problems) can also constitute a major threat to health. Such complacency can extend beyond those infectious diseases that have been successfully suppressed to embrace the concept that all infectious diseases are readily suppressed because of the advances of modern medicine. Shifting priorities, therefore, can allow for the reemergence, as well as the emergence, of diseases.

In May 1989, Rockefeller University, the National Institute of Allergy and Infectious Diseases, and the Fogarty International Center co-sponsored a conference on emerging viral agents. Although the conference focused on viruses, it spurred interest in the emergence and resurgence of *all* classes of infectious agents.

At the conference and in other forums, concern was expressed about the apparent complacency of the scientific and medical communities, the public, and the political leadership of the United States toward the danger of emerging infectious diseases and the potential for devastating epidemics. Recognizing these concerns, the Board on Health Sciences Policy of the Institute of Medicine (IOM) determined that the IOM could play a unique role by reviewing the relevant science, developing a research agenda, considering the implications for policy, and making specific recommendations for minimizing the public health impact of future emerging microbial threats. In mid-1989, a study proposal was developed and approved, and sponsors were secured. Thus, the 1989 conference served as an excellent prelude to the IOM study.

In February 1991, the IOM convened a 19-member multidisciplinary committee to conduct an 18-month study of emerging microbial threats to health. Committee expertise comprised the fields of epidemiology, virology, immunology, food safety microbiology, food toxicology, public health, molecular biology, cell biology, economics, microbial genetics, parasitology, infectious diseases, microbial pathogenesis, medical entomology and systematics, and bacterial physiology.

The charge to the Committee on Emerging Microbial Threats to Health was to identify significant emerging infectious diseases, determine what might be done to deal with them, and recommend how similar future threats might be confronted to lessen their impact on public health. The committee did not address biological warfare because this issue is already under study by another panel within the National Academy of Sciences.

The full committee held four meetings over the course of the study. At the first meeting, it was noted that a significant number of the members had ties to the biotechnology industry, which involved specific products such as diagnostic test kits and vaccines. Because the committee was not expected to make any disease- or product-specific recommendations, these ties were not considered to be conflicts of interest.

Also at the first meeting, the committee determined that, owing to the breadth of the topic, it would confine its work to emerging microbial threats to U.S. public health; it recognized, however, that even that topic could not be adequately addressed without considering emerging threats globally. The committee's recommendations thus target U.S. public health concerns, although they may have some relevance for the global population. The IOM published two earlier reports that bear on microbial threats outside the

United States: *The U.S. Capacity to Address Tropical Infectious Disease Problems* (1987) and *Malaria: Obstacles and Opportunities* (1991).

In addition to the meetings of the full committee, four task forces and a subcommittee met over the course of the study. The task forces provided additional information in four areas: bacteria, chlamydiae, and rickettsiae; viruses; protozoans, helminths, and fungi; and policy options. The subcommittee met to refine the committee's conclusions and recommendations.

For the purposes of this report, the committee makes an important distinction between infection and disease. Infection implies that an agent, such as a virus, has taken up residence in a host and is multiplying within it— perhaps with no outward signs or symptoms. In contrast, those who appear "sick" are said to have a "disease," and generally it is for these individuals that public concern is greatest. In fact, though, many more people usually are infected with the causative agent or exposed to the source of infection (such as an insect vector) than become ill. Controlling or limiting the disease depends in many cases on suppressing transmission. For example, although chronic carriers of hepatitis B virus or *Salmonella* bacteria may not be ill themselves, they are capable of transmitting infections to susceptible individuals and thus are a potential threat to public health.

Rather than organize the report around specific diseases, the committee decided to focus on factors that are implicated in the emergence of infectious diseases within the United States. The report begins with an executive summary, which reviews the main points of the committee's deliberations and presents its recommendations from Chapter 3. Chapter 1 provides background material for the general reader, lays out some of the reasons for optimism about the future, tempers that with information on some diseases that have recently emerged or that are emerging, and outlines the fundamental problems that must be addressed if we are to be prepared for the future. Chapter 2 defines "emerging microbial threats to health," identifies and discusses major factors in the emergence of such threats, and gives specific examples of situations in which these factors have been important to the emergence or reemergence of disease. The factors discussed are (1) human demographics and behavior, (2) technology and industry, (3) economic development and land use, (4) international travel and commerce, (5) microbial adaptation and change, and (6) breakdown of public health measures. Chapter 3 considers past and current efforts to address emerging threats in the context of recognition and intervention; it includes the committee's recommendations for approaching current and future emerging microbial threats. The report is written in large part as background for the general reader because the committee believes that the public needs to understand the importance of these threats.

It is this committee's considered opinion that the next major infectious agent to emerge as a threat to health in the United States may, like HIV, be a pathogen that has not been previously recognized. Therefore, rather than attempt to list and discuss all organisms that might pose a future threat, this report uses examples to illustrate principles involved in the emergence of contemporary infectious diseases and the resurgence of old diseases. It is the committee's hope that lessons from the past will illuminate possible approaches to prevention and control of these diseases in the future.

Joshua Lederberg, Co-chair   Robert E. Shope, Co-chair

Acknowledgments

In addition to the work of the committee and staff, the successful completion of a study such as this requires input from many people. The committee wishes to express its sincere gratitude to those who participated in the various task forces (see Appendix A) and prepared background papers: Scott Halstead of the Rockefeller Foundation, D. A. Henderson of the Office of Science and Technology Policy, Jonathan Kaplan and William Reeves, Jr. of the Centers for Disease Control, James LeDuc of the U.S. Army Medical Research Institute of Infectious Diseases, Llewellyn Legters of the Uniformed Services University of the Health Sciences, and Thomas Monath of OraVax, Incorporated. The contributions of these individuals, who gave generously of their time and expertise, were critical to the preparation of this report.

The committee also thanks those who gave presentations to its members: Deborah Keimig of the Armed Forces Medical Intelligence Center; Mitchel Cohen, Joseph Davis, Samuel Dooley, Jr., Walter Dowdle, Robert Gaynes, James Hughes, Brian Mahy, Joseph McDade, C. J. Peters, William Reeves, Jr., William Roper, and Stephen Thacker of the Centers for Disease Control; John Gingrich of the Defense Pest Management Information Analysis Center; Anthony Fauci of the National Institutes of Health; D. A. Henderson of the Office of Science and Technology Policy; and Thomas Monath of OraVax, Incorporated. These presentations contributed useful information and insightful consideration of issues related to emerging microbes.

The committee gratefully acknowledges the following who provided tables, graphs, funding data, and other information critical to the committee's deliberations: Marcia Lane of the American Association of Blood Banks; Brooke Whiting of the Association of American Medical Colleges; Janet Shoemaker of the American Society for Microbiology; Anthony Robbins of the Boston University Medical Center; Carmine Bozzi, Louisa Chapman, Nancy Cox, David Dennis, Robert Gaynes, Philip Horn, James Hughes, Robert Kaiser, Lauri Markowitz, Charles McCance, Peter Schantz, Carl Schieffelbein, and Dixie Snider, Jr. of the Centers for Disease Control; Jonathan Mann of the Harvard AIDS Institute; John Mekalanos of the Harvard Medical School; Gerald Meyers of Los Alamos National Laboratory; Marta Glass, Michael Gottlieb, James Meegan, Mona Rowe, Christine Stone, Tina Suhana, and Karl Western of the National Institutes of Health; Daniel Lahn of the National Vaccine Program Office; Lyman Roberts of the Office of the Surgeon General, U.S. Army; Jean-Marc Olivè of the Pan American Health Organization; Charles Clements of SatelLife; Francis Cole, Jr., and Stephen Speights of the U.S. Army Medical Research and Development Command; Roy Widdus of the U.S. Commission on AIDS; Maridette Schloe of the University of California, Los Angeles; Sam Joseph of the University of Maryland, College Park; Charles Hoke of the Walter Reed Army Institute of Research; and C. J. Clements, Marjorie Dam, and Akira Shirai of the World Health Organization.

We owe special recognition and thanks to Stanley Oaks, study director, who helped organize the committee, guided us through the study process, and assumed major responsibility for the preparation of this report, and to Elizabeth Meyer, research associate, whose many contributions included preparing meeting summaries, collecting and cataloging references, and the drafting of case studies, charts, tables, appendices, and several of the boxes scattered throughout the report. We also thank April Powers, Linda Clark, Lisa Jager, and Mary Jane Ball, project assistants, who helped with meeting planning and logistics, prepared briefing materials, and provided general committee support. Special thanks are owed to Greg Pearson, consultant editor/writer, who worked to incorporate the many pieces of written material into a coherent draft and who prepared the executive summary. Others within the Institute of Medicine who were instrumental to the work of the committee are Ruth Ellen Bulger and Polly Harrison, directors of the Divisions of Health Sciences Policy and International Health, respectively.

This study took place during a period of transition at the Institute of Medicine. Samuel Thier was president of the IOM at the initiation of the study. Following his move to Brandeis University in the fall of 1991, Stewart Bondurant became acting president. In January 1992, Kenneth Shine was designated president-elect; he assumed his full responsibilities in July 1992. The committee offers its sincere gratitude to these leaders and to Enriqueta Bond, the IOM executive officer, who provided guidance and advice during this critical period.

Joshua Lederberg, Co-chair   Robert E. Shope, Co-chair

Contents

EMERGING INFECTIONS

Microbial Threats to Health in the United States

Executive Summary

Disease-causing microbes have threatened human health for centuries. The Institute of Medicine's Committee on Emerging Microbial Threats to Health believes that this threat will continue and may even intensify in coming years. The committee's report, which is summarized here, describes key elements responsible for the emergence of infectious diseases; it also presents recommendations that, if appropriately implemented, should allow the United States to be better prepared to recognize and respond rapidly to these public health threats.

What are the factors, operating both singly and in combination, that are contributing to the emergence of such pathogens? Like other living organisms, infectious agents are subject to genetic change and evolution. This quality is manifested by their ability to infect new hosts, by alterations in their susceptibility to antimicrobial drugs, and by changes in their response to host immunity. Alterations can also occur in geographic ranges; in some cases, modern transport has led to rapid movement of agents throughout the world. The human host has changed as well. We have adopted new types of personal behavior and new food-processing methods that may enhance transmission of some microbes. New diseases and modern medical treatments may result in immunosuppression and thus increase susceptibility to pathogenic microorganisms. Moreover, in recent years, the human population has experienced rapid growth and increased mobility resulting in intrusion into new ecological settings. These changes in infectious agents and human populations favor exposure to new pathogens and more efficient transmission of recognized microbes.

Other changes are also affecting disease emergence. For example, some infectious agents exist in vertebrate reservoirs such as wild animals. These

1

agents, in some instances, have migrated and increased in number. Some microbes that are transmitted by insects or other vectors exhibit these characteristics as well; in addition, they may have become resistant to pesticides, which impedes efforts at control. Finally, the environment has changed and will continue to change. Humanity has altered the world's ecology through deforestation, urbanization, and industrialization, which some believe may lead to global climate change. Moreover, the world periodically experiences civil unrest and war, which can lead to regional breakdowns in sanitation, allowing microbes to flourish. Individually and collectively, these and other factors lead to the emergence and reemergence of microbial pathogens.

Infectious diseases remain the major cause of death worldwide (World Health Organization, 1992) and will not be conquered during our lifetimes. With the application of new scientific knowledge, well-planned intervention strategies, adequate resources, and political will, many of these diseases may be prevented by immunization, contained by the use of drugs or vector-control methods, and, in a very few cases, even eradicated—but the majority are likely to persevere. We can also be confident that new diseases will emerge, although it is impossible to predict their individual emergence in time and place. The committee believes that there are steps that can and must be taken to prepare for these eventualities. Its recommendations address both the recognition of and interventions against emerging infectious diseases.

RECOGNITION

The key to recognizing new or emerging infectious diseases, and to tracking the prevalence of more established ones, is surveillance. A well-designed, well-implemented surveillance program can detect unusual clusters of disease, document the geographic and demographic spread of an outbreak, and estimate the magnitude of the problem. It can also help to describe the natural history of a disease, identify factors responsible for emergence, facilitate laboratory and epidemiological research, and assess the success of specific intervention efforts.

The importance of surveillance to the detection and control of emerging microbial threats cannot be overemphasized. Poor surveillance leaves policymakers and medical and public health professionals with no basis for developing and implementing policies to control the spread of infectious diseases. The committee does not know whether the impact of human immunodeficiency virus (HIV) disease could have been limited if there had been an effective global infectious disease surveillance system in place in the late 1960s or early 1970s. However, without such a system in place, we would have little chance for early detection of emerging diseases in the future.

Current U.S. disease surveillance efforts include both domestic and international components. Domestically, the bulk of federal disease-reporting requirements (individual states also require reporting) are implemented through the National Notifiable Diseases Surveillance System, established in 1961 and administered by the Centers for Disease Control (CDC). The CDC also operates a domestic influenza surveillance program that supplies epidemiological information to public health officials, physicians, the media, and the public.

Notwithstanding such programs, the United States has no comprehensive national system for detecting outbreaks of infectious disease (except for food- and waterborne diseases). Outbreaks of any disease that is not on CDC's current list of notifiable illnesses may go undetected or may be detected only after an outbreak is well under way. Emerging infectious diseases, with the exception of those reportable diseases that reemerge, also are not detected through established surveillance activities. Another problem is the lack of coordination among the various U.S. government agencies, or between government agencies and private organizations, involved in these efforts. The effectiveness of U.S. domestic surveillance could be vastly improved by designating an agency or central coordinating body as a focus for such activities.

The committee recommends the development and implementation of strategies that would strengthen state and federal efforts in U.S. surveillance. Strategy development could be a function of the Centers for Disease Control (CDC). Alternatively, the strategy development and coordination functions could be assigned to a federal coordinating body (e.g., a subcommittee of the Federal Coordinating Council for Science, Engineering, and Technology's [FCCSET] Committee on Life Sciences and Health,[1] specifically constituted to address this issue. Implementation of the strategies would be assigned to the appropriate federal agencies (e.g., CDC, National Institutes of Health, U.S. Department of Agriculture). Approaches for consideration could include simplifying current reporting forms and procedures, establishing a telephone hotline by which physicians could report unusual syndromes, and using electronic patient data collected by insurance companies to assist in infectious disease surveillance.

---

[1]The FCCSET is a federally appointed body of experts that serve on seven standing committees and act as a mechanism for coordinating science, engineering, technology, and related activities of the federal government that involve more than one agency. In addition to conducting cross-cutting analyses of programs and budgets, the various committees and their subcommittees (interagency working groups) examine wide-ranging topics with the goal of reaching consensus on fundamental assumptions and procedures that can guide the actions of the participating agencies in achieving their mission objectives more effectively.

A second major domestic disease surveillance effort is the National Nosocomial Infections Surveillance System (NNISS), which currently gathers data from approximately 120 sentinel hospitals and is operated by CDC's Hospital Infection Program. Although nosocomial diseases constitute an important share of the burden of disease in this country, the system has several major limitations. For example, it cannot correct for differences among participating hospitals in diagnostic testing, intensity of surveillance, and provisions for postdischarge surveillance. The requirement that NNISS member hospitals have at least 100 beds, and the relatively small sample of hospitals that are included in the system, are also potential sources of bias. Current plans call for improvements in the dissemination of NNISS data, the inclusion of a surveillance component for immunosuppressed patients, and the addition of more sentinel hospitals, among other efforts.

The committee recommends that additional resources be allocated to the Centers for Disease Control to enhance the National Nosocomial Infections Surveillance System (NNISS) in the following ways:

1. Include data on antiviral drug resistance.

2. Include information on morbidity and mortality from nosocomial infections.

3. Increase the number of NNISS member hospitals.

4. Strive to make NNISS member hospitals more representative of all U.S. hospitals.

5. Evaluate the sensitivity and specificity of nosocomial infection surveillance activities performed in NNISS member hospitals.

6. Determine the reliability of antimicrobial susceptibility testing performed in NNISS member hospitals.

Considerable effort and resources are being expended on the various surveillance activities in which U.S. government agencies and the private sector participate. Much of this information, however, is not readily accessible. There is currently no single database from which a physician, researcher, health care worker, public health official, or other interested party can obtain information on disease incidence, antibiotic drug resistance, drug and vaccine availability, or other topics that might be relevant to infectious disease surveillance, prevention, treatment, and control.

The committee recommends that the U.S. Public Health Service develop a comprehensive, computerized infectious disease database. Such a database might consolidate information from more specialized sources, such as the National Nosocomial Infections Surveillance System (NNISS), the National Electronic Telecommunications System for Surveillance (NETSS), and the influenza surveillance system; it could also include

additional information, such as vaccine and drug availability. As an alternative, expansion of currently available databases and provisions for easy access to these sources should be aggressively pursued. The implementation of such a program should also encompass expanded efforts to inform physicians, public health workers, clinical laboratories, and other relevant target groups of the availability of this information.

U.S.-supported overseas laboratories have played a historic role in the discovery and monitoring of infectious diseases. The United States and other nations first created these disease surveillance posts, many of them in tropical and subtropical countries, to protect the health of their citizens who were sent to settle or administer recently acquired territory. After World War II, there was a second blossoming of such surveillance activities. The Fogarty International Center was established, as were several overseas laboratories staffed by Department of Defense personnel. Privately funded activities, like those of the Rockefeller Foundation Virus Program, were also important contributors to infectious disease surveillance at the international level.

Over the past two decades, a number of these facilities have been closed or are no longer operating with U.S. oversight. Nevertheless, although its efforts are substantially reduced from previous levels, the United States still maintains an international presence in infectious disease surveillance and research. As is the case in related domestic efforts, however, international infectious disease surveillance activities undertaken by U.S. government agencies remain largely uncoordinated and in need of a strategy to focus them in appropriate areas, such as emerging diseases.

The committee recommends that international infectious disease surveillance activities of U.S. government agencies be coordinated by the Centers for Disease Control (CDC). To provide the necessary link between U.S. domestic and international surveillance efforts, the body that is established for this purpose should be the same as that suggested earlier in the recommendation on domestic surveillance. Alternatively, a federal coordinating body (e.g., a subcommittee of the Federal Coordinating Council for Science, Engineering, and Technology's [FCCSET] Committee on Life Sciences and Health, specifically constituted to address this issue) could be assigned the coordinating function. Implementation of surveillance activities, however, should remain with the appropriate federal agencies (e.g., the CDC, Department of Defense, National Institutes of Health, U.S. Department of Agriculture).

The efforts of multilateral international organizations, such as the World Health Organization (WHO), are critical in coordinating infectious disease surveillance worldwide. The WHO is a focal point for surveillance data on several globally important infectious diseases; it also operates a number of surveillance networks around the world, composed of selected "collaborating centers," that report and investigate outbreaks of specific diseases, such as influenza and HIV disease. The WHO is often involved in early investigative efforts related to newly emerging or reemerging infectious diseases (e.g., Ebola, Lassa, yellow, and dengue fevers).

Current U.S. and international surveillance efforts are certainly of great value in detecting known infectious and noninfectious diseases. They fall short, however, in their ability to detect emerging infectious diseases. There has been no effort to develop and implement a global program of surveillance for emerging diseases or disease agents.

The committee believes that an effective global surveillance network on emerging infectious diseases is an essential element in efforts to combat microbial threats and that it should have four basic components:

1. a mechanism for detecting (using clinical presentation as the criterion) clusters of new or unusual diseases or syndromes;
2. laboratories capable of identifying and characterizing infectious agents;
3. an information system to analyze reportable occurrences and disseminate summary data; and
4. a response mechanism to provide feedback to reporting agencies and individuals and, if necessary, to mobilize investigative and control efforts of local and international agencies.

A global surveillance network should also comprise such elements as locally staffed surveillance centers to promote regional self-reliance and train local personnel, links to academic centers and other regional facilities involved in basic research, a clinical arm for hospital-based surveillance and drug and vaccine trials, an effective specimen collection and transport system, and an active system of data analysis and dissemination, with feedback to those providing data. Models that may offer useful lessons for the design of such a network include the WHO's global influenza surveillance network and its collaborating centers for specific diseases, the Pan American Health Organization's (PAHO) polio eradication program, and earlier infectious disease initiatives, such as the WHO smallpox eradication campaign and the Rockefeller virus program.

The committee recommends that the United States take the lead in promoting the development and implementation of a comprehensive global infectious disease surveillance system. Such an effort could be undertaken through the U.S. representatives to the World Health Assembly. The system should capitalize on the lessons from past successes and on

the infrastructure, momentum, and accomplishments of existing inter-national networks, expanding and diversifying surveillance efforts to include known diseases as well as newly recognized ones. This effort, of necessity, will be multinational and will require regional and global coordination, advice, and resources from participating nations.

INTERVENTION

The recognition of an emerging infectious disease is the first component of response, but what follows that recognition may, in fact, determine the final impact of an emerging disease on the public's health. Effective inter-vention against such diseases necessitates coordinated efforts by a variety of individuals, government agencies, and private organizations. The com-mittee believes that the current U.S. capability for responding to microbial threats to health lacks organization and resources. The recommendations in the subsections below address these deficiencies.

The U.S. Public Health System

In the United States, principal responsibility for protecting the public's health rests with the 50 state health departments, or their counterparts, and more than 3,000 local health agencies. At the federal level, the national focus for disease assessment is the CDC. A 1988 Institute of Medicine (IOM) report, *The Future of Public Health*, described the U.S. public health system as being in a state of disarray that has produced "a hodgepodge of fractionated interests and programs, organizational turmoil among new agencies, and well-intended but unbalanced appropriations—without coher-ent direction by well-qualified professionals." It is the committee's view that there has been little positive change in the U.S. public health system since the release of that report. The recent rapid increases in the incidence of measles and tuberculosis are evidence of these continuing problems.

Steps have now been taken to address inadequacies in programs for these diseases, but these responses are reactive, not proactive. It is the committee's belief that the *prevention* of infectious diseases must be stressed if the health of this nation's inhabitants is to be maintained or improved. Greater efforts directed at the recognition of and responses to emerging public health problems, particularly emerging infectious diseases, would help achieve this goal.

The problems of the U.S. public health system are attracting the atten-tion of policymakers. Recently, the U.S. Public Health Service published a set of strategies for improving disease surveillance, epidemiology, and com-munication, three key areas of weakness cited in the 1988 IOM report. A number of these strategies are particularly relevant to the emerging disease issues addressed by this committee. If implemented, these suggested improvements will, in part, respond to recommendations made in this report.

Research and Training

Many of the factors that are responsible for, or that contribute to, the emergence of infectious diseases are now known. Yet our understanding of these factors and of how they interact is incomplete. We are a long way from being able to develop strategies to anticipate the emergence of infectious diseases and to prevent them from becoming significant threats to health. The committee nevertheless sees this kind of development as a desirable long-term goal and concludes that research to achieve it should be strongly encouraged.

In July 1991, the National Institute of Allergy and Infectious Diseases (NIAID) convened a task force on microbiology and infectious diseases to identify promising research opportunities and to recommend research strategies for future NIAID programs. The committee has reviewed the January 1992 NIAID task force report, and it believes that its studies and the work of the task force are complementary. Consequently, the committee fully supports the conclusions and recommendations of the NIAID task force.

The committee recommends the expansion and coordination of National Institutes of Health-supported research on the agent, host, vector, and environmental factors that lead to emergence of infectious diseases. Such research should include studies on the agents and their biology, pathogenesis, and evolution; vectors and their control; vaccines; and antimicrobial drugs. One approach might be to issue a request for proposals (RFP) to address specific factors related to infectious disease emergence.

Several programs support research and training related to the epidemiology, prevention, and control of infectious diseases. Whether they involve U.S. or foreign scientists, have a broad or narrow focus, all of these programs contribute to the international capability to recognize and respond to emerging infectious diseases. The Rockefeller Foundation's International Clinical Epidemiology Network trains junior medical school faculty from developing countries in the discipline of epidemiology. After their training, these individuals return to their home countries, where they become part of a medical school-based training unit that helps evaluate the availability, effectiveness, and efficacy of health care.

Recently, the NIAID consolidated the International Collaboration in Infectious Disease Research (which allows U.S. scientists to develop overseas work experience) and the Tropical Disease Research Units (which focus on six diseases cited by the WHO as major health problems in the tropics) programs, as well as several other efforts in international health under one new initiative, the International Centers for Tropical Disease Research.

The CDC currently supports research and training in the area of infectious diseases through its National Center for Infectious Diseases. Earlier efforts by the agency, however, may have valuable components that deserve revisiting. For example, from the mid-1960s to the early 1970s, the CDC administered an extramural program that awarded grants to academic and other institutions for research in infectious disease prevention and control. The committee has concluded that this now defunct program filled a need for support in a critical area of research.

The committee recommends increased research on surveillance methods and applied control strategies; on the costs and benefits of prevention, control, and treatment of infectious disease; and on the development and evaluation of diagnostic tests for infectious diseases. Reinstating and expanding (both in size and scope) the extramural grant program at the Centers for Disease Control, which ceased in 1973, would be one important step in this direction. Similarly, the Food and Drug Administration's (FDA) extramural grant program should be expanded to place greater emphasis on the development of improved laboratory tests for detecting emerging pathogens in food.

An adequate supply of well-trained, experienced epidemiologists is critical to the nation's surveillance efforts. CDC's Epidemic Intelligence Service (EIS) provides health professionals with two years of training and field experience in public health epidemiology. The EIS is the model as well for another evolving program, the joint CDC/WHO Field Epidemiology Training Program (FETP), which places field-oriented epidemiologists in countries that need to develop and implement disease prevention and control programs. Current and former EIS officers and FETP graduates are important sources of information on emerging diseases and constitute a personnel nucleus for a global surveillance network. The distribution of these epidemiologists, however, is restricted because of the limited number of program graduates each year.

The committee recommends the domestic and global expansion of the Center for Disease Control's (CDC) Epidemic Intelligence Service program and continued support for CDC's role in the Field Epidemiology Training Program.

The seven overseas medical research laboratories maintained by the U.S. Department of Defense are the most broadly based international facilities of their kind supported by the United States. In addition to being well situated to recognize and study emerging disease threats, the facilities are valuable sites for testing new drugs and vaccines, because they are located in areas of the world in which the diseases of interest are endemic.

The committee recommends continued support—at a minimum, at their current level of funding—of Department of Defense overseas infectious disease laboratories.

In the area of training, previous studies have noted shortages of medical entomologists, clinical specialists trained in tropical disease diagnosis, prevention, and control, biomedical researchers, and public health specialists. The National Health Service Corps scholarship program, created in 1972, underwrites the costs of medical education in return for medical service in underserved areas of the United States. The committee is unaware of any similar program directed at individuals who wish to train for careers in public health and related disciplines. Such a program might attract those who otherwise would not consider careers in public health.

The committee recommends that Congress consider legislation to fund a program, modeled on the National Health Service Corps, for training in public health and related disciplines, such as epidemiology, infectious diseases, and medical entomology.

Vaccine and Drug Development

Vaccines and antimicrobial drugs have led to significant improvements in public health in the United States and in many other nations during the latter half of this century. Despite this encouraging history, the committee is concerned that many of the vaccines and drugs available today are the same ones that have been used for decades. It believes that there is a need to review the present vaccine and drug armamentaria with a view toward improving availability and "surge" capacity, as well as safety and efficacy.

VACCINES

Advances in immunology, molecular biology, biochemistry, and drug delivery systems have stimulated major new initiatives in vaccine development. As a result, the generation of vaccines that will come into use in the next decade is likely to be different from previous vaccines. For example, some will contain more than one highly purified antigen and will rely on new delivery methods. For all their potential, however, vaccines should not be viewed as magic bullets for defeating emerging microbial threats to health. The potential value of vaccination and the speed with which vaccines can be developed depend on many factors, such as the existing scientific knowledge of the agent (or a similar organism), its molecular biology, rate of transmission, pathogenesis, how the human immune system responds to natural infection, and the nature of protective immunity.

Economic factors may also impede vaccine development, because it requires an extensive, up-front investment in research. Most vaccine manufacturers (and policymakers) are reluctant to make the necessary financial commitment since few vaccines are highly profitable and strict federal safety and efficacy requirements make the risk of failure a very real possibility. Vaccine developers must also take into account the extra costs that may arise from liability claims for injuries or deaths blamed on vaccines. This concern has forced a number of vaccine manufacturers out of the marketplace.

Industry might be encouraged to assume a greater role in vaccine development if it was asked to participate in a public/private sector collaboration, similar to NIH's National Cooperative Vaccine Development Groups, whose focus is HIV disease vaccines. Another alternative might be to offer industry various economic incentives, such as minimum guaranteed purchases, to conduct its own development work.

Given the various disincentives to vaccine development for more common pathogens, the development of vaccines for emerging microbes is even more problematic. There may be potentially catastrophic consequences if the development process is left entirely to free enterprise. The committee thus believes that a comprehensive strategy is urgently needed. To bring a new vaccine rapidly from the research laboratory into general use—a necessary criterion if one hopes to prevent or control an emerging infectious disease—will require an integrated national process that

• defines the need for a vaccine, its technical requirements, target populations, and delivery systems;

• ensures the purchase and use of the developed product through purchase guarantees and targeted immunization programs;

• relies as much as possible on the capability of private industry to manage the vaccine development process, through the use of contracted production, if necessary;

• utilizes the capacity of the NIAID to manage and support basic, applied, clinical, and field research, and of the CDC and academia to conduct field evaluations and develop implementation programs;

• is centrally coordinated to take maximum advantage of the capabilities of the public and private sectors; and

• is prepared for the possible rapid emergence of novel disease threats, such as occurred in the 1918-1919 influenza pandemic.

The committee recommends that the United States develop a means for generating stockpiles of selected vaccines and a "surge" capacity for vac-

cine development and production that could be mobilized to respond quickly to future infectious disease emergencies. Securing this capability would require development of an integrated national process, as described above. The committee offers two options for implementation of this recommendation:

1. Develop an integrated management structure within the federal government and provide purchase guarantees, analogous to farm commodity loans, to vaccine manufacturers that are willing to develop the needed capacity.

2. Build government-supported research and development and production facilities, analogous to the National Cancer Institute's program for cancer therapeutics and the federal space, energy, and defense laboratories. The assigned mission of these new facilities would be vaccine development for future infectious disease contingencies.

ANTIMICROBIAL DRUGS

The usefulness of antimicrobial drugs can be ensured only if they are used carefully and responsibly, and if new antimicrobials are continually being developed. The development of drug resistance by microorganisms, as well as the emergence of new organisms, will require replacement drugs to be in the "pipeline" even while existing drugs are still effective. The establishment of public/private sector alliances, along the lines of the National Cooperative Drug Development Groups at the NIH, may be desirable to ensure the continued development of effective antimicrobial drugs.

The committee recommends that clinicians, the research and development community, and the U.S. government (Centers for Disease Control, Food and Drug Administration, U.S. Department of Agriculture, and Department of Defense) introduce measures to ensure the availability and usefulness of antimicrobials and to prevent the emergence of resistance. These measures should include the education of health care personnel, veterinarians, and users in the agricultural sector regarding the importance of rational use of antimicrobials (to preclude their unwarranted use), a peer review process to monitor the use of antimicrobials, and surveillance of newly resistant organisms. Where required, there should be a commitment to publicly financed rapid development and expedited approval of new antimicrobials.

Vector Control

The United States and other developed countries have been able to free themselves to a remarkable degree from the burden of vector-borne diseases by using a variety of methods of vector control. These methods include the spraying of chemical pesticides, application of biological control agents, destruction or treatment of larval development sites, and personal protection measures, such as applying repellents or sleeping under bednets.

For a disease agent that is known or suspected to be transmitted by an arthropod vector, efforts to control the vector can be vital for containing or halting an outbreak. This is true even for those vector-borne diseases, such as yellow fever or malaria, for which there is or may eventually be an effective vaccine. For most vector-borne infectious diseases, the onset of winter dampens transmission; it can even, in some cases, eliminate the vector or infectious agent. The exceptions are pathogens that can survive in humans for long periods and produce chronic infection (e.g., malaria and typhus). A sudden drop in cases of an unidentified disease at the start of winter may be the first epidemiological evidence that the disease is vector borne.

Although many local and regional vector-control programs can effectively combat small and even medium-size outbreaks of vector-borne disease, they are not equipped to deal with outbreaks that are national in scope. For example, regional vector-control programs cannot declare a health emergency or bypass the many legal restrictions that now limit the use of certain pesticides that are potentially useful agents for control. That authority rests with health and environmental agencies at the state and federal levels. The lack of a sufficient stockpile of effective pesticides, which might be required in the event of a major epidemic, continues to be a serious problem.

The committee recommends that the Environmental Protection Agency develop and implement alternative, expedited procedures for the licensing of pesticides for use in vector-borne infectious disease emergencies. These procedures would include a means for stockpiling designated pesticides for such use.

A growing problem in vector control is the diminishing supply of effective pesticides. Federal and state regulations increasingly restrict the use and supply of such chemicals, largely as a result of concerns over human health or environmental safety. In addition, the 1972 Federal Insecticide, Fungicide, and Rodenticide Act (FIFRA; Public Law No. 92-516) requires that all pesticides used in the United States be re-registered by 1997, a procedure that requires manufacturers to submit additional safety data. Some pesticide manufacturers have chosen not to re-register their products because of the expense of gathering necessary safety data. Partly as a result, many effective pesticides developed over the past 40 years are no longer available in the United States.

The Environmental Protection Agency (EPA) further restricts the use of pesticides through the Endangered Species Protection Plan, which prohibits the application of a wide range of pesticidal chemicals within the habitat of any endangered species. EPA has developed an emergency exemption procedure to allow pesticide use in restricted areas when the possibility of an outbreak of a vector-borne disease is great. This procedure, however, is extremely cumbersome and time-consuming, and the committee believes that it is essentially useless if followed as prescribed, since emergency approval of a pesticide is likely to come after the critical period during which its use could avert an outbreak.

As with vaccines, there is little economic incentive for firms to develop new pesticides for public health use, primarily because such use is a very small fraction of the total pesticide market. Pesticide development is now driven mainly by the demands of agriculture. Moreover, as pesticide development has become more specialized, there are fewer compounds available that have both agricultural and public health uses. The committee feels strongly that pesticide development for public health applications needs to be given some priority.

The committee recommends that additional priority and funding be afforded efforts to develop pesticides (and effective modes of application) and other measures for public health use in suppressing vector-borne infectious diseases.

Public Education and Behavioral Change

Public policy discussions and scientific efforts sometimes focus on vaccine and drug development to the exclusion of education and behavioral change as means for preventing and controlling outbreaks of infectious disease. This is unfortunate, because it is often only by changing patterns of human activity—from travel, personal hygiene, and food handling to sexual behavior and drug abuse—that the spread of disease can be halted.

Even when scientists and public health officials rely on and encourage education and behavioral change to prevent or limit the spread of infectious disease, the public may not be convinced of its necessity. Although scientists may see emerging microbes as a very real threat to public health, the average citizen may be unaware of the potential danger or may consider those dangers to be less important than other health risks, like heart disease and cancer. In such instances, a carefully conceived media campaign may have a beneficial effect on behavior that affects disease transmission.

The committee recommends that the National Institutes of Health give increased priority to research on personal and community health practices relevant to disease transmission. Attention should also be focused on developing more effective ways to use education to enhance the health-promoting behavior of diverse target groups.

*   *   *   *   *

It is the committee's hope that this report will be an important first step in highlighting the growing problem of emerging microbial threats to health and focus attention on ways in which the United States and the global community will attempt to address such threats, now and in the future. The committee strongly believes that the best way to prepare for the future is by developing and implementing preventive strategies that can meet the challenges offered by emerging and reemerging microbes. It is infinitely less costly, in every dimension, to attack an emerging disease at an early stage—and thus prevent its spread—than to rely on treatment to control the disease.

In some instances, the measures that this report proposes will require additional funds. The committee recognizes and has wrestled with the discomforts that such recommendations can bring—for example, the awareness that there are other compelling needs that also justify (and require) increased expenditures. But policymakers and the public alike must realize and understand the potential magnitude of future epidemics in terms of human lives and monetary costs. The 1957 and 1968 influenza pandemics killed 90,000 people in the United States alone. The direct cost of medical care was estimated to be $3.4 billion (more than three times the NIAID budget for fiscal year 1992) and the total economic burden to be $26.8 billion[2]—almost three times the total NIH budget for fiscal year 1992. A more current example offers a similar lesson. The recent resurgence of TB (from 22,201 cases in 1985 to 26,283 cases in 1991, or 10.4 per 100,000 population), after a steady decline over the past several decades, will be costly. Every dollar spent on TB prevention and control in the United States produces an estimated $3 to $4 in savings; these savings increase dramatically when the cost of treating multidrug-resistant tuberculosis is factored in. We also have a recent example of what results when early prevention and control efforts are lacking. The costs of AIDS/HIV disease—in human lives as well as dollars—have been staggering, and the end is not yet in sight. The objective in the future should be earlier detection of such emerging diseases, coupled with a timely effort to inform the population about how to lower their risk of becoming infected.

Obviously, even with unlimited funds, no guarantees can be offered that an emerging microbe will not spread disease and cause devastation. Instead, this committee cautiously advocates increased funding and proposes some more effective ways for organizations—domestic and international, public and private—as well as individuals—both health professionals and the lay public—to work together and, in some cases, combine their resources. These efforts will help to ensure that we will be better prepared to respond to emerging infectious disease threats of the future.

---

[2]Figures are in 1992 dollars.

1

Background

Infectious disease epidemics and pandemics have occurred throughout human history. Progress in medical science has made us less vulnerable to their devastation now than at any point in the past. Nevertheless, the nation's current experience with the human immunodeficiency virus (HIV) and acquired immunodeficiency syndrome (AIDS) is a sobering reminder that serious microbial threats to health remain and that we are not always well equipped to respond to them.

As we approach the twenty-first century, it must be remembered that large segments of the world's population still struggle against bacterial, viral, protozoal, helminthic, and fungal invaders. Before addressing the current situation, two past experiences are worth highlighting: the plague pandemic of the mid-1300s and the influenza pandemic of the early 1900s. Both demonstrate the potential danger of uncontrolled infectious disease.

PLAGUE

Plague, caused by the bacterium *Yersinia pestis*, has ancient roots. In the *Iliad*, for example, Homer makes reference to a plague-like illness prevalent during the Trojan War (1190 B.C.) that he noted was associated with the movement of rats into populated areas (Marks and Beatty, 1976). We know now that plague bacteria are transmitted to humans by fleas whose primary hosts are rodents. Rats, ground squirrels, rabbits, and, occasionally, even house cats can harbor infected fleas. The last great epidemic of plague occurred early in this century in India (causing more than 10 million deaths) (Mandell et al., 1990).

Bubonic plague, the most common form of the disease, is acquired directly from the bite of an infected flea. Other, less common forms of plague include pneumonic, which can develop from the bubonic form and is spread directly from person to person by the respiratory route; septicemic; and meningeal, or plague meningitis. Bubonic plague derives its name from the characteristic swollen lymph nodes (called buboes) in the groin, axilla, and neck areas. Untreated bubonic plague is fatal in half of all cases; untreated pneumonic plague is invariably fatal.

Plague is probably best known because of its role in the Black Death (so called because of the gangrenous extremities often seen in those with advanced disease), a devastating pandemic that swept through much of Asia and Europe during the Middle Ages. Some 20 million people, representing 20 to 25 percent of Western Europe's total populace, are thought to have died during a four-year period (McEvedy, 1988). In large European cities during the peak of the epidemic, people died in such great numbers that few were left to bury the dead. An accurate count of plague victims—especially the poor, who lived in the most crowded conditions—was impossible.

The Black Death arrived in Europe from central Asia in 1346, probably by the "Silk Road," a trading route from Asia to Europe. It reached Italy by ship from Caffa (McEvedy, 1988). Like many pandemics, its spread was made possible by the devices of transportation. Medical historians believe that the plague bacillus was endemic in the marmot population of Central Asia. It is likely that Mongol invaders who killed marmots for their fur inadvertently extended the range of the *Y. pestis*-infected rodents and their fleas. The Mongols often rode long distances in a single day and may thereby have transported an occasional infected rat or some fleas as they moved along the trade routes toward Europe (McNeill, 1976).

In the late 1890s, bubonic plague appears to have been introduced into San Francisco by infected rats traveling aboard an Asian merchant ship. In 1900, a small outbreak of the disease developed in the Chinese population of San Francisco. That same year, ground squirrels were found to be infected; soon the plague bacillus had infected most of the area's burrowing rodents (McNeill, 1976). Plague infection is now enzootic in much of the rodent population in the western United States, Mexico, and Canada.

Thanks to modern sanitation and the availability of antibiotics and pesticides, another occurrence of the Black Death seems unlikely. Still, an outbreak is not out of the question, particularly in regions, including the western United States and parts of South America, Africa, and Asia, where wild rodent populations are persistently infected with the plague bacillus. Isolated cases of plague are reported to this day in various parts of the world, including the United States. Crowding and poor sanitation, if they occur in or near areas where rodent plague is enzootic, could provide conditions for the reemergence of this once devastating bacterial illness. Current legal restrictions on the use of most pesticides in recreational and wildlife areas limit our ability to control plague in the event of an epizootic.

INFLUENZA

Influenza, like plague, has caused illness and death among humans for hundreds of years. Given this history, it is somewhat disconcerting that today many people consider this viral disease an unpleasant but basically harmless illness. A diagnosis of influenza nowadays often generates little more than sympathy from one's friends and family, yet one need look no further than the early 1900s to realize the seriousness of the threat that can be posed by this pathogen.

Although influenza pandemics have varied in the severity of their impact, all have caused widespread disease and death. This was especially true of the 1918 influenza A pandemic, which claimed more than 20 million lives worldwide in less than a year and ranks among the worst disasters in human history. In the United States alone, it is estimated that one in four people became ill during the pandemic and that 500,000 died. Mortality from influenza and pneumonia was estimated as 4.8 per 1,000 cases in 1918, three times that of immediately preceding years.

The symptoms of infection with influenza virus are familiar to nearly everyone: fever, chills, headache, muscular aches, and cough. Although most people recover fully within a week, even during pandemics, the elderly, the very young, and those with chronic diseases are at risk of death from the viral infection itself or from complications resulting from secondary bacterial pneumonia. (This kind of pneumonia is responsible for most influenza deaths in persons over the age of 60.)

The origin of the 1918 influenza pandemic remains in doubt, but it may have begun with a mild but sizable outbreak of illness in the United States early in that year, concurrent with the final stages of World War I. The outbreak was confined primarily to military camps and crowded workplaces and was distinctive, in retrospect, because of the large number of young adults who died of the disease. Overall, however, the initial mortality rate was low, and in many places the outbreak passed without comment. Indeed, what turned out to be the first wave of the pandemic was recognized only after the second wave had passed.

The first wave swept across North America in March and April and then subsided almost as rapidly as it had appeared; the infection moved on to Europe, where it first reached epidemic levels in France in April 1918. Over the following several months, influenza spread throughout the whole of Europe. European-based fighting forces found themselves losing the service of significant numbers of troops to what became popularly known (except in Spain) as the Spanish flu, owing to its high incidence in Spain.

Although only 2 to 3 percent of those who fell ill died, the unusually high fatality rate among previously healthy young adults meant the loss of a disproportionate number of society's most productive members. This first wave spread rapidly, encircling the globe in less than five months.

The disease resurfaced in a more virulent form in the United States in August of 1918, causing large numbers of deaths in many U.S. cities as it spread from the East Coast to California. Health authorities reacted by requiring citizens to wear masks in public places and by taking other steps that were presumed to prevent the spread of disease. Many of these efforts were not put in place, however, until the worst of the epidemic had passed.

A third wave, in the spring of 1919, completed what is usually described as the Great Pandemic, although substantial influenza mortality in 1920 might have been the result of the same outbreak (Kilbourne, 1987). The 1918 influenza pandemic affected such a large number of people over such a wide geographic area that it has been the focus of a number of studies (Hoehling, 1961; Crosby, 1976; Osborn, 1977; Neustadt and Fineberg, 1978; Kilbourne, 1987).

Although the 1918 pandemic ranks as one of the single most devastating outbreaks of infectious disease in human history, the technology of the time did not permit the virus to be isolated. Thus, no sample of the causative influenza strain is available for study, which means that the virus's remarkable virulence and transmissibility have not been investigated using the tools of modern molecular virology. Serological evidence suggests, however, that a virus antigenically similar to the 1918 influenza virus persists to this day in swine.

Since the 1918 pandemic, there have been two major global outbreaks of influenza A in the twentieth century—in 1957 and 1968. Significant but less serious pandemics occurred in 1947 and 1977. A potentially serious outbreak appeared imminent in 1976 but, for reasons that are still not clear, never materialized. Some see this 1976 episode as evidence of a failure to judge correctly the threat posed by a human pathogen. Others say that the experience simply points out how difficult it is to predict accurately the course of what could have been a devastating epidemic.

It is impossible to know when the next influenza pandemic will strike. Dangerous new pandemic influenza viruses are most likely to be the result of genetic reassortment of two different, existing influenza viruses. Fortunately, "successful" reassortments are rare. Even so, the danger of such recombinations is always present, and many scientists believe it is simply a matter of time before one occurs again. The lethal 1983 epidemic of avian influenza in chickens (caused by a point mutation in the H5N2 subtype) is a stark reminder that small changes in the viral genome can produce pathogens of exceptional virulence and transmissibility (Kawaoka and Webster, 1988).

OPTIMISM AND INDIFFERENCE

As will be made clear throughout this report, the number and variety of microbial threats to human health are daunting. Just as clear, however, is the fact that tremendous strides have been and continue to be made in the battle against infectious diseases. In particular, advances in medical science and public health practices have vastly improved our understanding of and ability to control many of these illnesses.

Penicillin, discovered in 1929 and eventually produced in a usable form during World War II, was the first of a multitude of new antibiotics that have saved the lives of many who otherwise would have succumbed to bacterial infections. Similarly, the development and mass production of effective vaccines against such diseases as measles, pertussis, diphtheria, and polio have prevented large segments of the population from contracting these and other very serious diseases. More recently, advances in biotechnology, in particular, genetic engineering, have made it possible to produce drugs, vaccines, and other therapeutic agents with increased specificity.

Also important in the battle against infectious disease have been interventions against arthropod vectors of disease agents. Pesticides have played a critical role in suppressing arthropod-borne diseases in the United States and abroad. Unfortunately, excessive agricultural use of some pesticides has resulted in the destruction of nonpest insects and, in some cases, in food and water contamination. Public health use of these chemicals can also cause resistance in the very insects they are intended to kill. In the United States, these environmental and public health concerns led to a 1972 ban on the agricultural use of DDT, a broadly effective and inexpensive means of controlling many insect pests. Ten years later, U.S. production of the chemical ceased altogether, and there was a dramatic worldwide drop in its use. Increasingly, insect resistance and legal restrictions on pesticide use are hindering efforts to control disease-carrying vectors with the repertoire of potentially available chemicals.

One of the most effective ways of preventing epidemics of arthropod-borne diseases has been to eliminate the sites in which the vectors breed and develop. This approach was attempted inadvertently as long ago as the sixth century B.C., when the Greeks and Romans undertook major engineering projects to drain marshy swamps in an effort to control outbreaks of fever, which it is now believed were due to malaria. General William C. Gorgas, a U.S. Army physician and engineer, effectively controlled malaria and yellow fever during construction of the Panama Canal (1904–1914) through a combination of drainage and larviciding (Gorgas and Hendrick, 1924). Another example is the eradication of *Aedes aegypti* from extensive areas of the Western Hemisphere by intensive control of the domestic water sources of this vector. Unfortunately, when such programs were ended, either for economic reasons or because limitations had been put on the use of pesticides, vector populations grew to pre-eradication levels (Soper et al., 1943).

Historically, advances in U.S. public health have come as a result of one or more major health crises—usually in the form of an epidemic or the fear of one. In the nineteenth century, for example, state and local authorities were willing to spend relatively large sums on sanitary and quarantine measures during epidemics, but once the danger was past, funds were eliminated and the health regulations fell into neglect. Fortunately, that pattern has changed somewhat; in its place, we have established and now maintain a system of health regulations and sanitary measures that generally protect the health of the U.S. population. Over time, however, systems deteriorate, and enforcement of regulations may become more lax. It is essential, therefore, that we continue vigorous efforts to prevent the introduction of infectious agents.

Sanitation and Hygiene

The practices of public sanitation and personal hygiene have dramatically reduced the incidence of certain infectious diseases. In the United States, the mistaken notion that exposed refuse was somehow responsible for outbreaks of yellow fever led to early efforts at sanitary control. In 1796, for example, the New York Medical Society declared that local conditions, especially the "intolerable stench" around the city's docks and the filth around slaughterhouses, were primarily responsible for outbreaks of epidemic fever, including yellow fever (Duffy, 1990). Laws were passed to establish a permanent health office to enforce quarantine regulations and to authorize the cleanup of city streets.

Clean water supplies and their protection from human and other wastes are now fundamental public health principles. Where good sanitary practices are followed, many diseases that once were epidemic, including cholera, are successfully controlled. The same may be said for personal hygiene. Hand washing is an effective method of preventing the spread of many infectious agents, including cold and enteric viruses. Similarly, safe food-handling practices, including proper storage, cleaning, and preparation, have resulted in fewer cases of bacterial food poisonings, among other benefits. The pasteurization of milk, which was instituted to prevent the transmission of bovine tuberculosis to humans, has been equally effective against other diseases such as brucellosis and salmonellosis.

Quarantine

The use of quarantine, another approach to controlling infectious diseases, dates back at least to the Middle Ages. The name itself derives from efforts in the mid-1400s by the Republic of Ragusa to prevent the spread of bubonic plague (McNeill, 1976). The republic, on the eastern shore of the Adriatic, required incoming ships to set anchor at sites away from the harbor. The ships' occupants were then required to spend 30 days ("trentina," later extended to 40 days, or "quarantina") in the open air and sunlight, a practice thought to preclude the spread of plague.

The earliest quarantine requirements in America were established in 1647 by the Massachusetts Bay Colony, specifically for ships arriving from Barbados. Other colonial settlements followed suit, with the goal of preventing the spread of yellow fever and smallpox (Williams, 1951). Quarantine proved to be an appropriate tool for controlling smallpox, an infectious viral disease spread easily from person to person, but the practice was ineffective in combating the spread of yellow fever, a mosquito-borne viral disease. In 1799, Congress granted authority for maritime quarantine to the secretary of the treasury and directed that state health laws (including quarantine of ships) be observed by customs officers.

In 1876, as a result of the failure of the Treasury Department to exercise its quarantine authority, U.S. Surgeon General John M. Woodworth proposed a national quarantine system. The proposal called for inspecting all incoming ships, conducting medical examinations of passengers and crews, and detaining under quarantine those thought to be infected. (The length of the quarantine was to be based on the incubation period of the specific disease in question.) These regulations were to be enforced by the Marine Hospital Service, the forerunner of the present U.S. Public Health Service (PHS).

Historically, there is no question that, as a public health measure, quarantine was relied upon more heavily than its practical value warranted. Detainment and isolation were extreme inconveniences to those affected; there was a stigma attached to being quarantined; the detection, restraint, and isolation of suspected cases of diseases that required quarantine were costly; and, because of the stigma, people failed to report their disease. Consequently, although quarantine was useful in controlling isolated outbreaks of human disease, and is still of value in combating epidemics of animal disease (if the animals thought to be infected are subsequently killed), for the most part quarantine policies did more harm than good.

Following World War II, the belief that the practice was of little use to modern disease control efforts began to gather support. A 1966 PHS advisory committee stated that "it is no longer possible to have confidence in the idea of building a fence around this country against communicable diseases, as is the traditional quarantine concept. The increasing volume and speed of international travel make this unrealistic" (Advisory Committee on Foreign Quarantine, 1966).

Following a reorganization of the PHS in 1967, the responsibility for quarantine was shifted to the Centers for Disease Control (CDC). For several years following that shift, CDC's Foreign Quarantine Division (currently the Division of Quarantine) operated 55 domestic quarantine stations and had a sizable presence abroad. Since then, this number has been greatly reduced, in line with modern epidemiological concepts and technologies. Last year, 7 domestic stations remained open, and in early 1992, the San Juan, Puerto Rico, station was reopened with a staff of one (C. McCance, Director, Division of Quarantine, Centers for Disease Control, personal communication, 1992).

Currently, the United States does not require immunizations for entry within its borders. The master of a ship or commander of an aircraft, however, must radio immediately to the quarantine station at or nearest the port of arrival to report any death or illness among passengers or crew. This procedure allows for the arriving carrier to be handled in a controlled manner. To supplement the few remaining quarantine stations, U.S. Immigration and Naturalization Service and U.S. Customs Service inspectors have been trained to inspect all passengers and crew for signs and symptoms of communicable diseases at ports to which CDC staff have been assigned. Persons who are suspected of being ill are referred to them; if the port has no such personnel, CDC staff at the nearest quarantine station are called. The agency has contract physicians at all ports of entry for medical backup. Certain animals, shipments of etiologic agents, and vectors of human diseases are required to have import permits, and their mode of shipment must conform to requirements.

Prior to 1985, CDC listed 26 diseases that invoked its authority to detain, isolate, or provisionally release persons at U.S. ports of entry. Today, only 7 such diseases are listed: yellow fever, cholera, diphtheria, infectious tuberculosis, plague, suspected smallpox, and viral hemorrhagic fevers. Over the past decade, this authority has been used only three times (C. McCance, Director, Division of Quarantine, Centers for Disease Control, personal communication, 1992).

Smallpox

The most heartening evidence of humankind's ability to triumph over infectious diseases is the eradication of smallpox. A systemic viral disease characterized by fever and the appearance of skin lesions, smallpox is believed by some to have been responsible for the death of more people than any other acute infectious disease. It has also been one of the most feared of all contagious diseases.

Like plague, smallpox was an ancient affliction. There is good reason to think that the Egyptian pharaoh Ramses V died of the disease in the mid-twelfth century B.C. (Fenner et al., 1988; Behbehani, 1991). A disease considered to be smallpox was mentioned in Chinese writings dating to the third century A.D. (Fenner et al., 1988).

Smallpox probably originated in either Egypt or India and over the ensuing centuries became endemic in both countries. The disease spread, eventually becoming pandemic, as explorers, soldiers, and others infected by the smallpox virus traveled to all parts of the globe. Smallpox was introduced into Mexico by the Spanish army in 1520, killing 3.5 million Aztec Indians (more than half the population) during the brief span of two years. By the late 1500s, the disease had also decimated the populations of South America. In Europe alone, during the seventeenth and eighteenth centuries, smallpox killed about 400,000 persons every year (Fenner et al., 1988; Behbehani, 1991). As late as the 1950s, there were some 50 million cases of smallpox worldwide each year. By 1967, the year that saw the start of the worldwide smallpox eradication program, between 10 and 15 million cases were reported annually (Fenner et al., 1988).

North America was not spared. The disease was introduced into Massachusetts by European settlers in 1617 and spread rapidly. Between 1636 and 1698, six major epidemics in Boston had caused a substantial number of deaths. Native Americans, like indigenous populations in other parts of the world, had never been exposed to the smallpox virus and were particularly hard hit; between one-half and two-thirds of the Plains Indians had died of smallpox by the time of the Louisiana Purchase. The practice of quarantine, instituted for the first time in the American colonies in a misguided effort to prevent the spread of yellow fever, was used with some success in the seventeenth century in the battle against smallpox. Nevertheless, epidemics during the eighteenth century sometimes affected as much as a third of the population. By 1785, smallpox had spread west to California and north to Alaska (Fenner et al., 1988).

The observation, perhaps as early as the tenth century in China, that uninfected people could be protected against smallpox infection by a process termed "variolation" offered the first hope that the disease could be controlled. In variolation, material from the pustule of an individual with smallpox was scratched into the skin of an uninfected person. In most instances, this procedure produced a self-limiting disease and, importantly, an immune reaction that protected those who had been variolated from future smallpox infection. Occasionally, people who were variolated would develop severe disease and die; furthermore, they could transmit the disease to others. Overall, however, variolation was blamed for only about a tenth as many deaths as were caused by naturally acquired smallpox. Variolation was introduced into the American colonies by Cotton Mather and was used extensively during the Revolutionary War.

Edward Jenner, an English physician, was aware that persons who worked with cows developed cowpox (a mild disease) but did not get smallpox. In

1796, Jenner inoculated a boy with cowpox lymph taken from a sore on a milkmaid. The child developed a mild local reaction. Six weeks later, he inoculated the boy with pus from a patient with smallpox. It produced no significant reaction; the boy was immune to the dreaded disease. Jenner used cowpox to immunize others against smallpox, a procedure called vaccination, which later became the means to prevent and subsequently eradicate the disease.

By the mid-1800s, Jenner's method of vaccinating against smallpox was being used in most parts of the world. The resulting steady decline in smallpox incidence was significant. In 1920, in the United States, more than 110,000 cases of smallpox were reported. By 1940, because of vaccination, fewer than 3,000 cases were reported. The last case of smallpox in the United States occurred in 1949 (Fenner et al., 1988).

Epidemic outbreaks of smallpox continued elsewhere, however, especially in countries lacking adequate health infrastructure and the economic means to support an immunization program. In 1967, a year in which there were some 2 million deaths worldwide from the disease (Fenner et al., 1988), the World Health Organization (WHO) initiated a global program to eradicate smallpox. The program combined widespread immunization in epidemic areas and extensive case-finding (surveillance and containment of disease outbreaks). During the program's 10-year life, much was learned about the importance of quality control in vaccine production and the need for flexibility in implementing a large-scale disease-control effort. Disease surveillance was key to the triumph over smallpox and is discussed more fully later in this report. The last naturally acquired case of smallpox was reported in Ethiopia in 1977.

Poliomyelitis

Currently, the Pan American Health Organization (PAHO), the WHO regional office for the Americas, is leading an effort to eradicate poliomyelitis (polio) from the Western Hemisphere. Begun in 1985, the PAHO polio eradication and surveillance program had three goals: achieving and maintaining high levels of vaccine coverage; intensifying surveillance to detect all new cases; and aggressively controlling outbreaks of disease. More than 20,000 health facilities are currently included in the program; 80 percent of them report weekly to a central facility.

By the end of 1991, it was evident that the program was succeeding. In that year, wild poliovirus was isolated from only eight persons in the Americas, whereas in 1986, there were more than 900 confirmed cases. All of the 1991 isolates were from children and were wild type 1 poliovirus (De Quadros et al., 1991). Importantly, by the end of that year, transmission of wild poliovirus seemed localized to one country, Peru. The program's ultimate goal of eradication of polio from the Americas thus appears to be closer and closer to achievement.

Several aspects of the program have helped it to succeed. The most important has been active feedback to data contributors. Not only do participating hospitals and clinics receive a weekly bulletin that summarizes and analyzes the data received by the central PAHO office each week (an activity greatly facilitated by the network of computers on which the surveillance system is based), but response teams are dispatched to outbreak areas for epidemiologic investigation within 48 hours of an outbreak report. Probably the second most important strength of the polio surveillance system is that it includes laboratory facilities, staffed with trained scientists, as well as clinical facilities. These laboratories are well supplied and equipped (all of the laboratories work with DNA probes; several have polymerase chain reaction [PCR] technology) and are able to exchange specimens as well as data.

The polio surveillance network is financed largely by its host countries, with substantial contributions from PAHO, the U.S. Agency for International Development (USAID), and the InterAmerican Development Bank (IADB). Support also comes from Rotary Club International and the CDC.

TROUBLE AHEAD

Balanced against this history of progress is the reality of a world still very much engaged in confronting the threats to health posed by a broad array of microbes. Medical and epidemiological uncertainties make it impossible to obtain an exact count of the number of infectious diseases that afflict human populations at any point in time. The evidence suggests, however, that humankind is beset by a greater variety of microbial pathogens than ever before. Some of this, of course, may be due to our increased ability to recognize or identify microbes.

Focusing on the past two decades is instructive. During this period, scientists have identified a host of apparently "new" infectious diseases, such as Lyme disease, that affect more and more people every year. Researchers are also discovering that a number of widely occurring diseases, whose exact causes had until recently remained a mystery, are probably the result of microbial infection. Peptic ulcer, a familiar and widespread condition, fits into this category (a recently described bacterium, *Helicobacter pylori*, is the probable cause), as does cervical cancer (strongly associated with human papillomavirus infection). The potentially infectious origins of other syndromes, such as atherosclerosis, rheumatoid arthritis, and chronic fatigue syndrome, are being pursued.

The incidence of a number of known infectious diseases is escalating, including some that were once considered under control. The reasons for the escalation vary but include the waning effectiveness of some approaches to disease control and treatment, changes in the ways human beings interact with the environment, and the fact that certain individuals have become more susceptible to infection. These circumstances explain the reemergence of, among other diseases, malaria and tuberculosis.

Finally, the introduction of disease agents into the United States from other parts of the world continues. HIV, whose place of origin is thought by many to be Africa, was the most dramatic because of its long incubation period, rapid spread, and initially unknown classification (see Chapter 2). There are other, less well-known examples. For example, malaria has been introduced in southern California and Florida (see Chapter 2), and dengue has appeared in southern Texas. Although both diseases were rapidly recognized and controlled, they are continually being introduced into this country by travellers from the tropics and thus remain constant threats.

A deadly, hemorrhagic disease of crab-eating monkeys, imported in 1990 to Reston, Virginia, received considerable media attention (see Chapter 2). Scientists at the U.S. Army's Research Institute of Infectious Diseases determined that the causative agent was a virus closely related to the fatal Ebola virus of Zaire and Sudan. (In Africa in 1976, 50 to 90 percent of those infected with the Ebola virus died.) The Reston virus, as it became known, was found to have infected veterinarians and other individuals caring for the monkeys, but fortunately this strain did not make people sick. Nevertheless, the episode illustrates well the potential of foreign disease agents to enter the United States.

Clearly, despite a great deal of progress in detecting, preventing, and treating infectious diseases, we are a long way from eliminating the human health threats posed by bacteria, viruses, protozoans, helminths, and fungi. The following brief snapshots of current and potential threats to health give a sense of the scope and magnitude of the challenges ahead.

Lyme Disease

Lyme disease is now the most common arthropod-borne disease in the United States. Since 1980, when only a handful of cases were reported, the incidence of the disease in the United States has grown steadily. In 1991, 9,344 cases of Lyme disease were reported to the CDC (D. Dennis, Chief, Bacterial Zoonoses Branch, Centers for Disease Control, personal communication, 1992). There is good reason to believe that these numbers are a significant underestimate. Epidemic Lyme disease is also a growing problem in Europe. In Germany alone, more than 30,000 new cases occur each year (Matuschka and Spielman, 1989). Cases have also been reported in China, Japan, South Africa, and Australia (Jaenson, 1991).

Lyme disease, which can evolve into a debilitating illness, is accompanied by an extraordinarily wide range of symptoms, many of which mimic other disease syndromes. The disease was initially named *erythema migrans* for the distinctive skin lesion that results from the bite of the spirochete-carrying ticks. Diagnosis of the condition, especially during its early stages, is difficult. Treatment relies on antibiotics, but this approach becomes less effective as the disease progresses. The disease is caused by infection with *Borrelia burgdorferi*, a spirochete, and it is transmitted by certain ticks in a complex cycle that also involves mice and deer.

The emergence of Lyme disease is directly linked to changes in land use patterns. In the eastern United States (and in Europe) during the seventeenth, eighteenth, and much of the nineteenth centuries, vast expanses of land were cleared for farming. In the United States during the 1900s, however, much of the East Coast underwent reforestation, in large part owing to the decline of the small farm and the shift of agriculture to the Midwest. New-growth forest now provides an ideal habitat for deer.

Reforestation was accompanied by increased residential development in wooded, suburban areas. The resulting proximity of people, mice, deer, and ticks has created nearly perfect conditions for the transmission of the Lyme disease spirochete to human hosts. Although people are becoming aware of the risk of contracting Lyme disease, ecological trends that favor the survival of reservoir and vector hosts continue. There is little reason to think that the upward climb in incidence will level off or decline soon.

Peptic Ulcer

Few, if any, infectious disease specialists 10 years ago would have predicted an infectious etiology for gastritis, peptic ulcer, or duodenal ulcer disease. Yet there is now considerable evidence that a bacterium, *Helicobacter pylori*, infects gastric-type epithelium in virtually all patients with these conditions.

H. pylori was identified initially as an unknown bacillus in biopsies of involved areas of active chronic gastritis (Warren and Marshall, 1983). Evidence that *H. pylori* infection is the cause, and not the consequence, of gastritis and ulcers is of several types. First, acute infection with *H. pylori* in humans results in chronic superficial, or type B, gastritis (Dooley et al., 1989). Second, *H. pylori* infection is not associated with other types of gastritis, which would be expected if it were merely infecting already damaged epithelium (O'Connor et al., 1984). Third, antimicrobial therapy directed against *H. pylori* has been shown to heal gastritis and duodenal ulcers in infected patients at least as effectively as acid-suppressive therapy (Glupczynski et al., 1988; Morgan et al., 1988; Rauws et al., 1988). Fourth, gastritis developed following experimental ingestion of *H. pylori* by human volunteers (Morris and Nicholson, 1989). Finally, recurrence of duodenal ulcers has invariably followed and not preceded recurrence of *H. pylori* infection (Logan et al., 1990).

Antibiotic treatment of gastritis, peptic ulcer, and duodenal ulcers associated with *H. pylori* currently is experimental. Results to date indicate that combinations of antibiotics are required to suppress or eradicate the bacterium.

Helicobacter pylori may also be associated with an increased risk of gastric carcinoma (Parsonnet et al., 1991; Nomura et al., 1991). The finding raises the possibility that this cancer, one of the world's most common, could be mitigated by screening for and treating *H. pylori* infection.

Malaria

Malaria, which had been eliminated or effectively suppressed in many parts of the world, has greatly increased in incidence over the past two decades. This parasitic disease results in some 1 million deaths each year, mostly among children, and is becoming increasingly difficult to treat and prevent. Many previously effective drugs no longer work against strains of the parasite that have become resistant. Particularly distressing is resistance to chloroquine, once the treatment of choice for the most severe form of malaria. Equally troubling is that a growing array of once-potent pesticides are no longer effective against mosquitoes that harbor the parasite. The use of other, still effective pesticides is often restricted.

Malaria occurs both in the tropics and, less frequently, in the temperate zones of the world. The disease was a major problem for early European settlers of North America. As recently as the early 1900s, half a million cases of malaria were recorded each year in the United States.

Currently, some 1,200 cases of malaria are diagnosed in the United States annually. The vast majority are individuals entering the country for the first time or returning from foreign travel. A very small number of cases are the result of direct transmission involving indigenous mosquitoes. Most of these have occurred among Mexican agricultural workers living in California in substandard conditions. The largest outbreak since 1952 involved 30 people in San Diego County in 1988. That experience and others like it, in conjunction with the rapid rise in drug-resistant strains of the malaria parasite, raise the possibility of even larger outbreaks in the future (see Chapter 2).

Malaria continues to pose a serious threat to the U.S. military. There were 500,000 cases of malaria among U.S. soldiers during World War II (Ognibene and Barrett, 1982; D. Robinette, Senior Program Officer, Medical Follow-up Agency, Institute of Medicine, personal communication, 1991), and more than 80,000 cases were diagnosed in American troops in Vietnam from 1965 to 1971 (Canfield, 1972). Troops sent to the Middle

East during the Persian Gulf War in 1991 were at risk of contracting malaria, which is endemic in western Saudi Arabia, Yemen, Oman, northern Iraq, and parts of the United Arab Emirates (Gasser et al., 1991). Fortunately, only six cases were diagnosed during the conflict (L. Roberts, Entomology Consultant, Office of the Surgeon General, U.S. Army, personal communication, 1992).

Dengue

Dengue affects more people worldwide than any other arthropod-borne disease except malaria. More than 2 billion people are at risk, and in some Asian cities virtually every child has been infected by age 12. A small but significant percentage of those infected with dengue virus have severe disease, with hemorrhagic fever and shock.

Epidemiologically, dengue hemorrhagic fever/dengue shock syndrome (DHF/DSS) has become an increasingly important international disease. During the first half of the 1980s, 804,000 cases were reported, more than during the previous 25 years. Another 993,000 cases were reported from 1985 through 1989 (Halstead, 1990). Also troubling is the fact that by the early 1990s, *Aedes aegypti* mosquitoes, the primary vector for dengue virus transmission to humans, had returned in large numbers to most of Central and South America, presenting abundant opportunity for new epidemics.

In 1985, another potential dengue vector, *Ae. albopictus*, was found to be established in the southern United States; it had been introduced in used tires imported from Japan. This mosquito, commonly known as the Asian tiger mosquito, has spread rapidly across the South and established itself as a permanent resident. Although it has not been found to carry dengue in the United States, it has other troubling features. Eastern equine encephalitis (EEE) virus was recently isolated from *Ae. albopictus* mosquitoes collected in and around a tire dump in Polk County, Florida, demonstrating the ability of this imported mosquito to carry a native virus (Centers for Disease Control, 1992d). EEE virus is perpetuated in nature in a cycle that includes primarily marsh-nesting and shore birds and the strictly bird-feeding mosquito *Culiseta melanura*. These *Ae. albopictus* mosquitoes probably acquired the virus by feeding on infected birds.

Tuberculosis

Tuberculosis (TB) was the leading cause of death from infectious disease in the United States and Western Europe until the first decade of this century, and it remained the second leading cause from that time until the advent of antimicrobial drugs in the 1950s (Rich, 1944; Waksman, 1964; Dubos and Dubos, 1987). At present, TB kills more people worldwide than any other infectious disease (Caldwell, 1987; Murray et al., in press). Each year, according to the WHO, 8 million new cases of clinical TB are diagnosed, and 2.9 million people die of the disease. In the United States, until 1985, TB incidence had been in decline for more than three decades. Between 1986 and 1991, however, 28,000 more cases were reported than were predicted to occur based on past experience.

TB is a bacterial disease whose principal manifestation is destruction of lung tissue; it is spread primarily through the respiratory route by patients with active pulmonary disease. One out of every 10 to 12 healthy individuals infected with the tubercle bacillus develops clinical disease. The case fatality rate of untreated TB in people with clinical disease is 50 percent, and their average life span is six months to two years.

Multiple factors are contributing to the rise in cases of TB. Of major importance are increased poverty and a growing number of homeless individuals and families, substance abuse, a deteriorating health care infrastructure for treating chronic infectious diseases, and the HIV disease pandemic (perhaps the most significant factor at present). Complacency within the medical community and among the public at large and shortages of the drugs used to treat TB are additional factors in the increase.

TB is difficult to treat. Multidrug therapy is invariably necessary, with the drugs administered over at least six months to effect a clinical cure and prevent the emergence of drug-resistant organisms. Where health care infrastructure is adequate and compliance with treatment is maintained, cure rates should exceed 90 percent, even in HIV-infected individuals who have TB, providing resistant organisms are not present. When treatment is either inappropriate or inadequate, resistance to one or more of the treatment drugs often develops. The increased finding of resistant organisms reflects a major breakdown in the social and health care infrastructures.

When multidrug-resistant TB is present, case fatality rates can exceed 80 percent in immunocompromised individuals (see Chapter 2). The presence of multidrug-resistant organisms puts not only TB-infected individuals but also health care workers, social workers, corrections officials, families, and contacts at risk of contracting a disease that is difficult or essentially impossible to treat. Multidrug-resistant TB now represents a major threat to health in the United States.

In the 1950s, with the advent of antituberculosis drugs, TB became one of several newly treatable infectious diseases. The common assumption regarding such diseases has been that drugs that have been effective in treating them will continue to be so. Current experience with TB is causing many to question that assumption. Other organisms that have developed resistance to frontline drugs (probably for some of the same reasons) are also signaling the possibility of trouble ahead. Penicillin-resistant streptococcal Group A and Group C infections and penicillin-resistant pneumococcal infections have been documented, as have vancomycin-resistant staphylococcal and enterococcal infections. Without more careful prescription of antimicrobials by physicians and more consistent compliance with treatment regimens by patients, pathogenic bacteria are likely to undergo mutations that will enable them to resist available antibiotic therapy.

NEXT STEPS

It is unrealistic to expect that humankind will win a complete victory over the multitude of existing microbial diseases, or over those that will emerge in the future. This will be true no matter how well stocked our armamentaria of drugs and vaccines, no matter how well planned our efforts to prevent and control epidemics, and no matter how advanced our basic science and clinical understanding of infectious diseases. Microbes are ranked among the most numerous and diverse of organisms on the planet; pathogenic microbes can be resilient, dangerous foes. Although it is impossible to predict their individual emergence in time and place, we can be confident that new microbial diseases will emerge.

Still, there are many steps that scientists, educators, public health officials, policymakers, and others can and should be taking to improve our odds in this ongoing struggle. With diligence and concerted action at many levels, the threats posed by emerging infectious diseases can be, if not eliminated, at least significantly moderated. To achieve this goal, however, a number of fundamental problems must be addressed. These problems fall into four broad categories:

• *Perceiving the Threats*: The emergence of HIV disease has stimulated a high level of interest in the scientific, medical, public health, and policymaking communities. By and large, however, awareness of and concern about the threats to human health posed by other emerging and reemerging microbial diseases remain critically low. A small minority, mainly infectious disease specialists, have for years warned of the potential for serious epidemics and our lack of preparedness for them. In what can only be called a general mood of complacency, these warnings have gone largely unheeded.

• *Detecting the Threats*: Surveillance is the primary means by which the incidence of established diseases is monitored and outbreaks of new diseases are detected. The domestic disease surveillance network in the United States is being scaled back as a result of fiscal problems in many states, raising concerns about its ability to perform a vital public health function. Equally worrisome, the existing international surveillance networks are focused on little more than a handful of well-defined diseases, and U.S. involvement in this worldwide effort is diminishing. Epidemiological knowledge of most globally important diseases is incomplete at best; for many there is very little information.

• *Understanding the Threats*: Despite progress in basic and applied infectious disease research, gaps remain in our knowledge about most bacteria, viruses, protozoans, helminths, and fungi. These scientific "blind spots" have slowed or prevented efforts to understand the variety of factors responsible for disease emergence and reemergence. The diversion of funds for emergencies or, in some cases, inconsistent levels of funding have made it especially difficult to address the full range of research opportunities and needs.

• *Responding to the Threats*: Once emerging microbial threats are detected, responses to them are often feeble. Diseases that appear not to threaten the United States directly rarely elicit the political support necessary to maintain control efforts. U.S. support for surveillance, control, and research activities in other countries is extremely limited. Here, as in other nations, failure to sustain domestic efforts to control infectious diseases is an equally serious problem. Ill-informed decision making can prevent accurate assessments of the actual danger posed by microbial threats to health, and it can slow or even halt steps to address an emerging disease problem. Ironically, these same forces can produce an overresponse to less serious situations. Finally, profit and liability concerns have undercut the market incentives for manufacturers of vaccines, drugs, and pesticides to develop and distribute needed supplies to the most impoverished populations both in the United States and in other countries.

History has shown and this committee believes that the threat from the emergence of infectious diseases is not one to be taken lightly. The development of a strategy for addressing emerging infectious disease threats requires that we understand the factors that precipitate the emergence of these agents and the resultant diseases. These factors are examined in Chapter 2.

2

Factors in Emergence

Emerging infectious diseases are clinically distinct conditions whose incidence in humans has increased. For the purposes of this study, the committee has focused on diseases that have emerged in the United States within the past two decades. Emergence may be due to the introduction of a new agent, to the recognition of an existing disease that has gone undetected, or to a change in the environment that provides an epidemiologic "bridge." (For an example of an emerging disease, see Box 2-1.) Emergence, or, more specifically, reemergence, may also be used to describe the reappearance of a known disease after a decline in incidence. Although an infectious agent plays a role in any emerging infectious disease, other causative factors may be important as well.

BOX 2-1 A Deadly Form of Strep

It was a shock to many when renowned puppeteer Jim Henson died suddenly in May 1990. How could a healthy man in his early 50s be so easily felled by a case of pneumonia? Since his death, attention has focused on a deadly "new" form of streptococcal bacteria. This new bacterium belongs to a category of strep bacteria called "Group A," a subset of organisms familiar to many as the cause of acute pharyngitis (strep throat). The new strep A has been killing otherwise healthy people (like Henson), and doing so in a frighteningly rapid fashion. This was true for a 30-year-old Canadian man who got a splinter in his finger, which later became infected. Within six days he had become so ill that he was admitted to an intensive care unit and placed on a respirator. He died six weeks later of sepsis (disseminated infection) (Goldman, 1991).

The new strep A bacteria, like all streptococcal organisms, are typically inhaled, but they can also enter the body through a cut or scrape. The infection they provoke once inside the body is especially insidious: its early symptoms are easily mistaken for signs of the flu. In several cases, the bacteria have overwhelmed their host with pneumonia, and in others, with kidney and liver damage before the infected person has sought treatment. So advanced, the infection is extremely difficult to treat. Even if massive doses of penicillin succeed in killing the bacteria, there are no means available to counter the effects of the deadly toxin they produce—which actually causes the pneumonia and tissue damage.

Although reports of the first cases of fatal infection with the new strep A appeared in the medical literature in 1989 (Stevens et al., 1989), health problems associated with the streptococcus family of bacteria are not new. In the days before antibiotics, they were responsible for widespread outbreaks of scarlet fever and rheumatic fever. Nor are these bacteria rare. Strep throat is so common an ailment among children that it could almost be considered a rite of passage.

Much about the new strep A remains a mystery. Some scientists—noting the similarity between the toxin secreted by the new strep A and the toxin once seen with scarlet fever—believe that this bacterium is an old microbe making a comeback. Others consider this highly virulent form of strep the result of a recent bacterial mutation.

Whatever its origin, the new strep A deserves attention. Experts strongly encourage people to seek immediate medical care if they become very ill (high fever, sore throat) in a sudden fashion, especially if they have recently suffered a cut or burn.

Although cases of infection with this new, deadly microbe remain quite rare, their increasing incidence in the past two years is cause for concern. A vaccine for streptococcal infections is in development, but researchers estimate that it will not be ready for public use for at least another three years. In the meantime, the Centers for Disease Control is working to track the new strep A more closely, with the hope of learning more about the bacterium and how to stop it.

Table 2-1 is a list of emerging infectious agents, categorized by type of organism. Appendix B provides more detailed information on each of these agents. The committee recognizes that this list is continually expanding, mainly as a result of the growing numbers of immunocompromised individuals. Therefore, it may not contain all organisms that fit the definition above.

Once a new pathogen has been introduced into a human population, its ability to spread becomes a critical factor in emergence. The same is true for agents that are already present in a limited or isolated human population:

TABLE 2-1 Part 1: Examples of Emergent Bacteria, Rickettsiae, and Chlamydiae

Agent	Related Diseases/Symptoms	Mode of Transmission	Cause(s) of Emergence
Aeromonas species	Aeromonad gastro-enteritis, cellulitis, wound infection, septicemia	Ingestion of con-taminated water or food; entry of organism through a break in the skin	Immunosuppression; improved technology for detection and differentiation
Borrelia burgdorferi	Lyme disease: rash, fever, neurologic and cardiac abnormalities, arthritis	Bite of infective *Ixodes* tick	Increase in deer and human populations in wooded areas
Campylobacter jejuni	Campylobacter enter-itis: abdominal pain, diarrhea, fever	Ingestion of contami-nated food, water, or milk; fecal-oral spread from infected person or animal	Increased recognition; consumption of uncooked poultry
Chlamydia pneumoniae (TWAR strain)	TWAR infection: fever, myalgias, cough, sore throat, pneumonia	Inhalation of infective organisms; possibly by direct contact with secretions of an infected person	Increased recognition
Chlamydia trachomatis	Trachoma, genital infections, conjunctiv-itis; infection during pregnancy can result in infant pneumonia	Sexual intercourse	Increased sexual activity; changes in sanitation
Clostridium difficile	Colitis: abdominal pain, watery diarrhea, bloody diarrhea	Fecal-oral transmis-sion; contact with the organism in the environment	Increased recognition; immunosuppression
Ehrlichia chaffeensis	Ehrlichiosis: febrile illness (fever, head-ache, nausea, vomiting, myalgia)	Unknown; tick is suspected vector	Increased recognition; possibly increase in host and vector populations
Escherichia coli O157:H7	Hemorrhagic colitis; thrombocytopenia; hemolytic uremic syndrome	Ingestion of con-taminated food, esp. undercooked beef and raw milk	Likely due to the development of a new pathogen
Haemophilus influenzae bio-group *aegyptius*	Brazilian purpuric fever: purulent con-junctivitis, high fever, vomiting, and purpura	Contact with dis-charges of infected persons; eye flies are suspected vectors	Possibly an increase in virulence due to mutation

TABLE 2-1 Part 1 *Continued*

Agent	Related Diseases/Symptoms	Mode of Transmission	Cause(s) of Emergence
Helicobacter pylori	Gastritis, peptic ulcer, possibly stomach cancer	Ingestion of contaminated food or water, esp. unpasteurized milk; contact with infected pets	Increased recognition
Legionella pneumophila	Legionnaires' disease: malaise, myalgia, fever, headache, respiratory illness	Air-cooling systems, water supplies	Recognition in an epidemic situation
Listeria monocytogenes	Listeriosis: meningoencephalitis and/or septicemia	Ingestion of contaminated foods; contact with soil contaminated with infected animal feces; inhalation of organism	Probably increased awareness, recognition, and reporting
Mycobacterium tuberculosis	Tuberculosis: cough, weight loss, lung lesions; infection can spread to other organ systems	Exposure to sputum droplets (exhaled through a cough or sneeze) of a person with active disease	Immunosuppression
Staphylococcus aureus	Abscesses, pneumonia, endocarditis, toxic shock	Contact with the organism in a purulent lesion or on the hands	Recognition in an epidemic situation; possibly mutation
Streptococcus pyogenes (Group A)	Scarlet fever, rheumatic fever, toxic shock	Direct contact with infected persons or carriers; sometimes ingestion of contaminated foods	Change in virulence of the bacteria; possibly mutation
Vibrio cholerae	Cholera: severe diarrhea, rapid dehydration	Ingestion of water contaminated with the feces of infected persons; ingestion of food exposed to contaminated water	Poor sanitation/ hygiene; possibly introduced via bilge-water from cargo ships
Vibrio vulnificus	Cellulitis; fatal bacteremia; diarrheal illness (occasionally)	Contact of superficial wounds with seawater or with contaminated (raw or undercooked) seafood; ingestion (occasionally)	Increased recognition

TABLE 2-1 Part 2: Examples of Emergent Viruses

Agent	Related Diseases/Symptoms	Mode of Transmission	Cause(s) of Emergence
Bovine spongiform encephalopathy (BSE) agent	Bovine spongiform encephalopathy in cows	Ingestion of feed containing infected sheep tissue	Changes in the rendering process
Chikungunya	Fever, arthritis, hemorrhagic fever	Bite of infected mosquito	Unknown
Crimean-Congo hemorrhagic fever	Hemorrhagic fever	Bite of an infected adult tick	Ecological changes favoring increased human exposure to ticks on sheep and small wild animals
Dengue	Hemorrhagic fever	Bite of an infected mosquito (primarily *Aedes aegypti*)	Poor mosquito control; increased urbanization in tropics; increased air travel
Filoviruses (Marburg, Ebola)	Fulminant, high-mortality hemorrhagic fever	Direct contact with infected blood, organs, secretions, and semen	Unknown; in Europe and the United States, virus-infected monkeys shipped from developing countries via air
Hantaviruses	Abdominal pain, vomiting, hemorrhagic fever	Inhalation of aerosolized rodent urine and feces	Human invasion of virus ecologic niche
Hepatitis B	Nausea, vomiting, jaundice; chronic infection leads to hepatocellular carcinoma and cirrhosis	Contact with saliva, semen, blood, or vaginal fluids of an infected person; mode of transmission to children not known	Probably increased sexual activity and intravenous drug abuse; transfusion (before 1978)
Hepatitis C	Nausea, vomiting, jaundice; chronic infection leads to hepatocellular carcinoma and cirrhosis	Exposure (percutaneous) to contaminated blood or plasma; sexual transmission	Recognition through molecular virology applications; blood transfusion practices following World War II (esp. in Japan)
Hepatitis E	Fever, abdominal pain, jaundice	Contaminated water	Newly recognized
Human herpesvirus 6 (HHV-6)	Roseola in children, syndrome resembling mononucleosis	Unknown; possibly respiratory spread	Newly recognized

TABLE 2-1 Part 2 *Continued*

Agent	Related Diseases/Symptoms	Mode of Transmission	Cause(s) of Emergence
Human immuno-deficiency viruses			
HIV-1	HIV disease, including AIDS: severe immune system dysfunction, opportunistic infections	Sexual contact with or exposure to blood or tissues of an infected person; vertical transmission	Urbanization; changes in lifestyles/mores; increased intravenous drug use; international travel; medical technology (trans-fusions/transplants)
HIV-2	Similar to above	Same as above	Same as above, esp. international travel
Human papillomavirus	Skin and mucous membrane lesions (often, warts); strongly linked to cancer of the cervix and penis	Direct contact (sexual contact/ contact with contaminated surfaces)	Newly recognized; perhaps changes in sexual lifestyle
Human parvovirus B19	Erythema infectiosum: erythema on face, rash on trunk; aplastic anemia	Contact with respir-atory secretions of an infected person; vertical transmission	Newly recognized
Human T-cell lymphotropic viruses (HTLV-I and HTLV-II)	Leukemias and lymphomas	Vertical transmission through blood/breast milk; exposure to contaminated blood products; sexual transmission	Increased intravenous drug abuse; medical technology (transfusion)
Influenza			
Pandemic	Fever, headache, cough, pneumonia	Airborne (esp. in crowded, enclosed spaces)	Animal-human virus reassortment; antigenic shift
Drift	Same as above	Same as above	Antigenic drift
Japanese encephalitis	Encephalitis	Bite of an infective mosquito	Changing agri-cultural practices
La Crosse and California Group viruses	Encephalitis	Bite of an infective mosquito	Increasing interface between human activity and endemic areas; discarded tires as mosquito breeding sites

continued on next page

TABLE 2-1 Part 2 *Continued*

Agent	Related Diseases/Symptoms	Mode of Transmission	Cause(s) of Emergence
Lassa	Fever, headache, sore throat, nausea	Contact with urine or feces of infected rodents	Urbanization/ conditions favoring infestation by rodents
Measles	Fever, conjunctivitis, cough, red blotchy rash	Airborne; direct contact with respiratory secretions of infected persons	Deterioration of public health infrastructure supporting immunization
Norwalk and Norwalk-like agents	Gastroenteritis; epidemic diarrhea	Most likely fecal-oral; alleged vehicles of transmission include drinking and swimming water, and uncooked foods	Increased recognition
Rabies	Acute viral encephalomyelitis	Bite of a rabid animal	Introduction of infected reservoir host to new areas
Rift Valley	Febrile illness	Bite of an infective mosquito	Importation of infected mosquitoes and/ or animals; development (dams, irrigation)
Ross River	Arthritis, rash	Bite of an infective mosquito	Movement of infected mosquitoes or people
Rotavirus	Enteritis; diarrhea, vomiting, dehydration, and low-grade fever	Primarily fecal-oral; fecal-respiratory transmission can also occur	Increased recognition
Venezuelan equine encephalitis	Encephalitis	Bite of an infective mosquito	Movement of mosquitoes and amplification hosts (horses)
Yellow fever	Fever, headache, muscle pain, nausea, vomiting	Bite of an infective (*Aedes aegypti*) mosquito	Lack of effective mosquito control and widespread vaccination; urbanization in tropics; increased air travel

TABLE 2-1 Part 3: Examples of Emergent Protozoans, Helminths, and Fungi

Agent	Related Diseases/Symptoms	Mode of Transmission	Cause(s) of Emergence
Anisakis	Anisakiasis: abdominal pain, vomiting	Ingestion of larvae-infected fish (undercooked)	Changes in dietary habits (eating of raw fish)

TABLE 2-1 Part 3 *Continued*

Agent	Related Diseases/Symptoms	Mode of Transmission	Cause(s) of Emergence
Babesia	Babesiosis: fever, fatigue, hemolytic anemia	Bite of an *Ixodes* tick (carried by mice in the presence of deer)	Reforestation; increase in deer population; changes in outdoor recreational activity
Candida	Candidiasis: fungal infections of the gastro-intestinal tract, vagina, and oral cavity	Endogenous flora; contact with secretions or excretions from infected persons	Immunosuppression; medical management (catheters); antibiotic use
Cryptococcus	Meningitis; sometimes infections of the lungs, kidneys, prostate, liver	Inhalation	Immunosuppression
Cryptosporidium	Cryptosporidiosis: infection of epithelial cells in the gastro-intestinal and respiratory tracts	Fecal-oral, person-to-person, waterborne	Development near watershed areas; immunosuppression
Giardia lamblia	Giardiasis: infection of the upper small intestine, diarrhea, bloating	Ingestion of fecally contaminated food or water	Inadequate control in some water supply systems; immunosuppression; international travel
Microsporidia	Gastrointestinal illness, diarrhea; wasting in immunosuppressed persons	Unknown; probably ingestion of fecally contaminated food or water	Immunosuppression; recognition
Plasmodium	Malaria	Bite of an infective *Anopheles* mosquito	Urbanization; changing parasite biology; environmental changes; drug resistance; air travel
Pneumocystis carinii	Acute pneumonia	Unknown; possibly reactivation of latent infection	Immunosuppression
Strongyloides stercoralis	Strongyloidiasis: rash and cough followed by diarrhea; wasting, pulmonary involvement, and death in immuno-suppressed persons	Penetration of skin or mucous membrane by larvae (usually from fecally-contaminated soil); oral-anal sexual activities	Immunosuppression; international travel
Toxoplasma gondii	Toxoplasmosis: fever, lymphadenopathy, lymphocytosis	Exposure to feces of cats carrying the protozoan; some-times foodborne	Immunosuppression; increase in cats as pets

those agents best adapted to human transmission are likely to be those that will emerge. Introduction of a disease-causing agent into a new host population and dissemination of the agent within the new host species can occur almost simultaneously, but they are more commonly separated by considerable periods of time. Changes in the environment and in human behavior, as well as other factors, may increase the chances that dissemination will occur.

For familiar, "old" agents, whose spread has been successfully controlled, reemergence is often the result of lapses in public health measures owing to complacency, changes in human behavior that increase person-to-person transmission of an infectious agent, or changes in the ways humans interact with their environment. The return of dengue fever into areas of South and Central America where previously *Ae. aegypti* had been eradicated and the resurgence of yellow fever in Nigeria, where more than 400 persons were estimated to have died between April 1 and July 14, 1991 (Centers for Disease Control, unpublished data, 1992), reflect the operation of these mechanisms.

THE CONCEPT OF EMERGENCE

Although specific agents are usually associated with individual diseases, historically it is the diseases that usually have been recognized first. With improved techniques for the identification of microbes, however, this situation is changing. The causative agents for many newly emergent diseases are often discovered virtually simultaneously with (or in some cases before) their associated disease syndromes. For this reason, the term *emerging microbial threat* as used in this report includes both the agent and the disease.

It is important to understand the difference between infection and disease. Infection implies that an agent, such as a virus, has taken up residence in a host and is multiplying within that host—perhaps with no outward signs of disease. Thus, it is possible to be infected with an agent but not have the disease commonly associated with that agent (although disease may develop at a later time).

In discussions about the emergence of "new" diseases, considerable debate has centered on the relative importance of de novo evolution of agents versus the transfer of existing agents to new host populations (so-called microbial traffic). It is sometimes presumed that the appearance of a novel, disease-causing microorganism results from a change in its genetic properties. This is sometimes the case, but there are many instances in which emergence is due to changes in the environment or in human ecology. In fact, environmental changes probably account for most emerging diseases.

For example, despite the fact that many viruses have naturally high rates of mutation, the significance of new variants as a source of new viral diseases has been hard to demonstrate, and there appear to be relatively few documented examples in nature. Influenza is probably the best example of a virus for which the importance of new variants (i.e., antigenic drift) can clearly be shown. Variants of the hepatitis B virus also have been shown recently to cause disease. However, cases like these are greatly outnumbered by instances of new diseases or outbreaks resulting from microbial traffic between species. Cross-species transfer of infectious agents is often the result of human activities.

The evolution of viruses is constrained by their requirement for being maintained in a host. It would therefore seem that new variants of nonviral pathogens, such as bacteria, would be more common than new forms of viral pathogens since nonviral organisms are less constrained by host requirements. However, most nonviral pathogens usually show a clonal origin (Selander and Musser, 1990; Musser et al., 1991; Tibayrenc et al., 1991a,b). That is, they appear to be derived from a single ancestor, suggesting that the evolution of a successful new pathogen is a relatively rare event. When it does occur, the new microbe probably originates in a single geographic area and is disseminated through channels of microbial traffic. One implication of this model is that the control of "new" diseases may be more likely if the new variant is identified early (e.g., by worldwide infectious disease surveillance) and steps are taken to prevent its further dissemination.

It is likely that emerging pathogens generally are not newly evolved. Rather, it appears that they already exist in nature. Some may have existed in isolated human populations for some time; others, including many of the most novel, are well established in animals. Infections in animals that are transmissable to humans are termed *zoonoses*. As discussed in Chapter 1, throughout history rodents have been particularly important natural reservoirs of many infectious diseases.

The significance of zoonoses in the emergence of human infections cannot be overstated. The introduction of viruses into human populations, for example, is often the result of human activities, such as agriculture, that cause changes in natural environments. These changes may place humans in contact with infected animals or with arthropod vectors of animal diseases, thereby increasing the chances of human infection. Argentine hemorrhagic fever, a natural infection of rodents, emerged as a result of an agricultural practice placing humans in close proximity to the rodents. Marburg, Machupo, Hantaan, and Rift Valley fever viruses are also of zoonotic origin, as, arguably, is human immunodeficiency virus (HIV). Yellow fever, whose natural cycle of infection takes place in a jungle habitat and involves monkeys and mosquitoes in tropical areas of Africa and South America, is probably an ancient zoonosis. Jungle yellow fever occurs when humans interpose themselves in the natural cycle and are bitten by infected mosquitoes. Yet there is also urban yellow fever, in which the same virus is transmitted among humans by other mosquitoes (e.g., *Aedes aegypti*) that have adapted to living in cities. It is generally believed that the movement of people through the slave trade and maritime commerce disseminated yellow fever, dengue, and chikungunya viruses, as well as *Ae. aegypti*, from Africa to other tropical areas. *Ae. aegypti* is still widespread in many urban areas of the southeastern United States, although the last yellow fever epidemic in a major U.S. city was in New Orleans in 1905.

Although the odds are low that a randomly chosen organism will become a successful human pathogen, the great variety of microorganisms in nature increases those odds. For example, field sampling and disease surveillance efforts have now identified more than 520 arthropod-borne viruses, or arboviruses (Karabatsos, 1985). The disease potential of most of these viruses is unknown, but nearly 100 have been shown to cause human disease (Benenson, 1990). In spite of the demise of the Rockefeller Foundation arbovirus program in 1971, and although only a few laboratories are actively searching for new pathogens in animals and arthropods, new viruses are being discovered every year (see Box 2-2).

One example of a recently discovered zoonotic virus is Guanarito, the cause of Venezuelan hemorrhagic fever. In the fall of 1989, an outbreak of an unusually severe and sometimes fatal disease was detected in the state of Portuguesa in central Venezuela. Patients presented for treatment with prolonged fever, headache, arthralgia, diarrhea, cough, sore throat, prostration, leucopenia, thrombocytopenia, and hemorrhagic manifestations. Physicians in the region initially diagnosed the disease as dengue hemorrhagic fever (DHF). During one period, from early May 1990 through late March 1991, 104 cases of the disease were recorded. Slightly more than a quarter of these patients, most of them adults, died (Salas et al., 1991).

All of the cases of the DHF-like illness occurred in the Municipio of Guanarito in Portuguesa State, or in adjoining areas in Barinas State. The Municipio of Guanarito, population 20,000, is located in the central plains of Venezuela, a major food-producing region. The outbreak was confined to the municipio's roughly 12,000 rural inhabitants, who either farm or raise cattle (Salas et al., 1991).

In the fall of 1990, a virologist from the Venezuelan Ministry of Health sent serum samples from several patients who were suspected to have DHF to the Yale Arbovirus Research Unit (YARU) at Yale University School of Medicine. No virus could be isolated after routine culture of the sera in mosquito cells (the standard method for recovery of dengue viruses).

In early 1991, a member of the YARU staff visited Venezuela while on a trip to South America collecting dengue virus isolates for an ongoing research project. In Caracas, the YARU staff member was given spleen cultures from two fatal cases of suspected DHF from the Guanarito area. Upon inoculation into newborn mice and Vero (monkey kidney) cell cultures at

BOX 2-2 Arboviruses

Worldwide, in 1930, only six viruses were known to be maintained in cycles between animal hosts and arthropod vectors like mosquitoes, gnats, and ticks (Karabatsos, 1985). Only one of the recognized arboviruses (*arthropod-bo*rne viruses), yellow fever virus, caused disease in humans. The other five viruses were responsible for epizootics and major economic losses in domestic animals: bluetongue in sheep and cattle, Nairobi sheep disease, Louping ill in sheep, vesicular stomatitis in cattle, and African swine fever.

Later in the same decade, there was an explosion of newly emerged arthropod-borne diseases in North America. Western and eastern equine encephalomyelitis viruses caused major outbreaks with high case fatality rates in both equines and humans. St. Louis encephalitis virus was associated with more than 1,000 cases and 201 deaths in residents of Missouri. Subsequent research demonstrated that each of these viruses was maintained in a cycle dependent on mosquitoes and birds. When any of the viruses invaded the human population, an epidemic often ensued.

Since the 1930s, 86 additional arboviruses have been found in North America. Fortunately, only a few, such as the California encephalitis complex, Colorado tick fever, and the dengue fever viruses, have been consistently associated with human disease. However, all 86 viruses are distributed widely, and many have thus far been shown to cause only inapparent infections in humans. A shift in the virulence of the viruses or in human susceptibility could potentially alter the present equilibrium. Some experts warn that the arboviruses are "viruses looking for a human disease."

The threat of arboviral disease is not limited to North America. The 1985 *International Catalogue of Arboviruses* (Karabatsos, 1985) identified 504 arboviruses worldwide, 124 of which have been associated with a disease. It is of continuing concern that nonindigenous viruses might be introduced into the United States through travel and trade.

The rate of discovery of arboviruses reflects the intensity of the worldwide search by the Rockefeller Foundation, government agencies, and universities from 1950 to 1980. There has been a significant decrease in activity for such programs in recent years, as seen in the table below. Yet all the while, new arboviruses continue to be found whenever and wherever a search is made.

Period	Isolations	Period	Isolations
Before 1930	6	1960–69	209
1930–39	10	1970–79	129
1940–49	19	1980–89	22
1950–59	109	Total	504

SOURCE: Karabatsos, 1985.

YARU, these samples subsequently yielded two isolates of a previously unknown arenavirus, a family of viruses generally thought to be rodent-borne. The organism was distinct from Lassa, Junin, and Machupo viruses, the other arenaviruses that are known to cause severe hemorrhagic illnesses in humans. The new agent has since been designated the Guanarito virus, and its associated disease has been labeled Venezuelan hemorrhagic fever (Salas et al., 1991).

Venezuelan health officials are now attempting to determine the risk factors, geographic distribution, and clinical spectrum of Guanarito virus infection and to update the incidence data on it. Studies are currently in progress at the U.S. Army Medical Research Institute of Infectious Diseases (USAMRIID) to develop an animal model for the disease and to evaluate possible therapeutic agents. In October 1991, scientists from YARU visited Venezuela to initiate a study to identify positively the rodent reservoir(s) of Guanarito virus.

Rodents have been implicated in a number of zoonotic infections, but the zoonotic pool also includes marine animals, such as seals, porpoises, and dolphins, which like humans are susceptible to outbreaks of infectious disease. Most such occurrences pass unnoticed, either because they occur far from shore or because the number of animals affected is too small to draw attention to the possibility of infectious disease. Occasionally, however, marine epidemics do attract attention, usually when large numbers of dead carcasses suddenly appear on a popular beach.

The most recent major epizootic, reported initially in harbor seals living in the waters off Europe and the United Kingdom, began in April 1988. Thousands of the animals died. The hardest-hit area was along Britain's East Anglian coast, where more than half of the native seal population is estimated to have died. The outbreak peaked in August and tapered off through late 1989. Few dead seals have since been reported in this area.

It now appears that the same or a similar disease was present in Siberian seals somewhat earlier than the European epizootic (Grachev et al., 1989). The disease was also found in porpoises (Kennedy et al., 1988) and in dolphins (M. Domingo et al., 1990). Extensive study of the European outbreak resulted in the isolation of the causative agent, a virus, which is similar to measles, canine distemper, and rinderpest viruses.

Occasionally, marine viruses cause disease in terrestrial mammals or humans. For example, a strain of influenza A virus (H7N7) led to epidemic outbreaks in seals in 1980 and caused conjunctivitis in humans who handled the affected seals (Webster et al., 1981). It has been suggested that vesicular exanthema of swine, a serious viral disease caused by a calicivirus, was introduced into pigs through feed that contained material from sea lions. Many caliciviruses of terrestrial mammals may have been introduced from marine sources (Smith and Boyt, 1990). Among human viruses, hepatitis E virus (the enterically transmitted non-A, non-B hepatitis that is usually waterborne and is widespread in tropical areas including parts of South America) has tentatively been classified as a calicivirus (Reyes et al., 1990).

There are also a number of established diseases whose link to an infectious agent has only recently been discovered. In addition to peptic ulcer, mentioned in Chapter 1, other diseases with a newfound link to a microbe include cervical cancer (associated with human papillomaviruses) and human T cell lymphotropic virus (HTLV)-I-associated myelopathy or tropical spastic paraparesis (resulting from infection with HTLV). Diseases for which possible links to infectious agents are under investigation include rheumatoid arthritis (parvovirus B19, HTLV-I); atherosclerosis (cytomegalovirus [CMV], herpes simplex virus [HSV]-1 and HSV-2, or *Chlamydia pneumoniae*); and insulin-dependent diabetes mellitus (coxsackievirus B5). Several of these examples are discussed later in this chapter.

Rather than categorize emerging microbial threats by type of agent—viral, bacterial, protozoal, helminthic, or fungal—this report classifies emerging threats according to the factors related to their emergence:

• Human demographics and behavior
• Technology and industry
• Economic development and land use
• International travel and commerce
• Microbial adaptation and change
• Breakdown of public health measures

The classification draws attention to the specific forces that shape infectious disease emergence (see Figure 2-1). These forces (i.e., factors in emergence) operate on different elements in the process of emergence. Some of the factors influence the acquisition of an emerging microbe by humans and other animals; others primarily affect the microbe's spread among populations. Although it is a difficult, if not impossible, task to predict the emergence of "new" infectious diseases/agents, it is helpful to understand the factors that facilitate the emergence and spread of infectious diseases in general. We must focus on what we *do* know: the infectious disease that will emerge or reemerge is likely to do so through one or more of the "facilitative pathways" diagrammed in Figure 2-1. An awareness of this system of pathways constitutes the first step to reasoned prevention and control of infectious diseases.

Many of the diseases addressed in this report have emerged because of a combination of factors. This is not surprising, given the often complex interactions of microbes, their human and animal hosts, and the environment. As much as possible, however, the committee has attempted to illustrate specific causes of emergence with diseases or agents whose emergence is primarily due to that one factor.

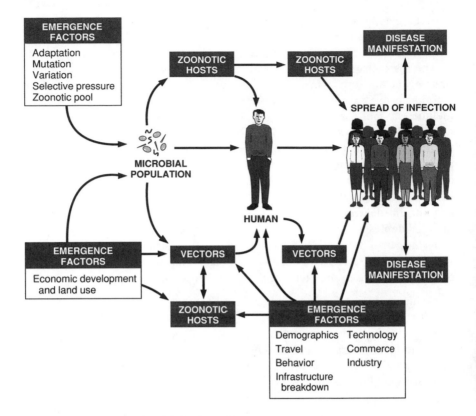

FIGURE 2-1 Schematic of infectious disease emergence.

HUMAN DEMOGRAPHICS AND BEHAVIOR

In the complex set of interactions that result in disease emergence, the human element—population growth, density, and distribution; immunosuppression; and behavior—plays a critical role. Increases in the size, density, and distribution of human populations can facilitate the spread of infectious agents; changes in the distribution of populations can bring people into contact with new pathogenic organisms or with vectors that transmit those organisms. Immunosuppression, a by-product of aging, the use of certain medications, diseases, or other factors, often permits infection by microorganisms that are not normally pathogenic in humans. Individual behavior, particularly sexual activity and the use of illegal drugs, contributes to the transmission of a number of diseases that have a major health impact on this and other countries.

Population Growth, Density, and Distribution

Until recently, most of the world's population lived in rural areas. In 1800, for example, less than 1.7 percent of people lived in urban communities. By 1970, however, more than a third of the world's people lived in urban settings. By the year 2000, that fraction is expected to rise to one-half (Dentler, 1977).

Not only are more people choosing to live in urban areas, but the size and density of many cities are also increasing, in part because of the overall population growth rate—each year the population of the world grows by approximately 70 million. High birth rates in many cities contribute to urbanization. By the end of the century, there will be 425 cities with a million or more inhabitants, an increase of 200 cities since 1985 (United Nations, 1985; World Resources Institute, 1986). Twenty-five cities are expected to have populations that exceed 11 million (Last and Wallace, 1992).

In many parts of the world, urban population growth has been accompanied by overcrowding, poor hygiene, inadequate sanitation (including wastewater disposal), and insufficient supplies of clean water. Urban development, with its attendant construction, emergence of slum areas and shanty towns, and infrastructure needs (e.g., water treatment and waste disposal facilities), has also caused ecological damage. These factors have created conditions under which certain disease-causing organisms and the vectors that carry them have thrived. The dengue viruses and their primary mosquito vector, *Ae. aegypti*, are one such example.

Dengue

There are four distinct serotypes of dengue virus, each of which can cause a spectrum of illnesses ranging from mild fever and general malaise (dengue fever) to shock and fatal hemorrhagic disease (dengue hemorrhagic fever/dengue shock syndrome [DHF/DSS]). Dengue typically is a disease of young children, although older children and adults can be affected. Dengue viruses are transmitted to humans by *Ae. aegypti* mosquitoes.

Although dengue fever has plagued tropical populations for hundreds of years, the more severe form of the disease, DHF/DSS, is relatively new. The first recognized epidemic of DHF/DSS occurred in Manila in 1953 (Hammon et al., 1960). Dengue fever is usually the result of primary infection with one of the four dengue virus serotypes. DHF/DSS occurs in people who have been infected with two or more serotypes. The global spread and mixing of dengue serotypes have been made possible by the movement of infected individuals from one area to another.

Over the past 15 years, outbreaks of dengue fever have become increasingly numerous and severe, especially in urban centers in the tropics. At the same time, epidemics of DHF/DSS have spread from Asia to the Americas. In the early 1980s, the disease arrived in Cuba, where it killed 158 Cubans in a major outbreak in 1981. The most recent epidemic took place in Venezuela in 1990; more than 3,100 cases of severe hemorrhagic disease were recorded, as well as 73 deaths (Gubler, 1991). There are currently endemic foci of DHF/DSS in the Caribbean and on the Yucatan Peninsula of Mexico.

Although the disease is concentrated in a small number of areas, worldwide incidence rates for DHF/DSS have skyrocketed. Since its appearance in 1956, there have been an average of 29,803 cases of DHF/DSS reported per year. Between 1986 and 1990, the average number of reported cases per year was more than 267,692 (Gubler, 1991). In Southeast Asia, DHF/DSS ranks as one of the leading causes of hospitalization and death among children.

Although the reasons for the increase in dengue activity and the changing disease pattern are not fully understood, the consequences of increased urbanization, densely populated areas, and poor sanitation play a significant role. These conditions favor the growth of mosquito populations. Dengue virus, which is short-lived in the human host, is best maintained in densely populated areas in which *Ae. aegypti* is abundant and susceptible individuals are concentrated. The lack of effective mosquito control in many tropical urban centers—a by-product of economic and political problems as well as indifference—has undoubtedly contributed to the dramatic rise in dengue infection worldwide.

The United States experienced dengue fever outbreaks in 1922 and 1945 (Langone, 1990). No cases of DHF/DSS have been reported to date, but imported cases of dengue fever occur annually in U.S. citizens who have returned from travel abroad. In 1990, for instance, 24 confirmed cases of imported dengue were reported to the Centers for Disease Control (CDC) (Centers for Disease Control, 1991c). Although *Ae. aegypti* and *Ae. albopictus* (a secondary vector) have become firmly established in much of the southeastern United States, epidemics of DHF/DSS, such as those seen in Cuba and Venezuela, are unlikely. The United States is less vulnerable because its standard of living is higher, houses are more likely to be screened, and discarded tires (see Box 2-3) and other containers that can breed *Aedes* are much less common than in many cities in the tropics. At present, the only effective way to limit the spread of dengue is to attack its principal vector, *Ae. aegypti*. Government-supported pesticide application programs, and efforts of private citizens to eliminate mosquito breeding sites (i.e., source reduction) near their homes, have been shown to work. The success of such source reduction efforts rests on public education programs.

Like the yellow fever vaccine, a reasonably priced dengue vaccine will be an important adjunct to vector control in stemming the spread of urban epidemics. Dengue vaccine development, however, has been complicated

BOX 2-3 Environmental Eyesore or Mosquito Nursery?

Both! Discarded tires are an eyesore to most, but to some mosquitoes they offer an ideal location to deposit their eggs. *Aedes aegypti* and *Ae. albopictus*, both vectors of diseases such as dengue fever, viral encephalitis, and yellow fever, prefer to lay their eggs in water that collects in containers. Discarded tires, which hold water no matter in what position they land and which do not typically harbor predators like fish or frogs, are perfect incubators for the eggs of these mosquitoes. And each year, the United States throws away a quarter of a billion tires and imports several million (mostly from Japan) to be retreaded and resold.

Not only do the mosquitoes find homes in discarded tires, but they also find transportation. When old tires are transported around the country by truck, mosquito eggs often go with them. Eggs then hatch hundreds of miles from where they were laid, and populations of adult mosquitoes can establish themselves in areas they might never have reached. *Ae. albopictus* actually "hitchhiked" to the United States in 1985 from Japan in a shipment of used tires. Already, this species has established itself as a resident.

Tires are not the only human-made accommodations favored by mosquitoes. Any container that holds water—an empty beer or soda can, a bucket, or flowerpot—that is left outside during the warm spring and summer months is an attractive egg-laying site for a female mosquito. Some mosquitoes will even breed indoors in a moist container in a basement, garage, or shed if given the opportunity. This is in part why aerial spraying of pesticides is not an effective way to control mosquitoes; the insects usually lurk (and lay their eggs) in damp hiding places that the chemicals cannot reach.

Thus, as innocuous as they may seem to many, discarded items like old tires and empty aluminum cans may play a role in the initiation and spread of mosquito-borne disease. Eliminating human-made breeding sites is a simple, logical way to reduce the chances of such disease.

by the dengue virus's four serotypes. Scientists do not expect that a vaccine will be available in the next 5 to 10 years.

Immunosuppression

Immunosuppression, a weakening of the immune system, can be caused by a number of factors, including the following:

- Inherited diseases
- Aging
- Prematurity (neonates)

- HIV infection
- Radiation treatment
- Immunosuppressive medications for transplantation, therapy of malignancy (chemotherapy), or treatment of autoimmune disease
- Malnutrition
- Pregnancy
- Severe trauma and burns
- Other concurrent infections
- Malignancy

Immunosuppression can result in disease in an individual who otherwise would have been able to fend off illness. Infections caused by typically nonthreatening organisms that take advantage of a person's weakened state are called *opportunistic infections*.

Although opportunistic infections have received a great deal of attention over the past decade with the onset of the HIV disease pandemic, they are not new. During the pandemics of influenza in the early part of this century, it was well understood that both the very young (who have immature immune systems) and the elderly (who have waning immune defenses and, often, concurrent disease) were in the greatest danger of succumbing to this viral disease. New medical treatments and technologies—for example, therapy for collagen-vascular diseases like rheumatoid arthritis and vasculitis, cancer chemotherapy, and organ transplantation—have created additional openings for opportunistic pathogens.

There is good reason to believe that opportunistic infections will continue to threaten human health. The mean age of the U.S. population continues to rise. More and more people are surviving into their eighties and nineties, when previously non-life-threatening infections become common killers. Suboptimal prenatal care for women of lower socioeconomic status, which often results in premature and disease-prone infants, will likely continue to be the norm. The number of people with AIDS will continue to grow as those who became infected years ago develop full-blown disease. The HIV-infected population serves as a particularly important point of surveillance for emerging opportunistic infections because of its size and because the immunosuppression that characterizes the disease is comprehensive.

In many cases, knowledge of the type and extent of a person's immune dysfunction makes it possible to predict the kinds of infections that person is likely to acquire. When immune deficiency is acute and general in nature, however, any number of infections are apt to result, often simultaneously and often with astounding intensity. Such is the case for people with HIV disease. It is not surprising that opportunistic infections account for 90 percent of all HIV disease-related deaths (Double Helix, 1990).

Opportunistic infections are often caused by naturally occurring organisms that reside in most individuals. These organisms typically are kept in check by a healthy immune system, and many of them—for example, certain types of digestion-aiding bacteria in the intestine—are actually beneficial to normal body function. Disturbances in the integrity of the gastrointestinal tract, often the result of chemotherapy or radiation therapy, can introduce intestinal bacteria into the bloodstream, which can ultimately lead to life-threatening infection. Prolonged therapy with antibiotics can suppress the normal, resident bacteria that tend to keep fungal organisms like *Candida* in check, and the fungi can initiate a potentially dangerous infection.

The definition of an opportunistic infection should also include those infections caused by organisms that are normally pathogenic in healthy hosts but that are more common or induce more severe infections in the immune-impaired host. For example, although a nonimmune, healthy person who comes into contact with varicella virus might develop, and recover from, chickenpox, a person with an impaired immune system has a good chance of dying from the infection.

"Reactivated" infections, another type of opportunistic infection, occur in people who were previously infected with an organism that the body was able to suppress but not eliminate completely. When the immune systems of these individuals weaken, the circulating organism has a chance to cause disease again, or, in many cases, for the first time. For example, an estimated 80 percent of Americans are infected with cytomegalovirus (CMV), a herpesvirus (National Institute of Allergy and Infectious Diseases, 1991b). The virus typically does not produce serious illness in healthy adults, but for transplant recipients, who receive immunosuppressive drugs to keep them from rejecting foreign tissue, CMV can be a life-threatening complication.

Tuberculosis (TB) is another example of an infection that can be reactivated during immunosuppression. The causative agent of TB, *Mycobacterium tuberculosis*, usually persists in the body long after primary infection. Although infection with this bacterium in a previously unexposed person is usually self-limiting, reactivated TB, which can occur years later, can cause life-threatening lung disease. In recent years, TB has stricken HIV-infected individuals with alarming severity, causing a rapidly disseminated disease involving organs throughout the body.

After declining steadily since the 1950s, the incidence of TB in the United States has recently begun to climb. Since 1986, reported cases have increased 16 percent (see Figure 2-2) (Snider and Roper, 1992). This trend is largely attributable to cases of TB among those infected with HIV. TB is also occurring with greater frequency among immigrants and refugees, substance abusers, the homeless, the medically underserved, and the elderly. The majority of the increase has been among racial and ethnic minorities (especially blacks and Hispanics), children and young adults, and immigrants and refugees.

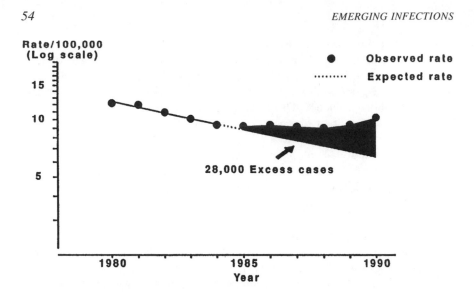

FIGURE 2-2 Incidence of tuberculosis, 1980 to 1990.
SOURCE: Center for Prevention Services, Centers for Disease Control.

The TB incidence rate among people infected with HIV is nearly 500 times the rate for the general population. In contrast to some fungal and other bacterial infections that occur only in the late stages of HIV disease, TB is a sentinel disease for HIV infection and tends to occur prior to other opportunistic infections, often before individuals realize they are HIV seropositive. In healthy individuals, pulmonary tuberculosis can be diagnosed and treated with relative ease (the cure rate is approximately 95 percent). In immunocompromised persons, however, the disease is often disseminated throughout the body, making it much more difficult to diagnose and treat.

Sexual Activity and Substance Abuse

The HIV disease pandemic is the most devastating outbreak of a sexually transmitted disease since the emergence of syphilis almost 500 years ago in Western Europe. Syphilis, a bacterial disease, spread rapidly during the late fifteenth and early sixteenth centuries, quickly reaching a prevalence of 20 percent in many urban areas (Hirsch, 1885). Scholars believe that the disease was disseminated by the sexual activities of soldiers, and heterosexual promiscuity was, and continues to be, the primary mechanism by which the infection is spread. The incidence of syphilis in the United States fell dramatically earlier in this century with the introduction of penicillin. Between 1985 and 1990, however, incidence almost doubled, most notably among heterosexuals who use crack cocaine (Centers for Disease Control, 1992f). A number of factors are associated with this rise, including multiple-partner sex to procure drugs, especially crack cocaine; inadequate health care among groups at risk; and declining educational levels among lower socioeconomic populations (Centers for Disease Control, 1991g).

The origin of HIV, the lentivirus (a member of the retrovirus family) that causes HIV disease and acquired immunodeficiency syndrome (AIDS), is not known. Viruses closely related to HIV have been present for hundreds, if not hundreds of thousands, of years in African nonhuman primates. Similar comparisons of human and nonhuman lentivirus isolates strongly suggest that HIV-2, the variant of HIV found primarily in persons from West Africa, may have infected humans following cross-species transmission from nonhuman primates (Gao et al., in press). This transmission could have occurred through bites of infected monkeys that were kept as pets, captured by trappers, or transported to other countries. Nucleotide sequence analyses show that HIV-2 and some isolates of simian immunodeficiency virus (SIV), an HIV-like virus, belong in the same subgroup; there are no data at present placing an SIV isolate from monkeys in the same subgroup as HIV-1. However, an SIV virus belonging to the same subgroup as HIV-1 has been isolated from chimpanzees. Yet if HIV-1-like viruses are present in nonhuman primates, it is possible that both HIV-1 and HIV-2 were occasionally, but infrequently, transmitted to humans and persisted in remote areas or in isolated individuals or populations for centuries. Although the earliest documented case of HIV infection was obtained from a serum sample collected in central Africa in 1959 (Garry, 1990), the country or continent in which the HIV disease epidemic began is not known. What is clear is that HIV and SIV arose through natural evolutionary processes.

The HIV disease pandemic initially escaped detection because of the disease's long incubation period (the time from infection to onset of life-threatening disease). After reservoirs of infection had been established in African and Western countries, HIV spread to all parts of the globe. In Africa, it is believed that HIV was transported by the movement of infected individuals from isolated rural communities to rapidly expanding cities. This urbanization was accompanied by changes in sexual behavior, which played a major role in the transmission of HIV among (primarily) heterosexual populations in Africa (Quinn et al., 1986). Preexisting infection with other sexually transmitted microorganisms, especially those that cause genital ulcers and local genital tract inflammation, probably facilitated heterosexual transmission of HIV (Hillman et al., 1989).

The early spread of HIV, particularly in the United States and Europe, was largely the result of high-risk sexual practices of some male homosexuals, and it was in this population that most of the early cases were seen. Within a short period, however, another major group of HIV-infected individuals emerged: intravenous substance abusers. The introduction of crack cocaine in the United States in the mid-1980s added another component to the complex epidemiology of HIV infection. Many persons who abuse crack cocaine use sex as a currency to support their habit. The result has been a striking rise in heterosexually transmitted syphilis, chancroid, and HIV infection. Although in the United States, HIV infection occurs predominately in male homosexuals and intravenous substance abusers, the rate of infection among non-substance-abusing heterosexuals is increasing.

The fact that HIV first established itself in the United States mainly among gay men has both negative and positive repercussions. On the negative side, rapid emergence was facilitated among those individuals who engaged in anal intercourse with multiple partners. On the positive side, unusual diseases related to HIV infection initially occurred in a specific subpopulation, and that specificity probably hastened recognition of the syndrome and its infectious nature. Had the first cases of AIDS occurred in a more diverse population, it is likely that discovery of the exact nature of the problem would have been slowed. Once the disease was recognized as a new entity with the potential for epidemic spread, the biomedical research community began a concerted effort to identify the etiologic agent. Collaborations were established between health care workers, who provided blood samples from patients, and researchers, who in turn isolated and defined properties of the virus so that blood tests could be generated and the development of drugs and vaccines could begin.

Unfortunately, the U.S. political sector was not as responsive to the crisis and by its slow response may have contributed to the explosive growth of the epidemic. A major reason for this hesitancy appeared to be the antipathy of some federal officials to the behaviors of those persons initially affected by HIV disease: gay men and substance abusers. In some instances, federal officials thwarted efforts to curtail the epidemic. For example, former Surgeon General C. Everett Koop has stated, "Even though the Centers for Disease Control commissioned the first AIDS task force as early as June 1981, I, as Surgeon General, was not allowed to speak about AIDS publicly until the second Reagan term. Whenever I spoke on a health issue at a press conference or on a network morning TV show, the government public affairs people told the media in advance that I would not answer questions on AIDS, and I was not to be asked any questions on the subject. I have never understood why these peculiar restraints were placed on me. And although I have sought the explanation, I still don't know the answer" (Koop, 1991).

More detrimental, however, was the government's continued resistance to proposed sex education programs designed to interrupt transmission of HIV (Koop, 1991). The federal government's recent revocation of funding for an approved five-year study of teenage sexual behavior (Marshall,

1991) indicates the continuing controversy and ambivalence that surrounds many aspects of the nation's response to HIV disease.

To date, no drug has been developed that can prevent or cure HIV infection, and it is not likely that a vaccine will be available soon. In many areas of the world, particularly Eastern Europe, India, and Southeast Asia, the numbers of cases of the disease are escalating rapidly. In Africa, the demographics of the pandemic are changing, with HIV-infected individuals moving away from cities and back to rural areas (R. M. Anderson et al., 1991). In Africa, Latin America, the Caribbean, and North America, HIV is infecting increasingly larger numbers of heterosexuals, intravenous substance abusers, and children (Centers for Disease Control, 1991a). In 1989, HIV disease passed heart disease to become the second leading cause of death in U.S. males aged 25 to 44, behind accidental and unintended injury (Centers for Disease Control, 1991e). Estimates now place the total number of adults worldwide who have developed HIV disease at more than 1 million and those who are infected with HIV at 10 million. The World Health Organization (WHO) estimates that as many as 40 million people could be infected with HIV by the year 2000 (World Health Organization, 1991).

TECHNOLOGY AND INDUSTRY

Notwithstanding all of their benefits, technology and industry may directly or indirectly cause the emergence of infectious diseases. Modern medicine has created situations that are ideally suited for the emergence of infectious agents. The food and agriculture industries work continually to prevent the introduction of pathogenic organisms into our food supply, but they are not always successful. Waterborne pathogens are controlled by the careful treatment and disinfection of drinking water, but breakdowns do occur and sometimes result in the spread of infectious disease.

Modern Medicine

Generally, people who enter the hospital expect that their health will be improved by the treatment they receive. For at least 1 out of 20 patients, however, this is not the case. Each year, an estimated 2 million individuals in the United States (about 5 percent of the total number hospitalized) suffer nosocomial infections—viral, bacterial, protozoan, and fungal infections that were not present or incubating at the time of hospital admission (Fuchs, 1979; Wenzel, 1988; Martone, 1990). The rates of nosocomial infections in developing countries may be 5 to 10 times higher (Wenzel, 1987).

The health and financial impacts of nosocomial infections in this country are staggering. More than 20,000 deaths annually are attributed to hospital-acquired infections, and patients who recover from these infections typically require 10 extra days of hospital care (Fuchs, 1979; Wenzel, 1988). Every year, hospital-acquired infections account for between $5 billion and $10 billion in additional medical-related expenses, most of which are due to excess hospital stays (Wenzel, 1987; Schaechter et al., 1989; Martone, 1990).

Although hospital sanitation has improved markedly since the late nineteenth century, when carbolic acid was first used as an antiseptic during surgery, nosocomial infections continue to challenge efforts to control them (Fuchs, 1979). Medical advances and antimicrobial resistance are at the heart of the struggle.

In February 1991, the CDC's Hospital Infections Division looked at 10-year trends in nosocomial infections using data collected through the National Nosocomial Infections Surveillance System (NNISS). The 1980s saw a tripling of the incidence of bacteremias (Ross, 1990) and a shift in the organisms that are most prevalent as the causes of nosocomial infections, from those that are generally susceptible to antimicrobials (e.g., *Proteus mirabilis*, *Escherichia coli*, and *Klebsiella pneumoniae*) to those that tend to be more refractory to treatment (e.g., *Enterobacter*, *Pseudomonas*, *Enterococcus*, and *Candida* species) (Schaberg et al., 1991). In addition, there appears to have been a significant increase in both the prevalence and variety of viral and fungal pathogens found to be causes of nosocomial infections (Ross, 1990). All of these observations implicate the hospital setting as a prime site for the emergence of microbial threats to health.

Many of the factors that increase the risk of infection in a hospital are inherent to any health care setting. Not only are persons with serious infections frequently admitted to hospitals, thus providing an intrahospital source of pathogenic organisms, but the proportion of people with increased susceptibility to infections is also greater in a hospital than in the general population. In addition, because health care institutions are not completely isolated from the community (employees, visitors, food, and supplies enter daily), patients are exposed to the same pathogens that circulate in the surrounding locale. Thus, nosocomial infections can be transmitted from staff to patients, from visitors to patients, and from patients to other patients. Infections can also be acquired from contaminated surfaces, such as floors, examining tables, or improperly sterilized instruments, and from the patient's own normal microbial flora, especially during invasive procedures.

Antimicrobial resistance, a problem in the treatment of many bacterial diseases, has particular relevance in the hospital setting. By their very nature, hospitals are filled with people who have increased susceptibility to infection. Also by nature, hospitals tend to use large quantities of antibiotics. (About a third of hospitalized patients receive such agents [Shapiro et al., 1979].) The combination of an immunologically vulnerable population and the widespread use of antibiotics is potentially risky, since the selective pressure exerted on microbes by the constant challenge of antimicrobial compounds favors the survival of organisms that are resistant to these drugs (Holmberg et al., 1987).

An organism's development of drug resistance through selective pressure usually begins with exposure to an antimicrobial drug. Antimicrobial drugs and other compounds designed to combat human pathogens work by killing or inhibiting the growth of susceptible microorganisms. Because of genetic variability, however, not every bacterium, virus, protozoan, helminth, or fungus is naturally susceptible to these drugs. The result is that the drugs leave untouched a small number of resistant microbes, effectively "selecting for" those organisms that can survive attack by the drugs. These resistant organisms pose a potentially serious threat to health. Although the role of selective pressure in antimicrobial resistance is clear, additional studies (using appropriate epidemiological and molecular biological methodologies) are needed to identify and investigate the risk factors that promote transmission of resistant pathogens in the hospital setting.

Many standard hospital procedures facilitate patient acquisition of nosocomial infections. The use of conventional medical devices is responsible for the greatest share of such infections: several hundred thousand cases of device-related disease occur each year. The most common of these (and the most frequent of all nosocomial infections) is urinary tract infection (UTI) (Harding et al., 1991). The great majority of hospital-acquired UTIs are the result of catheterization. In some cases, infection results from nonsterile insertion of the catheter; more frequently, however, it is the entry with the catheter of normal body bacteria (e.g., *E. coli* and *Staphylococcus* species, which are usually kept out of the bladder by the mucosal barriers of the urinary tract) that cause infection. Other devices, such as endotracheal tubes and mechanical ventilators, can cause infection in a similar fashion.

Pneumonia is the second most common hospital-acquired illness and the leading cause of death from nosocomial infection. Infections related to surgical wounds are the third most common type. Skin provides one of the body's natural defenses against microbial invasion, and it is also home to usually harmless staphylococcal bacteria. When the skin is broken, however, as happens during surgery or intravenous catheterization, staphylococci (including antibiotic-resistant hospital strains) can gain access to deeper tissues and cause infection. Bloodstream infections, the fourth most common type of nosocomial condition, occur when microbes make their way deep into the body—typically with the help of medical devices or the use of invasive procedures—and enter the bloodstream. On rare occasions, bloodstream infections, including transfusion-induced yersiniosis and HIV infection, can also result from the use of contaminated blood products (see Box 2-4) (Cover and Aber, 1989; Martone, 1990).

BOX 2-4   How Safe Is the Blood Supply?

Many of the 4 million people who receive a blood transfusion in the United States each year have concerns about contracting a communicable disease in the process. Like organs and other tissues that are transplanted, blood is a biological product that can host disease-causing microorganisms. Fortunately, however, blood that is donated today goes through a battery of tests designed to ensure that it is free of contamination by infectious agents. The American Red Cross (ARC) now tests donor blood for syphilis, hepatitis B and C, human T-lymphotrophic virus types 1 and 2 (HTLV-I and HTLV-II), HIV-1, and, recently, HIV-2 as well. HIV-2 currently ranks as the primary cause of HIV disease only in West Africa; yet as of September 1991, 31 people in the United States had been diagnosed with HIV-2 infection, making the virus a potential threat to the safety of the blood supply in this country (Johnston, 1991).

The Department of Defense (DOD) and the American Association of Blood Banks (AABB) recently took steps to protect the blood supply from contamination with another microorganism, the leishmania parasite. Found primarily in Africa and Asia, the parasite was found late last year in the blood of more than two dozen soldiers returning from the Persian Gulf War. Both the DOD and the AABB, as well as the ARC, plan to refuse donations until at least 1993 from all individuals—mainly members of the U.S. armed services—who have traveled to the Middle East since August 1990.

Many of the efforts made by blood banks to improve the safety of the blood supply have been tremendously successful. Thirty years ago, nearly one in three people who received a blood transfusion contracted some form of hepatitis; today, that risk has dropped to less than 1 in 100 (Russell, 1991). The chances of contracting HIV from a blood transfusion are considerably less than in the early 1980s, when AIDS was first identified. Prior to 1985, when testing for HIV in donor blood became widespread, more than 4,300 persons were infected by the virus through blood transfusions. From 1985 through December 1991, only 20 people have acquired HIV through transfusions (Centers for Disease Control, 1992e). The risk of HIV infection from a blood transfusion has been estimated at from 1 in 40,000 to 1 in 150,000 per unit of blood transfused, depending on the region from which the blood originated (Russell, 1991).

Safeguards against microorganism-contaminated blood unfortunately are not foolproof. As a result, doctors have become much more conservative about using transfusions. Most encourage patients to contribute their own blood prior to surgery whenever possible, and many doctors have sought new alternatives to transfusions altogether. Automated cell salvage techniques that can be used either during or after surgery to recover, cleanse, and return lost blood are one such alternative. Until the search for an effective blood substitute is successful (several companies appear to be close to developing a safe product), protecting the blood supply and its users from infectious disease remains a top priority.

Complex invasive procedures, such as tissue or organ transplantation, can also lead to nosocomial infection. The immunosuppressive drugs used to prevent the rejection of the foreign tissue or organ have the undesirable side effect of weakening the body's immune system. Often, these infections do not involve hospital microbes but pathogens from the donor tissue or pathogens that are already present in the recipient. Extensive testing of foreign tissue prior to transplantation guards against transmission of most such microbes. Latent agents, however, like the "slow" virus that causes Creutzfeld-Jacob disease, are extremely difficult to detect and may be inadvertently transferred to the transplant recipient in the seemingly normal tissue of the donor. Cases of HIV infection, hepatitis C, and CMV infection resulting from organ transplantation have all been documented, as have cases of Creutzfeld-Jacob, a degenerative brain disease, in recipients of transplanted corneas and human growth hormone (Lorber, 1988; Pereira et al., 1991).

HEALTH CARE DELIVERY

Changes in health care delivery over the past 20 years undoubtedly have had an impact on nosocomial infection rates. Rising health care costs play a key role. One cost-conscious health care strategy that appears to be contributing to the rise in cases of nosocomial infection is so called industrial management in hospitals. Industrial management is intended both to maximize the ratio of patients to nurses and to maintain pools of health care workers—particularly nurses—who can rotate frequently between two or more units of an institution. From the hospital's perspective, maximizing the ratio of patients to nurses is desirable because it decreases health care costs. At the same time, the practice can increase disease transmission by reducing the time available for proper sanitation and increasing the number of infected patients to whom a nurse is exposed.

Exacerbating the potential disease-producing quality of these problems is the increasing bidirectional transfer of patients between acute care and chronic care hospitals. The mixing of patients from acute care facilities (who tend to be severely ill) with residents of chronic care hospitals (who tend to have decreased immune function owing to aging or chronic illness, or both) is potentially risky. Compared with hospital-based programs, infection control programs in many long-term care facilities are rudimentary, at best. Unlike hospital-based programs, there are no standardized criteria for defining nosocomial infections in long-term care facilities; in addition, adequate studies designed to assess the efficacy of their surveillance and control measures have not been conducted. This state of affairs contrasts sharply with such efforts in acute care hospitals, which have received far more attention and federal funding.

The problem is likely to grow even more serious with time, given the Agency for Health Care Policy and Research's estimates that 43 percent of all those who turned 65 years old in 1990 will enter a nursing home at some point in their lives (Agency for Health Care Policy and Research, 1990).

In sum, hospitals and long-term care facilities can no longer be viewed as isolated epidemiological units but must be seen as part of a network of patient care facilities. This network makes it possible for nosocomial and community-acquired infections to be rapidly and widely spread.

PREVENTION OF NOSOCOMIAL INFECTIONS

Studies show, surprisingly, that even under the most sanitary of conditions, only about a third to a half of all hospital-acquired infections are preventable (Schaechter et al., 1989; Martone, 1990). Several factors "stack the deck" against infection control efforts. Little can be done to eliminate most of these risk factors, which include age (newborns and the elderly have limited immunity), severity of illness (related to length of stay, also a risk factor), and underlying diseases (latent infections or immune deficiencies) (Freeman and McGowan, 1978). Increased attempts at prevention for high-risk patients may be the only weapon against infection in these circumstances.

Two recent approaches to controlling hospital-acquired infections have been remarkably successful: CDC's 1987 "Universal Blood and Body Fluid Precautions" and hepatitis B vaccination. Under the universal precautions, blood and certain body fluids of *all* patients are considered potential sources of HIV, hepatitis B virus (HBV), and other blood-borne pathogens. The guidelines are a revision of a 1983 document that recommended special precautions (use of gloves and other protective barriers, and careful handling and disposal of needles and other sharp instruments) for blood and body fluids of patients known or suspected to be infected with blood-borne pathogens. The hepatitis B vaccine was licensed in 1982.

Statistics demonstrate the impact of these two infection control measures. A recent study by the Hepatitis Branch at CDC documented a 75 percent decrease in cases of hepatitis B among health care workers in four sentinel counties between 1982 and 1988 (Alter et al., 1990). The study's authors surmised that the decrease in cases was "probably a direct result of immunization with hepatitis B vaccine and of wider implementation of universal blood precautions" (Alter et al., 1990).

Although the hepatitis B story clearly can be counted as a victory for hospital infection control, new microbial threats are likely to surface in the future. Health care institutions are prime breeding grounds for new and more virulent strains of organisms and may well represent one of the most important sites of surveillance for new pathogens that will emerge to jeopardize health in the future.

Food Processing and Handling

The potential for foods to be involved in the emergence or reemergence of microbial threats to humans is great, in large part because there are many points in the food chain at which food safety can be compromised. This chain of events begins wherever crops or animals are raised; it proceeds through a complex system of manufacturing, distribution, and retailing and ends with the use of a food product by the consumer. Changes in any of a number of aspects of the farm-to-consumer chain, or inattention to food safety in general, can result in outbreaks of food-borne illness.

Although food containing viruses or parasites can cause illness (as can chemical contamination), the majority of individual cases of food-borne disease of known etiology in the United States are caused by bacteria. However, in more than half of the outbreaks of food-borne illness, the exact cause is unknown (Bean and Griffin, 1990). Although in many cases the lack of an exact cause reflects an incomplete investigation, at least some proportion of those outbreaks are likely to be the result of as yet unidentified food-borne pathogens.

There has been a substantial increase in our knowledge of food-borne diseases during the past 20 years, as reflected in an approximate tripling of the list of known food-borne pathogens. An important component of this increase in understanding is a better scientific grasp of the factors that allow microorganisms, and bacteria in particular, to cause human disease. Because of better methods of identifying food-borne pathogens, it has become clear that only certain strains of a bacterial species may cause food-borne illness.

For example, *Escherichia coli* is part of the natural intestinal flora of humans; its presence in a water sample has been used as evidence of fecal contamination by other pathogenic microorganisms. The majority of isolates of *E. coli* pose no threat to humans as food-borne pathogens. Researchers, however, have identified five distinct groups of *E. coli* that cause enteric disease. Based on the mechanism of pathogenesis of each group, they are designated enteroinvasive, enterotoxigenic, enteropathogenic, enteroadherent, and enterohemorrhagic *E. coli* (Archer and Young, 1988). The ability to detect these pathogenic isolates has been greatly enhanced by diagnostic tests that identify specific virulence-related genes or gene products such as toxins, adhesins, and cell-surface markers.

Improved epidemiologic surveillance has also played an important role in identifying microorganisms that cause food-borne disease. This was the

case for four outbreaks of human listeriosis, a bacterial infection that occurred in the United States, Canada, and Switzerland in the early to mid-
1980s. Careful monitoring of disease incidence data by medical facilities
allowed these epidemics to be detected, even though the actual number of
cases was relatively low. Subsequent epidemiologic investigations implicated cole slaw (Schlech et al., 1983), milk (Fleming et al., 1985), and soft
cheeses (Office of Federal Public Health, Switzerland, 1988; Linnan et al.,
1988) as the vehicle of infection. Of particular concern is that listeriosis,
caused by *Listeria monocytogenes*, is most often diagnosed in pregnant
women or their newborns and in immunosuppressed individuals, in whom it
can be fatal. The CDC has recently published recommendations for the
prevention of food-borne listeriosis; for those at high risk (immunocompromised individuals, pregnant women, and the elderly) the recommendations
cite additional foods to avoid (Centers for Disease Control, 1992h).

AGRICULTURAL CONDITIONS AND PRACTICES

Any change in the conditions or practices associated with the production
of agricultural commodities can affect the safety of the food supply. A
virtually uncontrollable factor, like the weather, can have a substantial impact. For example, drought can make grains more susceptible to mycotoxin-
producing fungi, and toxic fungal metabolites, such as aflatoxin, can threaten
the health of both humans and livestock. This particular risk has been substantially lessened by an ongoing U.S. Department of Agriculture (USDA)
program that monitors the status of major agricultural commodities. Once
identified, contaminated grain is destroyed.

New agricultural procedures can also have unanticipated microbiological
effects. For example, the introduction of feedlots and large-scale poultry
rearing and processing facilities has been implicated in the increasing incidence of human pathogens, such as *Salmonella*, in domestic animals over
the past 30 years. The use of antibiotics to enhance the growth of and
prevent illness in domestic animals has been questioned because of its potential role in the development and dissemination of antibiotic resistance
(Cohen and Tauxe, 1986; Institute of Medicine, 1989). Approximately half
the tonnage of antibiotics produced in the United States is used in the
raising of animals for human consumption. Thus, concerns about the selection of antibiotic-resistant strains of bacteria and their passage into the
human population as a result of this excessive use of antibiotics are realistic
(Institute of Medicine, 1989). It is conceivable that surveillance of feedlot
animals for the development of resistant organisms might be a means of
early warning for the emergence of newly drug-resistant pathogens.

Broad-based societal events indirectly related to agriculture may also
affect food safety. Recent concerns about bovine spongiform encephalopathy

(BSE) illustrate this point. In 1980, in England, the combination of increasing fuel prices and tighter restrictions on the use of organic solvents for lipid extraction led to changes in the processing of offal, the viscera and trimmings of butchered animals that are a major component of animal feed. The new methods do not appear to inactivate sufficiently the BSE agent, and increased incidence of BSE in domestic animals has been linked to offal. There is considerable controversy, at least in England, about whether the BSE agent may also infect humans (Dealer and Lacey, 1990, 1991; K. C. Taylor, 1991). To date, however, no human infections have been detected.

In addition to modifications of traditional farming methods, the introduction of new types of agriculture can have an impact on the emergence of microbial threats. Aquaculture and mariculture, for example, are rapidly becoming important methods of producing fish and seafood. Yet there has been relatively little effort to understand the potential microbial impact of this new technology. As aquaculture and mariculture farmers attempt to increase their yields of freshwater and marine animals, the stresses of overcrowding and overfeeding create ideal conditions for *Aeromonas hydrophila*, a common fish pathogen found in fresh and estuarine waters (Plumb, 1975; Hazen et al., 1978). Increasingly, *A. hydrophila*, *A. veronii* (biovariant *sobria*), *A. caviae*, *A. jandaei*, *A. trota*, *A. schubertii*, and *A. veronii* (biovariant *veronii*) are being implicated as causes of nosocomial, wound, waterborne, and food borne infections in humans (Daily et al., 1981; Buchanan and Palumbo, 1985; Hickman-Brenner et al., 1987, 1988; Janda and Duffcy, 1988; Carnahan et al., 1989; Carnahan and Joseph, 1991; Joseph et al., 1991; Samuel Joseph, Professor, Department of Microbiology, University of Maryland, personal communication, 1992). These bacterial infections are being found in immunocompromised individuals and those in otherwise poor health (W. A. Davis et al., 1978). Although there are a number of potential sources of infection with *Aeromonas* species, aquaculture and mariculture are probably the most common sources, since the incidence of these organisms in the products of these agricultural methods approaches 100 percent.

The use of human and animal fecal material to enrich pond cultures in parts of China and India raises additional concerns about the safety of some imported aquaculture products (Ward, 1989). Such practices may enhance the spread of pathogens transmitted by an oral-fecal route. In the Calcutta region of India, where this method of enrichment is used to raise prawns, a high incidence of non-O1 *Vibrio cholerae* contamination has been reported (Nair et al., 1991).

FOOD PROCESSING AND PRESERVATION TECHNOLOGIES

The application of new food processing and preservation technologies can have unexpected effects on the microbial safety of foods. Something as simple as a change in packaging can be important. For example, plastic overwraps for packages of fresh mushrooms were introduced in 1967 because they enhanced the keeping-quality of this highly perishable food. It was soon discovered, however, that the respiratory rate of mushrooms is so rapid that, even with a semipermeable plastic film, the oxygen in the pack is quickly depleted. This produces an anaerobic environment perfectly suited to *Clostridium botulinum*, the neurotoxin-producing bacterium that causes botulism (Sugiyama and Yang, 1975). The problem was remedied by punching two holes in the plastic film, which allowed sufficient oxygen transfer to prevent the growth of anaerobes and still permitted enough carbon dioxide accumulation to retard spoilage (Kautter et al., 1978).

Another example comes from China. It appears that the transportation of brined mushrooms in plastic bags in that country provided conditions favorable to the growth of *S. aureus* (Hardt-English et al., 1990). The resulting presence of staphylococcal enterotoxin brought a halt (which is still in force) in November 1989 to the importation of Chinese mushrooms into the United States.

New food preservation methods, such as modified atmosphere packaging (MAP), are being used with more frequency as U.S. consumers demonstrate a preference for *fresh* food products that have a minimum of processing and preservatives. MAP uses combinations of gases to suppress aerobic spoilage bacteria that create unpleasant odors and flavors (Seideman and Durland, 1984). Unfortunately, these gases may not discourage, and may even encourage, the growth of other pathogenic microorganisms that are not detectable by smell or taste (Post et al., 1985; Hintlian and Hotchkiss, 1986, 1987; Berrang et al., 1989; Ingham et al., 1990; Wimpfheimer et al., 1990; Hart et al., 1991).

One technology for ridding foods of microbial contaminants is ionizing irradiation. This approach was used for many years to sterilize medical equipment and supplies; at low doses, it can eliminate or control pathogenic bacteria, fungi, protozoa, and helminths in foods (Thayer, 1990). The technology is also highly effective for insect disinfestations. Ionizing irradiation to pasteurize or sterilize foods has been recommended as an effective tool for the control of food-borne diseases (Joint Expert Committee on Food Irradiation, 1980; Council for Agricultural Science and Technology, 1986; Thayer, 1990). It has been approved for various applications in more than 30 countries; this includes, recently, approval for eliminating insects from fruits, *Trichinella spiralis* from infected pork, and *Salmonella* from raw poultry. One of the unique characteristics of irradiation is that the appearance of foods processed in this way is not altered. Much of the controversy over the use of irradiation is the result of the misconception that treated foods are radioactive. Extensive research has unequivocally demonstrated that there is no induction of radiation in foods that are treated with isotope sources of ^{60}Co or ^{137}Cs, x-ray sources of up to 5 million electron volts (MeV), or accelerated electron beam sources of less than 10 MeV (Koch and Eisenhower, 1967; Becker, 1983). It should be noted, however, that irradiation is not a panacea. In dairy products, which contain lipids sensitive to oxidation, for example, taste is affected. Furthermore, the technique is generally considered much less effective for inactivating viruses, compared with its effectiveness with bacteria and other more complex pathogens (e.g., fungi).

DEMOGRAPHICS

There are several important, ongoing demographic changes in the United States that will have direct and indirect effects on the emergence of new food-borne microbial diseases. Foremost is the fact that, at least through the early twenty-first century, the population increasingly will be composed of the elderly, a group particularly susceptible to food-borne pathogens.

Population expansion and the accompanying demands on infrastructure can also affect the safety of the food supply. For example, when estuarine areas are developed for residential or recreational purposes, water treatment capacity often lags behind requirements imposed by the population increase. In some cases, potentially dangerous viral and bacterial pathogens are released into the water from sewage effluent and storm-drain runoff, where they are concentrated by shellfish and subsequently harvested and consumed, often with minimal processing. The closing of shellfish beds because of the presence of these pathogens has become a major public health and economic issue in a number of coastal regions. The problem is compounded by poaching from closed beds. Methods for testing water for human enteric viruses (e.g., hepatitis A and C, Norwalk virus, and caliciviruses) currently are inadequate (Institute of Medicine, 1991b).

CONSUMER ATTITUDES AND BEHAVIOR

In general, particularly in the developed world, the public expects its food supply to be safe. To a great extent this expectation has been met through the safe manufacturing and distribution of prepared foods. The extent of training that individuals receive in proper food handling and preparation is declining. Owing to changes in family structure and the roles of women, home economics courses are being deemphasized in schools, and the use of convenience foods and dining out is increasing. With these changes, assumptions about food safety may lead to complacency. Consumer inattention to appropriate steps for maintaining food safety in the home can easily overwhelm safeguards built into food production and processing.

COMMERCE

Historically, most foods have been produced and consumed locally. The internationalization of the food industry since World War II, made possible by the advent of refrigerated freighters, has changed this simple relationship. Now fresh fruits and vegetables that previously would have been available for only a few weeks can be obtained all year long. Wide-scale importation of food products has greatly increased dietary options for many consumers. At the same time, there is concern that these foods may come from regions in which hygienic practices are not on a par with those in the United States. With this concern in mind, the movement of the South American cholera epidemic into Mexico is being monitored closely by U.S. public health officials, since Mexico supplies the United States with much of its fresh produce during the winter months.

International trade has become so pervasive that it is virtually impossible to screen most of the food entering the country for known microbial hazards, let alone for new microbiological threats. This situation is likely to continue as political agreements remove barriers between trading partners. There is already virtually unrestricted movement of foods among the member nations of the European Economic Community, for example. Similarly, the U.S.-Canada-Mexico free-trade agreement is likely to lead to reduced inspection of imported foods, a subject that is currently being hotly debated. For foods entering the United States, as in Europe, there is likely to be increasing reliance on inspections conducted by the country of origin. This will necessitate the further development and implementation of international standards, such as the Codex Alimentarius of the Joint Food and Agricultural Organization/World Health Organization Food Standards Programme.

International commerce can affect food safety, even when the food itself is not being transported. This was the case in a 1986 outbreak of shellfish-related paralytic poisonings in South Australia and Tasmania. The poisonings were caused by *Alexandrium catenella*, *A. minutum*, and *Gymnodinium catenatum*, three dinoflagellate species not normally found in that part of the world. These marine plankton, which produce potent neurotoxins, are concentrated by shellfish as they filter particulate matter from seawater. The toxins do not affect shellfish, but they can cause serious neurological problems when consumed by warm-blooded animals. The likely source of the organisms was the bilge water of ocean-going freighters. Typically, bilge water is changed while ships are in port, releasing the microscopic stowaways. Studies have indicated that entire miniature ecosystems are transported around the world in this manner (Hallegraeff and Bolch, 1991; Jones, 1991).

DIET AND FOOD PREPARATION

New dietary habits also have had an impact on disease emergence. Immigration to the United States, in particular, the relatively recent heavy influx of peoples from Latin America and Asia, has introduced many U.S. residents to new foods. Although popular, some of these foods, or the ways in which they are prepared, can cause disease as a result of contamination by any number of organisms or their toxic byproducts. Ceviche—raw seafood served in lemon juice—and sushi—raw seafood and rice wrapped in seaweed—are perhaps the most obvious examples of ethnic foods that have been associated with disease transmission, in most cases caused by intestinal worms (helminths).

Trichinosis

Trichinosis, a generally self-limiting but potentially fatal disease caused by an intestinal roundworm that migrates to and encysts in striated muscle tissue, can be contracted from improperly prepared food. Trichinosis incidence in the United States had declined nearly every year since 1947 (Bailey and Schantz, 1990). As a result mainly of a single large outbreak of trichinosis, however, the incidence of the disease increased in 1990. The largest recent outbreak in this country occurred when uncooked, contaminated commercial pork sausage was consumed at a wedding reception. Ninety individuals, most of whom were Southeast Asian immigrants who customarily eat raw sausage, developed trichinosis (Centers for Disease Control, 1991i). Although the majority of cases of trichinosis still result from eating raw or insufficiently cooked commercial pork, consumption of insufficiently frozen or cooked wild game, particularly walrus and bear, has been increasingly associated with the disease, at least since 1975 (McAuley et al., 1991).

Anisakiasis

Cases of human anisakiasis, a food-borne disease, generally are caused by either of two species of nematode worms, *Pseudoterranova decipiens* and *Anisakis simplex*, commonly referred to as codworms and herring worms, respectively. Adult worms are found in marine mammals and release eggs that hatch in seawater; they are ingested by krill, which are eaten in turn by squid or fish. Larval-stage worms penetrate the bowel of the fish and encyst in the muscle. Humans contract anisakiasis by eating raw or partially cooked seafood containing nematode larvae.

Anisakiasis occurs most commonly in people living in coastal areas or areas in which the consumption of raw fish is customary. The fish most often responsible for anisakiasis are cod, pollock, halibut, rockfish, flatfish, mackerel, salmon, and herring. Although only 50 cases were documented in the United States from 1958 to 1988 (McKerrow et al., 1988), these figures probably underestimate the actual incidence of anisakiasis, which is not a reportable disease. In countries in which the consumption of raw seafood is common, anisakiasis is more prevalent. In 1984 in Japan, for example, 3,141 cases were reported (Oshima, 1987). With the current U.S. trend to encourage more people to eat fish for dietary reasons, it is important that the consumer be reminded to thoroughly cook the fish to preclude infection with nematodes, such as those that cause anisakiasis.

Water Treatment

Water that is untreated or that does not receive adequate processing can transmit infectious agents, such as bacteria (*Vibrio cholerae, Salmonella typhi*, enterotoxigenic *Escherichia coli*), viruses (hepatitis A virus and other enteroviruses, rotaviruses, Norwalk gastroenteritis viruses), and protozoan parasites (*Giardia lamblia, Cryptosporidium, Entamoeba histolytica*). A primary source for many of these pathogens is fecal contamination of source water that is subsequently inadequately treated, or similar contamination after treatment. Leakage of wastewater from septic tanks and other sewage disposal facilities into groundwater can also transmit infection. Fortunately, most water used in this country is effectively processed by municipal water treatment facilities.

In some instances, water is not treated. This is often the case with water from private wells or from natural springs. In 1989, for example, an outbreak of some 900 cases of gastroenteritis occurred in a new resort community in north-central Arizona. An investigation revealed that the source of the outbreak was tap water obtained from a deep well on the resort property. A Norwalk-like virus was apparently introduced into the well by a faulty sewage treatment facility nearby, whose untreated sewage passed through fractures in the sandstone and limestone fields surrounding the well (Lawson et al., 1991).

Water used for recreational purposes can also be the source of waterborne infectious disease outbreaks, caused by pathogens such as hepatitis A virus (Bryan et al., 1974) or *Shigella* (Blostein, 1991). Particularly in the southwestern portion of the United States, water used for recreation increasingly is actually reclaimed wastewater. Wastewater treated to remove undesirable organic and inorganic contaminants is also being used for irrigation, industrial processing, and nonpotable residential (watering lawns and trees, toilet flushing) and commercial (golf courses, for example) applications. Inadvertent ingestion of reclaimed water, which has undergone the same basic treatment as potable water (including disinfection), is not likely to cause waterborne disease. Reclaimed water used for drinking is more of a concern because of residual contamination.

Not unexpectedly, the higher the quality of source water entering water treatment facilities, the easier it is to produce safe water for drinking. Unfortunately, high-quality sources of potable water are increasingly difficult to locate and maintain. This is especially true for areas that depend on large watersheds, such as the Mississippi and Ohio rivers, which are often polluted with chemicals and biological wastes. To treat such polluted water adequately puts a heavy burden on water treatment plants. In many urban areas, the designed capacities of municipal water treatment facilities are being challenged by the growth in population; in addition, equipment or procedural breakdowns may allow inadequately treated water to reach the consumer.

Outbreaks of waterborne disease in the United States are uncommon because of the nation's extensive public health infrastructure. Public health authorities, however, are especially mindful of potential outbreaks following natural disasters, such as earthquakes and hurricanes, that can lead to contamination of municipal water supplies.

ECONOMIC DEVELOPMENT AND LAND USE

Dam Building and Rift Valley Fever

Until relatively recently, Rift Valley fever, which is caused by a mosquito-borne virus, occurred only in Africa south of the Sahara and was primarily a disease of sheep and cattle. Periodic outbreaks were prevalent in South Africa, Tanzania, Kenya, and, during the mid-1970s, in the Sudan.

The first major outbreak of human disease occurred in Egypt in 1977. An estimated 200,000 people became sick, and 598 died (Meegan and Shope, 1981). Death was usually associated with acute hemorrhagic fever and hepatitis. The outbreak also caused abortions in sheep and cattle, which resulted in a drastic shortage of red meat in the Cairo marketplace.

The Egyptian epidemic has been linked by some to the construction of the Aswan Dam. Completion of the dam, in 1970, required that 800,000 hectares of reclaimed land be flooded. The dam stabilized the water table in the Nile Valley, which caused water to puddle and to serve as breeding sites for mosquitoes. The mosquitoes, in turn, may have offered a conduit for the virus to enter Egypt from Sub-Saharan Africa, although this has never been proven.

Awareness of the possible association of Rift Valley fever with the ecologic change following completion of the Aswan Dam led scientists to examine the potential for outbreaks of the disease in other areas of dam construction. One such effort, started in 1977 by the U.S. Agency for International Development (USAID), focused on the Diama Dam, then under construction in the Senegal River Basin. Although Rift Valley fever had never been recognized in the region, surprisingly, a third of the local adult inhabitants were found to have antibodies to the virus (Tirrell et al., 1985). The pattern of infection indicated that the disease was endemic. Similar studies at the Institut Pasteur, Dakar, revealed widespread exposure to the virus among people and domestic animals in Mali and Mauritania, two of the countries bordering on the Senegal River. Early in 1987, the institute warned of "a potentially important risk of amplification of the virus in relation to the migration of domestic animal herds and human populations" in southern Mauritania (Digoutte and Peters, 1989).

Later in 1987, after the Diama Dam was activated, an epidemic of Rift Valley fever occurred near the village of Keur Macene, upstream from the new dam. The epidemic was associated with abortions in sheep and cattle, and severe human disease in 1,264 inhabitants. There were 244 deaths (Jouan et al., 1988). The association of this epidemic with prior construction of a dam paralleled the experience in Egypt 10 years earlier. Whereas in Egypt, Rift Valley fever virus was introduced into an immunologically virgin population, in Mauritania it was almost certainly endemic in people and livestock living near the site of the dam. Prior to 1987, the virus caused either inapparent infection or more serious disease in too few people to be recognized. Once the dam was activated, however, the ecology changed. Nonimmune people and their domestic animals who were already in, or entering, the areas became infected. Under these favorable circumstances, the disease rapidly reached epidemic proportions.

Mosquitoes indigenous to both Europe and North America are potentially capable of transmitting the Rift Valley fever virus. In Egypt, the virus demonstrated its capacity to be transported, and in both Egypt and Mauritania, the virus was able to cause epidemics when ecological changes favored mosquito breeding. In the United States, the virus could enter in the blood of an infected person or by way of an animal imported into a wildlife park or zoo. This is an admittedly unlikely possibility; nevertheless, should Rift Valley fever virus become established in vectors in this country, its control would require expensive, integrated efforts including vaccination of domestic livestock and extensive measures to kill vector mosquitoes.

Reforestation and Lyme Disease

The emergence of Lyme disease, caused by the spirochetal bacterium *Borrelia burgdorferi*, is intimately tied to changing land use patterns that date back over the past two centuries. Early in the 1800s, the eastern United States was rendered virtually treeless when vast tracts of land were cleared to make way for agriculture (Jorgenson, 1971; Cronon, 1983). Deforestation was enhanced by the prodigious quantities of wood needed for domestic fuel—as much as 20 cords were required each year for a New England home heated by open fireplaces. Additional wood was converted into charcoal for smelting iron and manufacturing glass. As the forests disappeared, so, too, did the deer population.

During the mid-1800s, agriculture in the United States began a monumental transition westward to the Great Plains, and the resulting abandonment of farms soon caused vast portions of the East to be retaken by forest. Unlike the relatively open primeval forest, however, this new woodland was choked with undergrowth and contained no predators large enough to regulate deer populations. Indeed, reforestation was so rapid that by 1980, the region was blanketed by four times as much woodland as in 1860, when less than a quarter of the land was forested (Thomson, 1977). Not surprisingly, deer in the eastern United States proliferated as their woodland habitat increased (Spielman, 1988). This rebound commenced during the early 1900s and became explosive during the past decade (Southeastern Cooperative Wildlife Diseases Study, 1922-1988).

At the same time that deer populations were increasing, people began to visit and to live in forested, rural areas, a trend that continues today. The resulting proximity of people, mice, deer, and ticks promotes human infection by the Lyme spirochete. This microbe is transmitted by the bite of certain *Ixodes* ticks (see Figure 2-3). The definitive host for these vectors is deer; the reservoir for the pathogen is the white-footed mouse.

Lyme disease is now the most common vector-borne disease in the United States. Cases of Lyme disease have been reported in all 50 states; 13 states reported more than 100 cases in 1990 (see Figure 2-4). Since 1982, 40,108 cases of Lyme disease have been officially reported to the CDC (D. Dennis, Chief, Bacterial Zoonoses Branch, Centers for Disease Control, personal communication, 1992). Diagnosis of Lyme disease is so frequent an occurrence for physicians who practice in areas in which transmission is intense, however, that many fail to take the time to report each case, and reporting efficiency within an endemic site tends to decline with time. For this reason, the official tally of cases of Lyme disease in the United States should be viewed as a highly conservative reflection of the actual state of affairs.

Lyme disease was originally called *erythema migrans* or *erythema chronicum migrans* because of the distinctive rash that migrates from the point at which the infecting tick attaches itself. Throughout the first half of the twentieth century, the condition was rarely seen and was diagnosed solely in a few residents of forested parts of northern Europe (Afzelius, 1921).

In the United States, the first case of what would later be called Lyme disease was reported in a resident of Wisconsin in 1969 (Scrimenti, 1970). Retrospective studies have since identified an even earlier apparent case, acquired in 1962 on Cape Cod in Massachusetts (Steere et al., 1986). The first recognized outbreak of Lyme disease occurred in coastal Connecticut

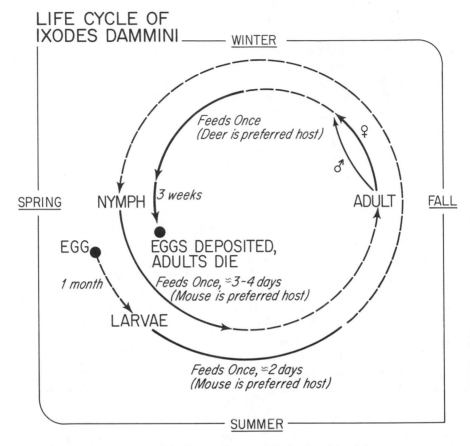

LIFE CYCLE OF
IXODES DAMMINI———— WINTER ————

*Feeds Once
(Deer is preferred host)*

♀
♂

SPRING   NYMPH *3 weeks*   ADULT   FALL

EGG●   ● EGGS DEPOSITED,
                    ADULTS DIE
1 month   *Feeds Once, ≈3-4 days
                    (Mouse is preferred host)*
        LARVAE

*Feeds Once, ≈2 days
(Mouse is preferred host)*

———— SUMMER ————

FIGURE 2-3 Life cycle of the Lyme disease tick, *Ixodes dammini.*
SOURCE: Spielman et al., 1985. Used with permission.

in 1975 (Steere et al., 1977). In 1975 and 1976, 51 people living in and
around the town of Old Lyme, Connecticut, suffered from a condition that
was tentatively diagnosed as juvenile rheumatoid arthritis and later as Lyme
arthritis, in recognition of the focus of the epidemic. The link between
Lyme arthritis and *erythema migrans* was established in the mid-1970s
(Steere et al., 1986). In recognition of the enlarging spectrum of the disease,
the term Lyme disease soon replaced Lyme arthritis.

Because Lyme disease initially was thought to be endemic only in south-
central Connecticut, travel to that part of the country was considered, until
the early 1980s, to be an essential criterion for diagnosis. Thus, residents of
other states who presented with symptoms consistent with Lyme disease
were not diagnosed as such unless a relevant travel history could be docu-

mented. The ironic result was that Lyme disease was not considered to have occurred in Massachusetts until the case criteria were changed in 1982. This confusion resulted in an inordinate number of diagnoses of spider-bite during the 1970s, before these skin lesions were correctly attributed to the bites of spirochete-infected *Ixodes* ticks.

Once deer and infected ticks become well established in a populated site, the risk of human Lyme disease increases rapidly. Such was the case in the New York vacation communities on Fire Island, which became notorious foci of Lyme disease during the late 1970s, registering an annual incidence of about 1 percent (Hanrahan et al., 1984). A similar rise in cases occurred between 1975 and 1983 on Great Island, Massachusetts, where the annual incidence came to exceed 5 percent (Steere et al., 1986). An epidemic outbreak in Ipswich, Massachusetts, began in 1980, the year after *Ixodes* ticks were first discovered on the carcasses of deer. By 1986, the annual incidence of Lyme disease in that community came to exceed 10 percent (Lastavica et al., 1989). Similarly explosive growth in the trend of human cases of Lyme disease has been noted elsewhere, particularly in parts of New York, New Jersey, Pennsylvania, Wisconsin, and Minnesota.

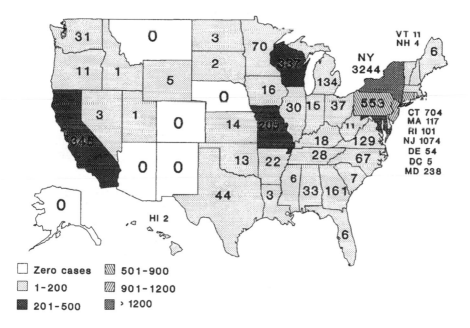

FIGURE 2-4 Distribution of Lyme disease in the United States, 1991.
SOURCE: D. Dennis, Division of Vector-Borne Infectious Diseases, Centers for Disease Control.

Epidemic Lyme disease is an increasing problem in Europe, fueled by a post-World War II trend of reforestation and proliferation of deer. Epidemic Lyme disease was first diagnosed in Europe in the mid-1980s, a few years after the epidemic was recognized in the United States (Matuschka and Spielman, 1989). Reports of Lyme disease in Europe rose rapidly, until by 1988, twice as many cases were reported there as in the United States (Matuschka and Spielman, 1989). At least 1,000 new cases occur annually in Sweden (Jaenson, 1991), and similar incidence levels have been reported in Switzerland and Austria. The comparable annual estimate of new cases for Germany is much higher—between 30,000 and 60,000 cases (Matuschka and Spielman, 1989). Indeed, *Borrelia*-specific antibody is said to be detectable in some 7 percent of German residents. This extraordinarily high frequency of Lyme disease may be related to the large number of Central Europeans who live in forested areas and visit the forests for recreational purposes.

Lyme disease has been reported in many temperate parts of the world, including northeastern China, Japan, South Africa, and Australia (Jaenson, 1991). Unconfirmed, anecdotal reports of Lyme disease have been received from tropical Africa and South America.

A variety of etiologically distinct infectious agents are transmitted by the same ticks and maintained in the same rodents that perpetuate the agent of Lyme disease (Spielman, 1988). In the United States, babesiosis, a malaria-like disease caused by *Babesia microti*, has been diagnosed in people living in or near the same areas in which Lyme disease is prevalent. In human hosts, both of these infections can be fatal. Simultaneous infection is common.

Global Warming

Although it is still a controversial issue, the potential effects of global warming on disease transmission must be considered. This is particularly true for diseases caused by mosquito-borne viruses, since temperature increases in cooler climates may enlarge areas suitable for mosquito breeding. Unfortunately, it is currently impossible to predict accurately the effect of warming on disease emergence. This does not mean, however, that the issue should not be addressed. It is thus disturbing to note the apparent lack of interest in global warming as a possible contributor to public health crises on the part of funding agencies and environmental groups.

According to the best estimates obtainable from mathematical modeling, the earth's temperature could increase by as much as 5°C by the year 2050 (National Research Council, 1992). Should this occur, the distribution of disease vectors and the organisms they transmit might very well change. Research has shown that replication of virus in the mosquito is temperature dependent (Hardy et al., 1983). A warmer planet would likely enhance the transmission of some viruses, while slowing or halting the transmission of others. For example, in the western United States, the geographical distribution of St. Louis encephalitis virus might expand north into areas in which transmission typically is blocked by cool temperatures (Hess et al., 1963). At the same time, the range of western equine encephalitis virus might shift from the southern part of the country northward, to cooler, more temperate habitats.

Other possible effects of global warming, such as increased precipitation or a rise in sea level, could affect the distribution of vectors that rely on water to complete their life cycles. For example, some mosquito species might alter their range and thus come into contact with new viruses or hosts; other species might become extinct in certain areas.

A change in climate can also affect the survival of infectious agents, particularly viruses, outside their hosts. Humidity can favor or hinder the transmission of pathogenic agents. The seasonality of some human viral diseases (such as influenza A) may be due to climatic factors that exert an influence on the organism, its host, or both; sudden alterations in the climate could dramatically affect disease incidence.

The ability of infectious agents to adapt to changed conditions is considerable. Whether global warming occurring over an extended period of time would have any appreciable effects on these organisms, their distribution, or their ability to cause disease is unknown. Based on current knowledge, however, this committee believes that the impact of population growth (particularly when it leads to high population density) is likely to have a more predictable effect on the emergence of infectious diseases than the projected changes in global temperatures.

INTERNATIONAL TRAVEL AND COMMERCE

Travel

Travel, which involves the movement of people and microbes from one region to another, has always contributed to the emergence of infectious diseases. Whether new diseases emerge depends on the novelty of the microbe being introduced, its transmissibility, and the existence of an environment suitable for maintaining the disease and its agent. It is important to distinguish between transient introductions or acquisitions of novel diseases, which are common, and the establishment and propagation of a new pathogen, which are rare. Two examples of such establishment are syphilis and smallpox. According to the view that is still most widely held, syphilis is believed to have been introduced into Europe by sailors returning from the New World (Ampel, 1991). European explorers are believed to have introduced smallpox to the Americas (Crosby, 1972).

Until its global eradication in 1977, smallpox was frequently spread by travel. In 1940, nine years before the disease was eradicated in the United

States, there were nearly 3,000 cases reported in this country (Fenner et al., 1988), all of which occurred in or were the result of transmission from infected foreign travelers. The same pattern holds for dengue (see the earlier discussion), which is currently hyperendemic in parts of Asia and the Caribbean. In 1990, the U.S. Public Health Service (PHS) reported 102 suspected cases of imported dengue, although only 24 cases could be confirmed (Centers for Disease Control, 1991c).

Many other diseases common in other countries are periodically introduced into the United States by travelers. Lassa fever, an acute viral illness, is endemic to West Africa. It first came to the attention of U.S. health officials because of a series of epidemics in Africa between 1969 and 1974 (Carey et al., 1972; Monath et al., 1973; Fraser et al., 1974). Many of the original outbreaks, including almost all of the secondary cases, involved health care personnel who had cared for infected patients. The best known of these instances was an outbreak at an American mission hospital in Jos, Nigeria (Frame et al., 1974), which is the subject of a popular book, *Fever!* (Fuller, 1974).

Because Lassa fever is endemic to parts of Africa, sporadic introductions into the United States by travelers returning from that country are likely (see Box 2-5). However, since the virus is maintained in a rodent species not normally found in the United States, it is unlikely that the disease will become established in this country (barring the emergence of a suitable rodent host in the United States or changes in the host range of the virus). Nevertheless, each imported case of the disease has the potential to be followed by a significant number of secondary infections among close contacts.

MALARIA

Malaria, considered one of the greatest contemporary killers among infectious diseases, is no longer endemic to this country but is one of the diseases that is most frequently imported. The CDC reported 1,173 imported malaria cases in 1991 (Centers for Disease Control, 1992b). Figure 2-5 shows malaria incidence data for 1930 through 1990. During this period, there were four major peaks of malaria, including one that began in 1980. During this latest peak, virtually all of the cases were imported.[1]

---

[1]Blood transfusions are an occasional source. Spread of the disease as a result of needle sharing by heroin users led to an outbreak of 47 cases in California in 1971 (Friedman et al., 1973). In addition, two imported cases in 1990 were iatrogenic, occurring in patients with late-stage Lyme disease who went to Mexico for malariotherapy. Malariotherapy is not recognized in the United States but is available in some foreign countries as an unconventional treatment for spirochetal infections (e.g., syphilis and, in this case, Lyme disease) in which patients are inoculated with blood containing *Plasmodium vivax*, one of the four species of malaria parasites (Centers for Disease Control, 1990a). The fever resulting from the malaria infection is supposed to cure the individual by killing the spirochetes, but scientific proof of the efficiency of this procedure has not been demonstrated.

BOX 2-5 Imported Lassa Fever

In early 1989, a man who had visited Nigeria for a funeral became sick after returning to the United States. The patient was a 43-year-old mechanical engineer living in a Chicago suburb. Shortly after his return from Nigeria, he walked into a health clinic complaining of fever and sore throat. The area was in the midst of a winter influenza epidemic, and he was advised to take acetaminophen for the fever but was not otherwise treated. The symptoms worsened, and when he returned three days later, swollen lymph nodes and a phlegm-covered throat were noted, for which he was given penicillin. Five days later, his condition had deteriorated; his symptoms now included bloody diarrhea and facial swelling, and he had elevated liver enzymes.

An attentive specialist who saw the patient at a local hospital suspected a viral hemorrhagic fever after reviewing the patient's history. That history revealed that the patient had been in Nigeria for his parents' funerals until a few days before his illness began. His mother's death, of a febrile illness, had occurred two weeks before the patient's symptoms appeared, and was followed by his father's death from a similar illness 10 days later. The travel and disease history made the clinician suspect Lassa fever, a disease known to be endemic to Nigeria, and he called the CDC in Atlanta. The CDC was later able to confirm the diagnosis of Lassa fever by virologic methods. Ribavirin, the only drug presently available for this infection, was ordered for the patient, but he died of cardiac arrest before the drug arrived.

A total of 102 people had come into contact with the patient when he was likely to have been infectious. High-risk contacts (in this instance, immediate family who had had intimate contact, washed soiled linens, and shared utensils) were also placed on prophylactic ribavirin. Medium-risk contacts included a laboratory technician, the patient's nurse, and a physician who was not wearing gloves when he inserted an intravenous line into the patient.

None of the contacts became infected, a somewhat unusual circumstance in the case of this disease. The patient was undiagnosed for almost two weeks, during which time the virus could have been passed to the patient's care givers, to other patients of these care givers, and to family members. Transmitted primarily through direct contact with the blood or other bodily fluids of an infected person, Lassa has been suspected in some cases to be spread by airborne transmission. Had this been true in the Chicago case, the number of direct and indirect contacts in danger of contracting the disease could have been much greater.

The ease with which people can travel around the world today means that "exotic" diseases can move just as quickly. Physicians must be consistently aware of infectious diseases that originate in other parts of the world, and vigilant about obtaining a travel history for patients with undiagnosed illness, especially if it is accompanied by fever.

SOURCE: Holmes et al., 1990.

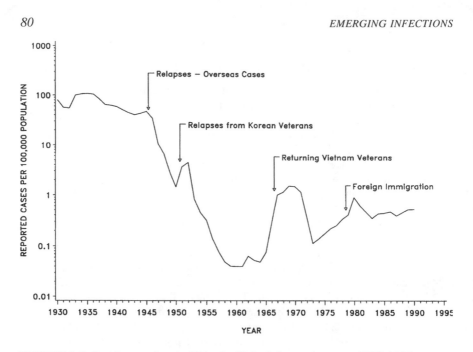

FIGURE 2-5 Incidence of malaria in the United States, by year, 1930-1990.
SOURCE: Centers for Disease Control, 1991h.

Until the mid-1970s, most cases of imported malaria in the United States
occurred in war veterans who had acquired the disease while on overseas
duty.

Outbreaks of nonimported (indigenous) cases of malaria, which appear
to be associated with infected migrant workers, have occurred in southern
California (mostly in San Diego County) and Florida (Branati et al., 1954;
Centers for Disease Control, 1991f). These outbreaks have been small and
so far relatively isolated, but the potential exists for the disease to become
reestablished in the United States, since competent mosquito vectors are
present in abundance. In fact, secondary cases in local contacts of individuals with imported disease are periodically recognized (Maldonado et al.,
1990; Centers for Disease Control, 1991f).

In the areas of California and Florida where malaria outbreaks have
occurred, sanitary facilities and housing are often substandard, a fact that
can complicate vector-control efforts as well as medical treatment. Finding
and treating illegal migrant workers infected with the malaria parasite are
especially hard. The demand for cheap migrant labor and the limited availability of housing and health care for these workers may mean that the

scenarios in California and Florida will be repeated in other areas of the country. One recent report documented two cases of malaria in New Jersey in which neither individual had traveled outside of the state (Malaria Branch, Centers for Disease Control, unpublished report, 1991). States in the Southwest and along the Gulf of Mexico are at particular risk for malaria because of their proximity to the border with Mexico, where many of the illegal immigrants gain access to the United States.

Commerce

The international transportation of goods has indirectly led to the emergence of a number of infectious diseases. Most often it is not the goods themselves that pose the problem. Rather, it is infected animals in the cargo hold of a plane or ship, or bilge water contaminated with potentially pathogenic microbes that can hitch a ride from one part of the world to another. As discussed later in this chapter, the current cholera epidemic in the Western Hemisphere appears to be the direct result of international shipping. Transportation also played a significant role in the emergence of plague in the United States in 1900 (see Chapter 1).

Viruses are a particular problem because of their wide distribution, the ecology of their vectors, and their potential to cause human disease. The current *International Catalogue of Arboviruses* (Karabatsos, 1985) lists more than 500 separate viruses, about a fifth of which are capable of causing human disease. In general, viral diseases are hard to diagnose because of their variety and the difficulties associated with working with them in the laboratory. Viruses are often maintained in nature through enzootic cycles of transmission. Human infection is not essential to their long-term survival, in fact, humans often represent a dead-end host. There are undoubtedly undetected viruses in rural areas of the United States and in remote corners of the world that could cause human disease. With continued movement of people into rural areas, environmental damage caused by development, and the transport of people and products between remote areas and more developed parts of the world, the stage has been set for the emergence of "new" viral diseases.

HANTAAN AND RELATED HANTAVIRUSES

The Hantaan virus and related hantaviruses are some of the most recently recognized causes of an emerging disease. This group of viruses causes hemorrhagic fever with renal syndrome (HFRS), which is known as epidemic hemorrhagic fever in China and Korean hemorrhagic fever in Korea. The prototype virus, Hantaan, was first isolated in 1976 (H. W. Lee et al., 1978) from the lungs of its natural reservoir host, the striped field mouse, *Apodemus agrarius*. Subsequent studies have identified antigenically related viruses that are also capable of causing acute, life-threatening human disease. These include Seoul virus, maintained in the domestic rat, *Rattus norvegicus* (Lee et al., 1982), and Puumala virus, maintained by the bank vole, *Clethrionomys glareolus* (Brummer-Korvenkontio et al., 1980).

Seoul virus causes a less severe form of HFRS, while Puumala virus is the cause of *nephropathia epidemica*, a disease commonly seen in Scandinavia, in the western portion of Russia, and, with increasing frequency, in Western Europe. Seoul virus is distributed virtually anywhere in the world where there are large, uncontrolled populations of *R. norvegicus* (LeDuc et al., 1986). This virus has been isolated and human infections documented in both North and South America (LeDuc et al., 1984, 1985; Childs et al., 1987; Glass et al., 1990). Undoubtedly, the present-day distribution of Seoul virus had its origin in international commerce and its unwanted rodent passenger, *R. norvegicus*.

The hantaviruses have also found their way into laboratory rodent colonies, in which they cause chronic, asymptomatic infections (LeDuc, 1987). Serious human disease and death have been documented in animal handlers, scientists, and others who unknowingly have been exposed to hantavirus-contaminated rat colonies. These problems continue to exist today, especially in Asia, where quality control of rodent breeding facilities is not as rigorously monitored as in the United States (Umenai et al., 1979; Desmyter et al., 1983; Lloyd et al., 1984).

The viruses have been spread in laboratory animals in several ways. Inbred strains of infected rats have been distributed to investigators around the world. Transplantable tumors, traditionally maintained in laboratory rats, have been the source of additional rodent and some human infections (Yamanishi et al., 1983). Continuous cell lines may also harbor the viruses, although examination of all rat-origin cell lines held by the American Type Culture Collection failed to identify any hantavirus contamination (LeDuc et al., 1985). The risk of contamination to reagents, such as monoclonal antibodies produced in infected rodent hosts, is currently unknown but clearly plausible. Recent studies have demonstrated that the common house mouse, *Mus musculus*, may harbor hantaviruses. Hantaviruses have been isolated from domestic mice in Texas (Baek et al., 1988) and in Yugoslavia (Diglisic et al., 1991; T. Avsic-Zupanc, Microbiologist, Institute of Microbiology, Medical Faculty of Ljubljana, Slovenia, personal communication, 1991).

Stopping the distribution of hantavirus-contaminated laboratory animals, cell cultures, or reagents is difficult, since there is no readily available commercial test for screening animals for infection. This issue is discussed more fully below.

The Filoviruses

In the late 1960s, a group of nonhuman primates was shipped from Uganda to Marburg, Germany, for use in vaccine development. The monkeys were infected with what was then an unknown virus, later to be named Marburg virus in recognition of the site of its discovery. Several animals died during shipment or immediately after arrival, and animal handlers and technicians were infected with this new virus. The resulting human disease was especially virulent, secondary cases occurred, and many people died (Martini, 1969).

Several years later, epidemics caused by another virus, later shown to be closely related to Marburg virus, occurred in Zaire and Sudan. These outbreaks claimed nearly 200 lives and almost completely eliminated medical support for the affected areas. The virus was later named Ebola virus, after the Ebola River which passes through the epidemic region. Marburg and Ebola are now recognized as members of the Filoviridae, a distinct family of viruses (Pattyn, 1978).

In 1989, the scenario of Marburg virus threatened to be repeated again, but this time in the United States. Scientists at the U.S. Army Medical Research Institute of Infectious Diseases (USAMRIID) at Fort Detrick in Frederick, Maryland, were notified of excessive mortality among nonhuman primates recently imported from the Philippines to a facility in nearby Reston, Virginia, just outside Washington, D.C. USAMRIID staff had recently investigated an outbreak of simian hemorrhagic fever, a disease known to cause substantial mortality among infected nonhuman primates, and the Reston officials suspected that the same disease was present in their colony. However, when virus isolates were obtained from sick or dead monkeys and examined by electron microscopy, virus particles of characteristic filovirus morphology were observed (Geisbert and Jahrling, 1990). Public health officials were immediately notified, since preliminary attempts to identify the virus suggested that it was the highly virulent Ebola virus (Jahrling et al., 1990). Only after considerable study was it determined that the virus isolated was a distinct, new filovirus, later named Reston virus.

Several people were infected with Reston virus during the epizootic; however, to date, none has suffered overt clinical symptoms. At present, the potential of the Reston virus to cause human disease is uncertain. Regardless of the characteristics of this particular virus, the episode clearly demonstrates the critical role played by international commerce in introducing an exotic pathogen into the United States.

Perhaps the greatest problem associated with international commerce and its relation to disease emergence is the lack of appropriate, widely available diagnostic tests to allow effective screening of animals (and products made in animals) that are destined for investigational use. In contrast to arthropod vectors of disease, which can be controlled through the judicious use of pesticides, it is not desirable to kill potential animal reservoirs of disease when the research being pursued requires that the particular animal remain alive. Those who work with imported biological materials need to be aware of the potential for contamination by infectious agents. Although it is generally not done, screening imported laboratory animals, cell lines, and transplantable tumors (including hybridomas used to make monoclonal antibodies) for exotic pathogens probably is the only effective mechanism to reduce the risk of emerging diseases.

MICROBIAL ADAPTATION AND CHANGE

Microbes are exceedingly numerous and diverse, but only a small fraction are capable of causing disease in animals or humans. To survive, most microbial species, whether pathogenic or not, must be well adapted to a particular ecological niche and must compete effectively with other microorganisms. Their small size and high surface-to-volume ratios facilitate rapid growth and extensive impact on their environment. Microbial pathogens can colonize animals, humans, and arthropods because they have acquired (or evolved) a number of genes and gene products that enable them to do so. These gene products are extremely varied, but they include factors involved in transmission from one host to another, in cell-surface attachment and invasiveness, in countering or suppressing specific and nonspecific host immune responses, in persisting or surviving inside and outside a host organism, and in resistance to antimicrobial drugs. Nonpathogens can become pathogens (a rare event), and low-virulence pathogens can become highly virulent through mutation, recombination, and gene transfer.

Because of the relatively small amount of DNA or RNA, or both, that they carry, their rapid growth rate, and large populations, microbial pathogens can evolve and adapt very quickly. These evolutionary mechanisms (Table 2-2) allow them to adapt to new host cells or host species, produce "new" toxins, bypass or suppress inflammatory and immune responses, and develop resistance to drugs and antibodies. The ability to adapt is required for the successful competition and evolutionary survival of any microbial form, but it is particularly crucial for pathogens, which must cope with host defenses as well as microbial competition. There are, for example, a number of determinants that can exert an influence on viral evolutionary events (Table 2-3). In fact, although hosts can help to drive the evolution of their parasites, the opposite is probably also true (Hamilton et al., 1990). Coevolution of pathogens and their animal and human hosts will continue to be a challenge to medical science because change, novelty, or "newness" is built into such relationships.

TABLE 2-2 Examples of Viral Evolutionary Mechanisms

Mechanism	Example	Reference
Point mutations	A single amino acid change can affect virulence; lethal chicken influenza	Kawaoka and Webster, 1988
Intramolecular recombination	Insertion of piece of genome; eastern equine encephalitis virus and Sindbis-like virus → western equine encephalitis virus	Hahn et al., 1988
Genetic reassortment	Origin of pandemic influenza viruses of 1957 and 1968; external protein gene(s) from animal virus	Scholtissek et al., 1978
Recombination and mutation	Evolution of live polio-virus vaccine following administration	Kew and Nottay, 1984
Biased hypermutation (uridine to cytosine transitions)	Evolution of SSPE virus from measles virus	Catteneo et al., 1989
Genetic rearrangement	Evolution of rubella virus	Dominguez et al., 1990
Recombination between deletion mutations	Regeneration of func-tional plant virus genome	Allison et al., 1990

NOTE: SSPE = subacute sclerosing panencephalitis.
Adapted from Kilbourne, 1991. Used with permission.

Natural Variation/Mutation

RNA VIRUSES

RNA viruses confront us with a paradox. On the one hand, their muta-tion rates are extraordinarily high (because unlike DNA viruses, RNA vi-ruses have no mechanisms for correcting errors made during replication). On the other hand, the clinical expressions of the diseases they cause (such as poliomyelitis and measles) have remained constant for centuries. Never-theless, analysis of RNA virus genomes reveals that each "virus" comprises a heterogenous mixture of mutants in variable proportions. Thus, any given strain or isolate is, in fact, polymorphic or represents a subset of the quasi-

TABLE 2-3   Evolution of New Viruses: Constraints and Opportunities

Constraints
  Extreme viral alterations are lethal
  There may be requirements for co-evolution of viral cellular proteins
  Virus survival requires a critical level of virulence
  Propagation in alien hosts tends to be attenuating
  Adaptation to ecological niches is exquisitely specific
  Penetration of human immunologic barrier usually requires major
    antigenic change
  Infection with nonhuman (zoonotic) viruses is sometimes but not
    always contagious
Opportunities
  High viral mutation rates
  Interviral genetic interaction
  Ecological change increasing opportunity for contact of man with vectors
    or viruses
  Changes in human behavior (e.g., sexual)
  Altered behavior of viruses in immunocompromised hosts

Adapted from Kilbourne, 1991. Used with permission.

species (E. Domingo et al., 1978). A virus, then, is identified as a consensus that reflects the predominating mutant(s) in a mixed population. Because predominating mutants seldom change, only unusual selective pressure by the host's immune response or other factors, such as host adaptation, will allow new mutants to gain ascendancy, resulting (rarely) in the emergence of distinguishably new viruses.

Influenza A Virus

Although influenza viruses mutate at a rate similar to other RNA viruses, they are unique in that they also evolve (undergo meaningful changes) relatively rapidly in nature. This is due to selective pressure on the virus from the large population of partially immune people, who have antibodies to the virus as a result of previous infections. To survive, the virus must undergo some degree of genetic mutation (or "antigenic drift"). This process is continuous and results in regional epidemics of influenza.

Much less frequently, the surface proteins—called hemagglutinin (H) and neuraminidase (N)—of the influenza virus undergo a radical change (an "antigenic shift") that creates a virus so different that no person possesses immunity to it. A pandemic of life-threatening disease results. Interestingly, the radical changes that have produced pandemic influenza viruses are rooted in the virus's acquisition of genetic material from animal influenza A viruses. Scientists have hypothesized that agricultural practices in Southeast

Asia (where most new strains of influenza arise) that put ducks, pigs, and farmers in close proximity may facilitate genetic shift in the virus (Scholtissek and Naylor, 1988; Langone, 1990; Morse, 1990). This theory is based on the idea that pigs have been infected by both an avian influenza virus and a human influenza virus. These viruses, while inside the pig, exchange genetic material, potentially resulting in a more virulent virus capable of initiating a pandemic if passed to humans.

To date, 14 distinct H and 9 distinct N influenza A antigens have been identified in birds and animals. Only three subtype combinations (representing three H and two N antigens) are known to cause disease in man: H1N1, H2N2, and H3N2. There have been two antigenic shifts in the influenza A virus since 1918: the first, in 1957, produced the H2N2 subtype; the second, in 1968, the H3N2 subtype. Antigenic drift and antigenic shift both challenge the immunity of human populations and require constant changes in the composition of influenza vaccine. Predicting the direction of these changes (based on worldwide surveillance data) is difficult.

Human Immunodeficiency Virus

A second example of RNA variability is HIV. HIV-1 and HIV-2, the two known HIV viruses, exhibit extensive genetic variability and exist in infected individuals as a complex mixture of closely related genomes, or quasispecies. These quasispecies undergo rapid genetic change such that the major viral form present in chronically infected persons differs over time. This continual change can result in alterations of those parts of the virus recognized by the human immune system; the effect of such alterations is to make the immune system less able to eliminate or suppress the virus.

It is likely that the extensive genetic variability of HIV-1 and HIV-2 will present major problems in the development of an effective vaccine. Because the differences between HIV-1 and HIV-2 are significant, a vaccine against one will probably not be effective against the other. More worrisome is the possibility that an HIV-1 or HIV-2 vaccine will not be effective against all quasispecies within that one subgroup. The quasispecies in any one person are closely related to each other but are different from those in someone else, raising the possibility that vaccines of different antigenic composition will be needed to prevent infection or disease in different individuals. Of additional concern is the fact that the majority of HIV isolates from other countries, such as Thailand and countries in Africa, differ substantially from strains found in the United States and Europe. It is highly probable that a widely effective HIV vaccine will need to be a composite of viral antigens from different regions of the globe or that multiple vaccines, targeted for specific regions, will need to be developed.

The mutability of HIV has been mentioned repeatedly during the HIV disease pandemic, raising questions about how broad a biological change the virus might undergo (Vartanian et al., 1991). It is important to make a distinction between point mutations—to which HIV is prone—and changes in pathogenic properties, such as initiation of infection, that would influence host range and mode of transmission. HIV does undergo frequent point mutations, especially in regions of the genome that are likely to be targeted by vaccines (Phillips et al., 1991). Although it is theoretically possible that such a change could alter its infective properties, the stability of other RNA viruses, with regard to host and organ specificity, indicates that this possibility is unlikely. Also reassuring is the general experience that evolutionary adaptation of pathogens tends toward lesser virulence.

DNA VIRUSES

Hepatitis B Virus

Hepatitis B is a DNA virus, but because it uses reverse transcriptase to replicate, it shares with RNA viruses the tendency to undergo significant and rapid genetic change. In recent years, a number of rare viral variants have been identified in patients infected with hepatitis B. These have generally fallen into two categories: variants with truncated protein products ("precore" and "pre-S" variants) and vaccine escape mutants.

The precore and pre-S variants have mutations in regions of DNA that immediately precede the coding sequences for certain viral proteins (core or surface protein, respectively). The mutations cause a truncated product to be manufactured and also appear to alter pathogenesis, especially in the case of precore variants (Neurath and Kent, 1988; Carman et al., 1991; Liang et al., 1991; Omata et al., 1991). The precore region of the hepatitis B virus is not required for the production of viral particles. Precore mutants thus are viable but lack the viral antigen known as HBeAg, which is a key component of some diagnostic tests. This variant was first isolated in patients in Italy and Greece who had an unusual form of severe chronic hepatitis but were negative for HBeAg (Carman et al., 1989; Carman et al., 1991). Since then, the precore variant has also been isolated from patients with fulminant acute hepatitis B infection (Carman et al., 1991; Liang et al., 1991; Omata et al., 1991).

In one study in Japan (Omata et al., 1991), nine patients with either acute fulminant hepatitis B infection (five patients) or severe exacerbation of chronic hepatitis B (four patients) were tested. Hepatitis B virus was successfully recovered from seven of the nine patients, and a precore variant with the identical nonsense (terminating) mutation was isolated. This variant was not found in 10 controls with acute, self-limited hepatitis B. In another study, the precore variant was found in sera from eight of nine patients who were negative for HBeAg and had fulminant hepatitis B infection, but not in sera from six other patients who had fulminant hepatitis B but were positive for HBeAg. Finally, a nosocomial outbreak of fulminant hepatitis B with five fatalities occurred in Haifa, Israel, in 1989. The outbreak was traced to an intravenous heparin flush bottle that had been contaminated after use in a patient who was a chronic hepatitis B carrier. The same hepatitis B precore variant was detected in each of the patients (Liang et al., 1991). In addition to the single nonsense mutation at nucleotide 1896 (seen in all the precore isolates that have been identified to date), there was an additional mutation at nucleotide 1901, which the authors speculated might be related to the especially high mortality caused by this variant.

A vaccine escape mutant, by contrast, generally does not cause altered pathogenesis but lacks a particular antigenic site, allowing it to infect hosts protected by immunization or passively acquired antibody in much the same way that antigenic drift occurs in influenza A. Hepatitis B vaccine has been used in Italy since 1982 to protect infants born to mothers who are chronic carriers of hepatitis B. The hepatitis B vaccine escape mutant was found during follow-up studies of this population (Carman et al., 1990). Of 1,590 vaccinees (infants and family contacts), 44 became positive for hepatitis B surface antigen, indicating that they had become infected with hepatitis B despite immunization and prophylactic hepatitis B hyperimmune globulin. Another 7 patients were identified later. Viral DNA from a patient (in the original group) chosen for detailed study demonstrated a variant that lacked a major antigenic determinant and was therefore no longer neutralized by hyperimmune globulin or (presumably) by vaccine-induced antibodies. The loss of the antigenic site was due to a point mutation that altered a single amino acid. The other apparent vaccine failures were not as thoroughly investigated. Although it is not known conclusively whether this mechanism accounted for the other cases, there were indications that at least some of the other vaccine failures were due to an escape mutant. The localization of these mutants to a particular geographic region (the Mediterranean) was puzzling. This may have been due to host immunogenetic factors or suboptimal immunization schedules, or to the use of both vaccine and immunoglobulin, which increases selective pressure favoring an escape mutant.

BACTERIA

Bacteria cause disease because they produce so-called virulence factors. Virulence factors have several roles in bacterial pathogenesis: they allow the bacteria to resist nonspecific host clearance mechanisms; they help the bacteria acquire nutrients necessary for growth and survival; they assist the bacteria to resist specific host immune mechanisms; and they provide the bacteria with a competitive advantage by inhibiting other microorganisms in the host.

The evolution, *ab initio*, of virulence by mutations would be an extraordinarily complex chain of events and is more often inferred as a natural process than observed in the laboratory. Resistance to antibiotics and to serum bactericidal factors, however, is a unit step often seen in experiments. More often, virulence genes can be characterized by their transmission from one cell to another.

Virulence factors vary from organism to organism and can often be transferred among receptive bacteria by bacteriophages and plasmids. This movement of genetic material is one way that bacteria cope with changes in their surroundings, such as the presence of antibodies or phagocytic cells. Bacteria may possess more than one virulence factor, including toxins (neuro-, entero-, endo-, cyto-, erythrogenic, etc.), enzymes, colonization factors, adhesins, bacteriocins, hemolysins, and cell invasion and drug resistance factors (see Table 2-4).

In addition to the versatility afforded by gene transfer, an unexpected plasticity has been found in bacteria that amplifies particular genes related to rapid growth or virulence (Terzaghi and O'Hara, 1990). Hence, salmonellae growing rapidly in rich media are genotypically different from those starved for specific carbon sources (Sonti and Roth, 1989). The same is true for cholera vibrios in their host environment compared with aqueous reservoirs (Mekalanos, 1983).

This plasticity has introduced new complications into the evaluation of pathogenicity of bacterial strains that have been stored in the laboratory, supporting the intuitions of a prior generation of medical bacteriologists. The underlying genetic mechanisms are still under study; it is not yet known whether they involve more than intense natural selection operating on large populations subject to modest rates of spontaneous mutation. Whatever the mechanism, the emergence of enhanced virulence potential is observed within time intervals measured in days or hours.

Brazilian Purpuric Fever

The most recent example of the emergence of a new disease that is likely to have been the result of a mutation causing enhanced virulence occurred in 1984. In that year, an outbreak of severe disease in 10 children, aged three months to eight years, occurred in a single town in São Paulo State in Brazil. Symptoms included high fever, vomiting, and abdominal pain, followed by the development of purpura and shock owing to vascular collapse. All 10 children died within 48 hours of the onset of the fever.

It was thought at first that the children had contracted meningococcal

TABLE 2-4 Representative Examples of Virulence Factors Encoded by Bacteriophages, Plasmids, and Transposons

Mobile Genetic Element	Organism	Virulence Factor
Bacteriophage	Streptococcus pyogenes	Erythrogenic toxin
	Escherichia coli	Shiga-like toxin
	Staphylococcus aureus	Enterotoxins A D E
		Staphylokinase
		TSST-1 toxin
	Clostridium botulinum	Neurotoxins C D E
	Corynebacterium diphtheriae	Diphtheria toxin
Plasmid	Escherichia coli	Enterotoxins LT, ST
		Pili colonization factor
		Hemolysin
		Urease
		Serum resistance factor
		Adherence factors
		Cell invasion factors
	Bacillus anthracis	Edema factor
		Lethal factor
		Protective antigen
		Poly-D-glutamic acid capsule
	Yersinia species	Intracellular growth factor
		Capsule production factor
	Yersinia pestis	Coagulase
		Fibrinolysin
		Murine toxin
Transposon	Escherichia coli	Heat-stable enterotoxins
		Aerobactin siderophores ?
		Hemolysin and x-pili operons ?
	Shigella dysenteriae	Shiga toxin ?
	Vibrio cholerae	Cholera toxin
		ZOT toxin
		ACE toxin

NOTE: TSST-1=toxic shock syndrome toxin-1; LT=heat-labile enterotoxin; ST=heat-stable enterotoxin; ZOT=zona occludens toxin; ACE=accessory cholera enterotoxin; ?=the DNA structure strongly suggests a transposon, but actual transposition has not been demonstrated.

SOURCE: J. Mekalanos, Department of Microbiology and Molecular Genetics, Harvard Medical School.

meningitis. Microscopic examination and culture of cerebrospinal fluid (CSF), however, were negative for *Neisseria meningitidis* (Centers for Disease Control, 1985). Within the next two years, additional outbreaks and isolated cases were reported in nine other towns in São Paulo State. It was also determined that a similar outbreak had occurred in May 1984, in the neighboring state of Paraná (Centers for Disease Control, 1985, 1986; Brazilian Purpuric Fever Study Group, 1987a,b). Subsequent epidemiologic investigation revealed that the majority of the children had developed purulent conjunctivitis (from infection by the bacterium *Haemophilus influenzae*, biogroup *aegyptius*), which had resolved prior to the acute onset of the high fever, vomiting, and abdominal pain.

No pathogenic organisms were cultured from blood or CSF in the first reported outbreak, probably because antibiotics had been administered before culture material was obtained (Centers for Disease Control, 1985). In subsequent outbreaks, however, *H. influenzae*, biogroup *aegyptius*, was isolated from blood or bloody CSF (Centers for Disease Control, 1986; Brazilian Purpuric Fever Study Group, 1987b; Irino et al., 1987). This was the first time this bacterium had been shown to produce invasive disease.

The disease, which became known as Brazilian purpuric fever, has since been reported in Central Australia. In one of two reported Australian cases, the organism was cultured from blood but not CSF (McIntyre et al., 1987). Other cases may have occurred, but because of the high prevalence of meningococcal disease in that part of the country, they were diagnosed as meningococcaemia. Brazilian purpuric fever may in fact have a wide geographic distribution. Parts of the world in which *Haemophilus* conjunctivitis is common, such as northern Africa (McIntyre et al., 1987), are potentially at risk for epidemics of Brazilian purpuric fever.

Selective Pressure and the Development of Resistance

The emergence of resistance in a known infectious agent may be a greater threat to public health than the emergence of a new disease. This is especially true if the agent causing the new disease is susceptible to currently available antimicrobial drugs or, if a vector is involved in transmission, the vector is susceptible to control strategies. If an emerging disease agent is resistant to currently available antimicrobials, the problem of control is considerably magnified, as it would be if an insect vector developed pesticide resistance. Thus, resistance to antimicrobials or pesticides is a critical factor in the emergence of infectious diseases.

RESISTANCE TO ANTIBIOTICS

An increasingly important contributor to the emergence of microbial threats to health is drug resistance. Microbes that once were easily controlled by antimicrobial drugs are, more and more often, causing infections that no longer respond to treatment with these drugs. Almost always, this resistance is the result of selective pressure.

There has always been resistance to antibiotics. No drug is universally effective against all bacteria, and as a drug is used, resistant organisms emerge from the initially susceptible population (Jacoby and Archer, 1991). For example, the fluoroquinolones, when first introduced, were broadly effective and had low toxicity. With increasing use, most methicillin-resistant *Staphylococcus aureus* (MRSA) have become quinolone resistant, as have increasing numbers of *Pseudomonas aeruginosa* and other gram-negative nosocomial pathogens. The only available drug effective against MRSA and other methicillin-resistant staphylococci is vancomycin. About the only pathogenic bacterium that has not developed resistance to at least one antibiotic is *Treponema pallidum*, the spirochete that causes syphilis. Treating resistant infections requires the use of more expensive or more toxic alternative drugs and longer hospital stays; in addition, it frequently means a higher risk of death for the patient harboring a resistant pathogen. Estimates of the cost of antibiotic resistance in the United States annually range as high as $30 billion (Phelps, 1989). Even with the continuing development of new drugs, resistance to antibiotics is an increasingly important problem with certain bacterial pathogens.

Drug discovery programs have been crucial to the development of more effective antibiotics. A recent survey of vice presidents at major U.S. and Japanese pharmaceutical companies, however, found that about half of those companies have decreased or recently halted their antibiotic research programs. These decisions were reportedly based on perceptions that market needs for antibacterial products have been "satisfied" and that the market is "saturated" (Shlaes et al., 1991).

Pneumococci

Streptococcus pneumoniae is the commonest cause of community-acquired bacterial pneumonia and is also implicated in meningitis, otitis, sinusitis, bronchitis, and peritonitis, among other infections. For many years, pneumococcus was consistently susceptible to relatively low doses of penicillin (minimal inhibitory concentrations [MIC] of 0.1 microgram per milliliter or less). In the past 25 years, increasing numbers of penicillin-resistant isolates have been reported. Of the more than 5,000 *S. pneumoniae* isolates submitted to the CDC between 1979 and 1987 as part of a 35-hospital surveillance system, 5 percent had MICs greater than or equal to 0.1 microgram per milliliter (Spika et al., 1991). In other parts of the world, the frequency of resistance is even higher: more than 20 percent in Chile, South Africa, and parts of Spain (Klugman, 1990) and as high as 58 percent in Hungary (Marton et al., 1991). Patients infected with such strains can fail to respond to penicillin treatment, and some penicillin-resistant strains are also resistant to chloramphenicol, clindamycin, erythromycin, tetracycline, and trimethoprim-sulfamethoxazole, thus leaving few options for therapy. Today, in some areas, pneumococcal susceptibility to antibiotics can no longer

be assumed. Isolates obtained from blood and spinal fluid samples of seri-
ously ill patients need to be tested for drug sensitivity.

Staphylococci and Enterococci

Infection with *Staphylococcus aureus* can cause a number of serious
conditions, including bacteremia, endocarditis, meningitis, osteomyelitis,
pneumonia, and urinary tract infection. Beta-lactamase-producing *S. aureus*
emerged soon after penicillin came into clinical use and now constitutes 90
percent of isolates. Beta-lactamase gives the organism the ability to inactivate beta-lactam antibiotics. Beta-lactams that are not inactivated by the
staphylococcal enzyme, like methicillin, nafcillin, oxacillin, cloxacillin, and
many cephalosporins, provided effective therapy until methicillin-resistant
S. aureus appeared. In 1990, 15 percent of all *S. aureus* isolates in the
United States were resistant to methicillin, and in critical care units the
frequency was often higher (Wenzel et al., 1991). These resistant organisms
are just as virulent as their methicillin-susceptible counterparts and can
cause life-threatening infections.

Although *S. aureus* is a frequent cause of infection associated with medical devices (artificial heart valves, joint replacements and other prosthetic
devices, and venous catheters), the coagulase-negative staphylococci have
become the most common cause of these infections in the past decade (Mandell
et al., 1990). Most of these organisms make beta-lactamase, and 40 percent
are resistant to methicillin and other beta-lactams, making vancomycin almost the sole effective agent for treatment (Jacoby, 1991).

Although a few vancomycin-resistant, coagulase-negative staphylococcal
isolates have been reported in Europe and the United States, vancomycin-
resistant enterococci may represent an even greater threat as an emerging
nosocomial pathogen. Outbreaks have been reported in several U.S. cities
within the past two years. Some strains (also resistant to ampicillin, gentamicin,
and teicoplanin) are resistant to all currently licensed antibiotics that are
recommended for treatment of serious enterococcal infections. This finding
is particularly worrisome, since these organisms are becoming a major cause
of nosocomial infections in this country.

Pseudomonas aeruginosa

Pseudomonas aeruginosa is an important cause of nosocomial infections, especially in the immunocompromised patient (Schaberg et al., 1991).
This organism has an outer cell membrane that can exclude various antibiotics, and it has many inactivating and modifying enzymes to counter
aminoglycosides, beta-lactams, and other antimicrobial agents. Although *P.
aeruginosa* is frequently susceptible to ceftazidime, resistance can arise by

mutations that result in the overproduction of its chromosomal beta-lactamase. Resistance can also emerge to imipenem and other carbapenems through production of a plasmid-mediated beta-lactamase (Watanabe et al., 1991) or by mutational loss of an outer membrane protein that is the major channel for imipenem entry (Trias and Nikaido, 1990). Other mutations affecting drug uptake confer resistance to virtually all aminoglycosides (Maloney et al., 1989), whereas resistance to fluoroquinolones can evolve through mutations that affect drug accumulation or DNA gyrase (Robillard and Scarpa, 1988).

Mycobacterium tuberculosis

After a decline in rates of infection over several decades, the United States is experiencing a disturbing increase in tuberculosis (TB). Compared with the incidence of many other diseases, 28,000 excess U.S. cases of TB in a seven-year period seems a relatively low figure (Fox, 1992). Because TB is highly contagious, however, it poses a profound threat to public health. TB bacteria are easily passed from person to person in airborne droplets formed when a person with active TB sneezes or coughs.

Even more alarming has been the rise of multidrug-resistant tuberculosis (MDRTB). Prior to 1984, about 10 percent of TB bacteria isolated from patients in the United States were resistant to even a single antibacterial drug. In 1984, 52 percent of patients were infected with tubercle bacilli resistant to at least one drug, and 32 percent were resistant to one or more drugs (Marwick, 1992). Outbreaks of MDRTB have been reported in 13 states. Ten percent of the recorded MDRTB cases to date have occurred in previously healthy people whose mortality rate—70 to 90 percent—has been nearly the same as that of immunosuppressed persons with MDRTB (Snider and Roper, 1992).

The CDC has released preliminary results of a joint study with the New York State Health Department showing that cases of drug-resistant TB have more than doubled since 1984 (Goodstein, 1991). CDC data from the first quarter of 1991 show that many of these drug-resistant strains are resistant to both of the frontline TB drugs, rifampin and isoniazid (Centers for Disease Control, unpublished data, 1992). Outbreaks of MDRTB have occurred in hospitals in Miami and New York City, as well as in the New York State prison system. In one hospital in New York City, the median interval between diagnosis of MDRTB and death was only four weeks. Additional clusters of MDRTB were reported to the CDC in 1990 and 1991 from Mississippi, Missouri, and Michigan (Centers for Disease Control, 1992g).

There are five frontline drugs known to be highly effective against My-cobacterium tuberculosis and five second-line drugs that can be used when resistance to one or more of the frontline drugs is detected. Ironically, in the United States, until April 1992, there were shortages of antituberculosis drugs, some of which are crucially needed when resistance to the frontline drugs rifampin and isoniazid is present (Centers for Disease Control, 1991j; Marwick, 1992). These shortages had occurred because several pharmaceutical companies had ceased production of these drugs.

Because of its persistence in the body, the tubercle bacillus is a notoriously difficult pathogen to control. Although bacille Calmette-Guerin (BCG) vaccine protects against severe tuberculous meningitis and disseminated TB in children (Benenson, 1990), its efficacy against pulmonary TB in adults has varied widely in different parts of the world. Treatment of conventional TB is effective, but expensive, requiring daily treatment with multiple drugs for a minimum of six months. There is a universal tendency among TB patients to stop taking their drugs when the drugs begin to have their beneficial effect or to take the medications only intermittently. When this happens, relapses are frequent and very often are caused by drug-resistant tubercle bacilli that have survived the initial course of treatment. The emergence of drug-resistant M. tuberculosis is in many ways an index of individual compliance with antituberculosis chemotherapy and of the inability of the health care infrastructure to ensure adequate treatment. Many public health agencies that once could play key roles in this process have had their budgets cut drastically in recent years and hence are unable to perform this crucial service.

MDRTB is extraordinarily difficult to treat, and a majority of patients do not respond to therapy. Total treatment costs for an individual with MDRTB can be as much as $150,000, ten times the cost of traditional treatment; the cost of the treatment drugs alone can be as much as 21 times as great (see Table 2-5). In an outbreak of MDRTB in 1990 in Forth Worth, Texas, the cost of treating 10 patients was $950,433. The budget available that year to the Fort Worth/Tarrant County, Texas, Tuberculosis Control Program was less than one-fifth that amount (Centers for Disease Control, 1990b).

The preferred treatment for classical TB consists of isoniazid, rifampin, and pyrazinamide. For patients whose tubercle bacilli are thought to be resistant to isoniazid, a fourth drug, ethambutol, should be added to the regimen until drug susceptibility results are known. Isolates of tubercle bacilli resistant to both isoniazid and rifampin, now representing about 20 percent in some cities, require specialized treatment with additional medications, which may include streptomycin and ciprofloxacin for almost two years.

The tubercle bacillus is a slow-growing organism. Three to six weeks are needed to grow the bacteria in the clinical laboratory, and an additional three to six weeks are needed to screen for antibiotic resistance. Such ex-

TABLE 2-5 Drug Costs per Course of Treatment for One Individual with Either Susceptible or Varying Levels of Drug-Resistant Tuberculosis

Level of Resistance and Drugs Used for Treatment	Course of Treatment	Cost of Drugs (1991 $)
Classical, susceptible tuberculosis		
INH, RIF, PZA	2 months	
followed by INH, RIF	4 months	277
or		
INH, RIF, PZA	6 months	495
INH or RIF resistant tuberculosis		
INH, RIF, EMB, PZA	2 months	
followed by RIF, EMB, PZA	10 months	2,113
or		
INH, EMB, PZA	16 months	2,769
INH + RIF resistant tuberculosis		
INH, RIF, EMB, PZA	2 months	
followed by EMB, PZA, STR, CIP	22 months	6,033

NOTE: INH=isoniazid; RIF=rifampin; PZA=pyrazinamide; EMB=ethambutol; STR=streptomycin; CIP=ciprofloxacin.

SOURCE: D. Snider, Jr., Division of Tuberculosis Control, National Center for Prevention Services, Centers for Disease Control.

tended laboratory procedures can result in a delay in diagnosis, which means that patients with unrecognized drug-resistant TB may be treated ineffectively and remain infectious for a longer period. In HIV-positive individuals, MDRTB usually causes death within 4 to 16 weeks after being diagnosed, which is often before laboratory tests on drug susceptibility and resistance can be completed.

There is no evidence that mutation rates in *M. tuberculosis* organisms have increased or that increased virulence is to blame for the recent deadly outbreaks of TB (Weiss, 1992). It is likely that drug-resistant forms of tuberculosis arose because of patient noncompliance with the 6- to 12-month regimen of antibiotics required to treat TB. Ineffective treatment regimens also play a role in the rising incidence of TB. To address noncompliance, some states with high TB rates are considering approaches to outreach, such as expanding directly observed therapy (DOT;) others may reestablish inpatient facilities similar to the TB sanatoria of the first half of this century. Standard treatment regimens for TB have also been updated. Instead of taking two or three antibiotics, TB patients now take four. Still, as noted earlier, the current shortages of antituberculosis drugs in the United States have made even standard treatment difficult.

RESISTANCE TO ANTIVIRALS

Some viral infections can be successfully controlled with currently available antiviral drugs. Unfortunately, as has been the case for antibiotics, resistance to antiviral drugs has been reported (see Table 2-6). Two examples of resistance are discussed below. Potentially effective new drugs undergoing preclinical and clinical testing may replace some antivirals that have been rendered unusable as a result of excessive patterns of resistance.

Despite the efforts of researchers to discover new, effective antiviral drugs, very few ever reach the point at which they become available to those who need them. Thousands of compounds may be screened before a single candidate with desirable antiviral properties and acceptable tolerance is found. Drugs that are potentially useful against viral infections fit into three categories: those that inactivate viruses (virucides); those that inhibit the replication of viruses within their host cells (antivirals); and those that work indirectly by augmenting or modifying the host's immune response to viral invasion (immunomodulators) (Hayden and Douglas, 1990). There are no clinically practical virucidal drugs at this time, since those currently available are toxic to host cells as well as viruses. Unlike those antibiotics that are bactericidal and can rid the patient of the organism, current antivirals only suppress viral replication. Ultimately, control of the viral infection relies on the individual's immune response.

TABLE 2-6 Antiviral Drugs for Which Resistance Has Been Demonstrated

Antiviral Agent	Antiviral Spectrum
Acyclovir	Herpes simplex virus
	Varicella-zoster virus
Amantadine/rimantidine	Influenza A
Dideoxycytidine	Human immunodeficiency virus-1
Dideoxyinosine	Human immunodeficiency virus-1
Foscarnet	Cytomegalovirus
	Herpes simplex virus
Ganciclovir	Cytomegalovirus
	Herpes simplex virus
Idoxuridine (topical)	Herpes simplex virus
Trifluridine (topical)	Herpes simplex virus[a]
Vidarabine	Herpes simplex virus[a]
Zidovudine	Human immunodeficiency virus-1

[a]Resistance to these drugs can be demonstrated in the laboratory but has not yet been documented in clinical isolates.

SOURCE: F. Hayden, Associate Professor of Internal Medicine and Pathology, Department of Internal Medicine, University of Virginia Hospital.

Antiviral drugs can interfere with viral invasion and replication at several specific points. For example, the drug can prevent the attachment of the virus to the host cell, or it may interfere with the assembly of new viruses within the host cell. Although many compounds that have antiviral activity exist or can be synthesized, most cannot be used because of toxicity, because they adversely affect a host cell function, or because they fail to reach concentrations required for antiviral activity in humans (Hayden and Douglas, 1990).

The emergence of antiviral resistance is not well understood. Primary resistance, which exists even before first exposure to a drug, is uncommon, although virus populations appear to consist of heterogenous mixtures of mutants with varying drug sensitivities. Emergence of resistant subpopulations, or de novo mutations creating drug resistance, occur because of selective drug pressure. The frequency and speed at which this occurs varies among virus-drug combinations and is heavily influenced by the type of infection and nature of the host. The usefulness of drug sensitivity assays in such situations is limited. The clinical significance of in vitro resistance is often unclear, a factor that complicates therapeutic decisions.

Antiviral resistance is linked to critical amino acid changes in viral proteins that are targets of drug action or responsible for drug metabolism. Individuals who are immunocompromised, with chronic or recurrent viral infections (particularly herpesvirus infections), often develop drug-resistant viruses. Because resistance to antiviral drugs appears to occur quite rapidly in such individuals, appropriate use and availability of drugs with alternative mechanisms of action are important. Sufficient data are not yet available, however, to recommend limitations on the use of antiviral drugs.

Acyclovir and Herpes Simplex Virus

Acyclovir, an antiviral that inhibits viral DNA synthesis, is the agent of choice for managing infections with herpes simplex virus (HSV). Resistance to acyclovir was a relatively uncommon event prior to the onset of the HIV disease pandemic. Previously, occasional resistance to acyclovir was seen in cancer patients or transplant recipients who were receiving treatment for HSV infection. Acyclovir-resistant HSV in HIV-infected individuals with advanced disease can cause extensive ulcerative lesions that may lead to progressively more serious HSV disease (Laughlin et al., 1991).

The occurrence of resistance does not appear to be linked to dosage or to treatment schedule. Even initial exposure to acyclovir can induce resistance. Most commonly, resistance is caused by a mutation in the virus that results in an inability to produce thymidine kinase, the enzyme toward which acyclovir is targeted. Foscarnet, an antiviral drug that inhibits viral DNA polymerase, is used in the treatment of acyclovir-resistant HSV (Laughlin et al., 1991). Currently, there is no evidence of person-to-person spread of this drug-resistant virus.

Zidovudine and Human Immunodeficiency Virus-1

Zidovudine, also known as azidothymidine (AZT), is effective in prolonging the survival and improving the quality of life of those infected with HIV-1, including those with AIDS, those with symptomatic HIV infection, and HIV-infected asymptomatic individuals. Zidovudine works by inhibiting the viral enzyme reverse transcriptase (RNA-dependent DNA polymerase) (Hayden and Douglas, 1990).

Unfortunately, resistance to the drug has been documented and appears to be associated with length of treatment (most isolates demonstrate reduced drug susceptibility after six months of treatment) and CD4-lymphocyte counts of less than 200 per cubic milliliter (Laughlin et al., 1991). Resistance develops gradually as the result of point mutations in the gene for reverse transcriptase; multiple mutations are necessary to confer high-level resistance (Laughlin et al., 1991).

RESISTANCE TO ANTIMALARIALS

Over the past 15 years, there has been a tremendous resurgence of malaria around the world and an increase in the percentage of cases caused by *Plasmodium falciparum*, the most virulent of the four human malaria parasites (Institute of Medicine, 1991a). Worldwide, as many as 2 million people will die from malaria in 1992, most of them children in Africa.

The seriousness of the worldwide increase in malaria incidence is heightened by the spread of parasites resistant to the available assortment of antimalarial drugs. Malaria parasites, like bacteria and viruses, can develop resistance to the drugs used to prevent or treat infection. And, as is the case with antibiotics, resistance is often the result of overuse or misuse of antimalarial drugs. However, unlike the case for antibiotics, the development of antimalarial drugs is not a high priority for U.S. pharmaceutical companies. Within the United States, this task is almost entirely the domain of the Walter Reed Army Institute of Research. Globally, the Special Programme for Research and Training in Tropical Diseases, a joint project of the United Nations Development Programme, the World Bank, and the World Health Organization, is an important participant in antimalarial drug development.

Resistance to quinine, the first antimalarial drug ever marketed, was initially reported in 1910 in Germans who developed malaria while working in Brazil (Peters, 1987). Since then, a number of other antimalarials have been developed, the most notable of which is chloroquine.

Resistance to chloroquine in *P. falciparum* was first reported in 1961 in two Colombian workers (Young and Moore, 1961) and has been partly to blame for the resurgence of malaria. Soon after this account, similar reports were received from Thailand, Vietnam, Cambodia, Malaya, and Brazil. By 1970, nearly 20 percent of all malarious regions had recorded cases of chloroquine-resistant *P. falciparum* malaria (Lepes, 1981). Today, there are only a few areas in the world where chloroquine is effective against this parasite.

Resistance to the newer antimalarials, such as mefloquine, is also occurring. In Thailand, for example, there is evidence of considerable *P. falciparum* resistance to the drug (Peters, 1990; Institute of Medicine, 1991a). This is of great concern, both because this drug has not been on the market for long (demonstrating the rapidity with which these parasites can adapt to the presence of the drug) and because the development of new antimalarial drugs to which the parasites are susceptible is not a rapid process; mefloquine was originally synthesized in the late 1960s and underwent 17 years of testing to demonstrate efficacy before being licensed (Institute of Medicine, 1991a).

Although *P. falciparum* causes the most severe type of malaria and is increasing in prevalence, *P. vivax* is responsible for the majority of malaria morbidity worldwide. It is of considerable concern, therefore, that *P. vivax* has also developed resistance to chloroquine, which was first reported in 1989 in Papua New Guinea (Rieckmann et al., 1989). Chloroquine-resistant *P. vivax* malaria has also been diagnosed in Indonesia (Schwartz et al., 1991). No one knows for certain how quickly and how far this resistance will spread. Because of the problem of resistance to chloroquine, travelers should seek the latest guidance on prophylaxis before going into malaria-endemic areas.

Given the distribution of malaria cases throughout the world, drug resistance is of much greater concern outside the United States than within it. Still, the potential for the reemergence of malaria in this country, and the role of drug resistance in such a scenario, cannot be overlooked. In the United States, as recently as the early 1900s, up to 500,000 cases of malaria occurred each year, most of them in the South (Institute of Medicine, 1991a). Currently, some 1,200 total cases of malaria both drug susceptible and drug resistant are reported each year in this country, almost all of which occur in individuals who have been infected in other parts of the world (so-called imported malaria). Small outbreaks of nonimported malaria, the result of mosquito transmission from imported cases, have also been reported (Maldonado et al., 1990; Centers for Disease Control, 1990c, 1991f). Thus far, the outbreaks have been quickly and easily contained. A continued increase in drug-resistant malaria throughout the world, however, may increase the number of cases of imported malaria, thereby improving the chances for malaria to regain a foothold in the United States.

VECTOR RESISTANCE TO PESTICIDES

Agriculture accounts for about 75 percent of the pesticides used in the United States. In 1987, approximately 407,000 tons of pesticides were applied in agricultural settings throughout the nation, of which about 89,500 tons were insecticides. About 10 percent of the pesticides used worldwide are applied for public health purposes, mainly to control malaria, filariasis, schistosomiasis, onchocerciasis, and trypanosomiasis (Moses, 1992).

This high volume of pesticide use for agricultural purposes has contributed to the development of resistance in infectious disease vectors, particularly mosquitoes. Public health use of insecticides has also played a role in the emergence of resistance, although not in the United States, where public health use of insecticides is not sufficiently regular to elicit the development of resistance.

Resistance, in the field, to a number of pesticides belonging to organochlorine, organophosphate, and other insecticide groups has developed in vector arthropods. In addition, recent evidence from laboratory studies points to the emergence of resistance in mosquito larvae to the delta endotoxins of the commercialized microbial control agents *Bacillus thuringiensis israeliensis* (Georghiou, 1990) and *B. sphaericus* (Rodcharoen and Mulla, in press). Although resistance to these agents has not yet been demonstrated in a field situation, the laboratory finding illustrates the strong potential for the development of such resistance.

New Understandings:
Microbes as Cofactors in Chronic Disease

Although medical science has been able to discern the causes of many diseases, the etiology of some that have a significant impact on the health of the U.S. population is still speculative, even after decades or more of research. The recognition that an "old" disease, with heretofore unknown causes, is associated with an infectious agent is one of the more interesting ways infectious diseases emerge. A number of diseases are now thought to be caused by microbial infection or to involve microbes as cofactors in pathogenesis. These include, but are not limited to, atherosclerosis, rheumatoid arthritis, insulin-dependent diabetes mellitus, Reye's syndrome, Kawasaki disease, systemic lupus erythematosis, and Alzheimer's disease. The final chapters on these diseases have not been written; it remains to be seen which, if any, will be determined with certainty to involve microbial agents. The examples below illustrate the relationships between some of these diseases and the infectious agents associated with them.

Human T-cell Leukemia Virus Types I and II

Isolation of the first pathogenic human retrovirus was reported in 1980 (Poiesz et al., 1980) and was soon followed by the isolation of a second, closely related but distinct virus (Kalyanaraman et al., 1982). These viruses subsequently became known as human T-cell leukemia virus types I and II (HTLV-I, HTLV-II); they are sometimes referred to as human T-lymphotropic viruses. Multiple isolates of the HTLVs have now been obtained, novel regulatory properties identified, and areas of endemicity throughout the world defined by seroepidemiological studies.

Although HTLV-II has not been linked definitively to a specific disease, HTLV-I has been shown to be etiologically associated with two very different diseases. The first, adult T-cell leukemia/lymphoma (ATLL), for which the virus is named, was first described in southern Japan (Uchiyama et al., 1977), where the virus is endemic. ATLL is a malignancy primarily of CD4+ (T-helper/inducer) lymphocytes, and in the leukemic phase, the HTLV-I provirus is monoclonally integrated into the DNA of neoplastic cells. The onset of disease occurs many years after the initial infection, and the most severe forms of the disease are characterized by generalized lymphadenopathy, visceral and cutaneous involvement, and bone lesions (Kuefler and Bunn, 1986). Effective treatment is not available, and death usually occurs within one year of diagnosis. Fortunately, only 2 to 5 percent of HTLV-I-infected persons develop ATLL (Murphy et al., 1989).

The second HTLV-I-associated disease is a neurological condition called tropical spastic paraparesis (TSP), which was first described in the Caribbean (Gessain et al., 1985). The same syndrome was subsequently described by doctors in Japan, who called it HTLV-I-associated myelopathy (HAM) (Osame et al., 1986). This disease, which is now usually referred to as TSP/HAM, begins with difficulties in walking and weakness and spasticity in the legs; it can also include back pain, sensory disturbances, urinary incontinence, and impotence in men. Disability progresses over several years, and eventually victims may become confined to a wheelchair. Because afflicted individuals have high concentrations of HTLV-I-specific antibodies in serum and spinal fluid (Osame et al., 1990), sometimes in association with an human leukocyte antigen (HLA)-linked high immune responsiveness to HTLV-I (Usuku et al., 1988), some investigators feel that TSP/HAM is an immunological disease triggered by the virus. As with ATLL, TSP/HAM occurs in a small percentage (about 1 percent) of HTLV-I-infected persons (Kaplan et al., 1990).

Interest in HTLV-I increased with the in vitro observation of several investigators that the efficiency of replication of HIV, the virus that causes

HIV disease and AIDS, increased in cells transformed by HTLV-I. The subsequent identification of persons in endemic areas, many with AIDS, who were infected with both HIV and HTLV-I (Cortes et al., 1989; Hattori et al., 1989) led to the speculation that interaction of these two viruses may potentiate disease progression. The prevalence of infection with both HIV and HTLV-I or HTLV-II is increasing in populations of intravenous drug abusers in the United States (Lee et al., 1991). This increase offers the possibility of a study group, albeit an unwanted one, in which to assess this additional risk for disease.

HTLV-I has also been implicated as a factor in other disease syndromes, including polymyositis, arthritis, infective dermatitis, mycosis fungoides, and multiple sclerosis (although the latter is controversial). In addition, HTLV-II was recently linked to chronic fatigue syndrome (DeFreitas et al., 1991). It is probable that the full spectrum of diseases and immunological abnormalities associated with the human retroviruses has yet to be delineated. It is also probable that additional human retroviruses exist but have not yet been discovered.

ATHEROSCLEROSIS

Atherosclerosis, commonly known as hardening of the arteries, is the result of an uncontrolled proliferation of arterial smooth muscle cells, which eventually can block the flow of blood through the vessel. This disease is the underlying cause of strokes and myocardial infarctions and results in more deaths in the United States (and in other industrialized countries) than any other single disease. The burden on the U.S. health care system is estimated to be in excess of $60 billion per year (Levi and Moskovitz, 1982; Kannel et al., 1984).

Although it is well known that smoking, high cholesterol levels, and elevated blood pressure are major risk factors for atherosclerosis, viruses can generate the pathologic events—cell destruction, metabolic changes within cells, and cell transformation—that precede the appearance of atherosclerotic lesions. This observation has led some researchers to conclude that a virus or viruses may play some role in the disease. Supporting this theory are reports that chickens can develop atherosclerotic lesions as a result of infection with an avian herpesvirus (Fabricant et al., 1978, 1980; Minick et al., 1979). In humans, two similar viruses, herpes simplex virus (HSV-1 and HSV-2) and cytomegalovirus (CMV), infect infants and young children worldwide. During infection, the viruses are often found in the blood vessels, potentially exposing the smooth muscle cells to their effects. In one recent study, CMV infection was demonstrated in patients with atherosclerosis; there was no evidence of either HSV-1 or HSV-2 infection in the same individuals (Melnick et al., 1990). Other studies have implicated

CMV, as well as HSV-1 and HSV-2 in human atherosclerotic disease (Benditt et al., 1983; Yamashiroya et al., 1988; Hendrix et al., 1989, 1990).

Recently, a bacterium, *Chlamydia pneumoniae*, was reported to play a potential role in the pathogenesis of atherosclerotic disease. The investigators examined the consequences of human infection with *C. pneumoniae* and found evidence, in the form of persistently elevated levels of anti-*C. pneumoniae* antibodies and immune complexes containing chlamydial lipopolysaccharide, that chronic infection with this bacterium was associated with increased risk for coronary heart disease. This risk was shown to be independent of those factors—age, smoking, total cholesterol to high-density-lipoprotein-cholesterol ratios, and hypertension—most often associated with atherosclerosis (Saikku et al., 1992). Because *C. pneumoniae* infection is fairly common and can be treated with antibiotics, a proven association of this organism with atherosclerosis and subsequent myocardial infarction could have a significant public health impact.

Human Papillomavirus

Papillomaviruses were described and associated with disease in the early to mid-1900s. Research on these viruses, however, suffered from the inability to grow them in cells in the laboratory. It was not until the 1980s that techniques to identify and characterize human papillomavirus (HPV) became readily available (deVilliers, 1989). In the past 10 years, more than 67 HPV types have been defined; the molecular biology of the virus has been developed in exquisite detail; and knowledge concerning molecular mechanisms of infection and disease has emerged (Reeves et al., 1989).

Epidemiological studies have shown that HPV infection (with HPV types 16 and 18) is the major risk factor for cervical cancer (Reeves et al., 1989), an important public health problem in the United States and the developing world. The American Cancer Society estimated that 13,000 new cases would occur in the United States in 1991, resulting in about 4,500 deaths (American Cancer Society, 1991). Most of these cases and deaths could have been prevented by appropriate screening and control programs. Cervical cancer is uniquely amenable to secondary prevention by screening and early treatment since it evolves through surgically curable premalignant stages to invasive disease over a 10- to 20-year period (Tabbara et al., 1992).

Other factors besides HPV infection, however, play a role in the development of cervical cancer. For example, a woman's risk of cervical cancer is directly related to the number of sexual partners she has had (the greater the number of partners the greater her risk) and inversely related to age at first intercourse (the younger her age, the greater the risk). It has only recently been recognized that male sexual behavior also influences cervical cancer risk. Spouses of women with cervical cancer are more likely to exhibit high-risk sexual behavior than spouses of women without the disease (Brinton et al., 1989). These behaviors undoubtedly increase the chance that the men will be exposed to sexually transmitted agents such as HPV. There is growing evidence that other venereal disease agents, such as HSV-2 and HIV, interact with HPV in a multiplicative fashion to boost the risks for cervical cancer (Hildesheim et al., 1991).

Women infected with HIV have at least a 10-fold increased risk for active HPV infection and a 12-fold increase in risk of cervical neoplasia (Laga et al., 1992). HPV infection and cervical disease also progress more rapidly and are more refractory to treatment in women with HIV infection. As the prevalence of heterosexually transmitted HIV increases among women, HPV infection and cervical disease will continue to emerge as major opportunistic complications. The strong association between HIV and HPV infection may involve interactions between the proteins of HPV and HIV, in addition to general immunosuppression.

For all of the apparent links between HPV infection and cervical disease, the relationship is not a simple one of cause and effect. For example, no study has found HPV in all cervical cancers, and a variety of studies have shown that 10 to 50 percent of healthy women are infected with HPV (Burk et al., 1986; Cox et al., 1986; Toorn et al., 1986; and Reeves et al., 1987). HPV infection can only be estimated by detecting viral DNA, and there is no single accepted criterion for judging the results of such testing. In addition, there is no clinically useful serological assay that can independently estimate past HPV infection. Well-standardized commercial kits can be used to diagnose HPV infection, but infection alone is neither sufficient nor necessary for cervical cancer. The condition appears to be brought on by a complex interaction of infections and demographic, behavioral, and hormonal risk factors. The only currently efficacious cervical cancer control strategy is secondary prevention—detecting and ablating preinvasive cervical intraepithelial neoplasia (CIN) lesions. New strategies based on HPV detection and Pap smear screening may be possible.

BREAKDOWN OF PUBLIC HEALTH MEASURES

The control of many infectious illnesses has occurred as societies themselves have become more advanced. Improvements in medicine, science, and public health have come only as a result of the complex growth and maturation of modern civilization. Many of the protections now in place, such as vaccination, proper hygiene, water and sewage treatment, and safe food-handling and distribution practices have vastly improved our ability to control infectious disease outbreaks.

Despite the appearance of security, however, there is only a thin veneer protecting humankind from potentially devastating infectious disease epidemics. Alone or in combination, economic collapse, war, and natural disasters, among other societal disruptions, have caused (and could again cause) the breakdown of public health measures and the emergence or re-emergence of a number of deadly diseases.

Inadequate Sanitation: Cholera

Cholera, a sometimes rapidly fatal diarrheal disease caused by the bacterium *Vibrio cholerae*, reached epidemic levels in South America in January 1991 for the first time in almost a century. Inadequate sanitation played a role in its reappearance, which occurred initially in several coastal cities in Peru; then the disease spread through much of the continent. A scattering of epidemic-related cases were reported later in the year in Central America and the United States. As of December 1991, there had been 366,056 reported cases of the disease and 3,894 deaths in these three regions (Pan American Health Organization, 1991).

It is believed that *V. cholerae* was first introduced into the harbor at Lima, Peru, through the dumping of bilge water by a ship arriving from the Far East. Once in the water, the bacteria rapidly contaminated the fish and shellfish, which were then consumed (often in the form of ceviche, a dish made with raw seafood that is popular in that part of the world). Following the initial seafood-related cases in humans, the organisms are thought to have been spread by fecal contamination of the water supply.

Epidemiologic investigations in Peru have implicated such contaminated municipal water supplies as the principal means by which the disease is now being transmitted. Based on a study by the U.S. Environmental Protection Agency (EPA) that showed a possible link between chlorination and cancer, Peruvian officials apparently ceased treating much of the country's drinking water in the early 1980s (C. Anderson, 1991). A paucity of hygienic food preparation practices also appears to have played a role.

The epidemic is traveling northward at a rapid rate; several cases have already been reported in the United States, originating from contaminated foodstuffs. U.S. public health authorities are maintaining a close watch on foods imported from South and Central America (the majority of fresh fruits and vegetables imported into the United States during the winter come from Mexico). In February 1992, at least 31 of 356 passengers and crew aboard a flight from Buenos Aires, Argentina, to Los Angeles, California (with a brief stopover in Lima) were diagnosed with cholera (18 in California, 9 in Nevada, 3 in Japan, and 1 in Argentina—1 person died). At least 54 other passengers reported having diarrhea of unknown etiology. This illustration demonstrates the ease with which this disease can be transported worldwide (Centers for Disease Control, 1992c).

Cholera can almost always be treated successfully with oral rehydration therapy, which replaces fluids and essential salts lost in diarrheal stools. Disease surveillance and maintenance of a clean water supply are the most effective methods of preventing disease spread. Currently available vaccines are of limited effectiveness.

Extensive transmission of cholera and other waterborne infectious diseases in the United States is highly unlikely, owing to the generally high standards required of U.S. municipal water and sewage treatment facilities. Outbreaks could occur, however, in areas with substandard water supplies and inadequate sewage disposal. Occasional cholera outbreaks in the United States are most often caused by fecal contamination of estuarine waters. Inadequately treated sewage can be taken up by the fin fish and shellfish harvested from these waters; their consumption can infect humans if the fish are prepared improperly. As coastal areas become increasingly crowded and water treatment facilities are overwhelmed or poorly maintained, a rise in cases of *Vibrio* infection is likely.

Complacency

There can be a delicate balance between maintaining control of a disease and the initiation of an epidemic. It is one thing to have this balance disrupted by essentially uncontrollable elements; it is quite another to have it go awry as a result of individual or organizational complacency.

Sometime in the 1950s, the attention given to acute infectious diseases by public health and medical officials, physicians, researchers, and others began to wane, and a shift in focus to chronic, degenerative diseases occurred. Much of the reason for this shift was the notion that infectious disease problems were becoming a thing of the past—science, medicine, public health, and an improved standard of living had brought most of these diseases under control. People were living longer and developing more chronic illnesses as a result. The emergence of HIV disease and AIDS swung the pendulum back to infectious diseases. HIV disease and the host of opportunistic infections that accompany it have severely challenged the scientific, medical, and public health communities, as well as politicians. Infectious diseases clearly are not a problem of the past.

Measles is highlighted here as an example of complacency regarding the control of infectious diseases. Tuberculosis is yet another example that has already been discussed in other sections of this report. There are certainly other diseases, however (including typhoid, diphtheria, whooping cough, tetanus, and louse-borne typhus) that may pose significant threats to health when complacency sets in.

INADEQUATE LEVELS OF IMMUNIZATION: MEASLES

Immunization against infectious diseases is one of the most effective ways of improving overall public health. Medical researchers have developed dozens of vaccines, a number of which have been incorporated into childhood vaccination programs. These programs have greatly reduced the health-related and financial impacts of a number of previously devastating diseases. However, if such programs falter or are carried out incompletely, diseases that are now relatively rare can reemerge as the killers they once were. This phenomenon is a danger to all countries, particularly those with poor or inactive immunization programs (see Table 2-7).

The incidence of measles, a highly communicable viral disease, declined rapidly in the United States after the introduction of an effective vaccine in 1963. There were some 500,000 reported cases each year during the 1950s, a number that had dropped to less than 2,000 by the early 1980s. In 1989, however, the number of measles cases began to climb, and by 1990, more than 26,000 cases were reported, the largest number since 1977 (Atkinson and Markowitz, 1991). What happened?

TABLE 2-7 Percentage of 1-Year-Olds Immunized Against Measles in the Americas in 1990

Country	Percentage	Country	Percentage
Panama	99	Belize	81
Anguilla	99	Nicaragua	81
British Virgin Islands	99	Turks and Caicos	81
Montserrat	99	Brazil	77
St. Kitts/Nevis	99	Paraguay	77
Chile	98	El Salvador	75
Dominican Republic	96	Jamaica	74
Argentina	94	Suriname	74
Cuba	94	**United States**[a]	**70**
Honduras	91	Guatemala	68
Antigua	89	Mexico	66
Barbados	87	Peru	64
Bahamas	86	Venezuela	64
Costa Rica	85	Grenada	63
Colombia	82	Ecuador	62
St. Lucia	82	Bolivia	53
Uruguay	82	Haiti	31

[a]Data are for 2-year-olds.
SOURCE: Bernier, 1991.

Measles vaccine induces immunity in more than 95 percent of individuals over one year of age (R. M. Davis et al., 1987). The requirement that school-age children in the United States present evidence of measles vaccination in order to be admitted to school was largely responsible for the dramatic reduction in the incidence of measles in the 1960s, 1970s, and early 1980s. Vaccination levels in preschool-age children, however, were lower than for those attending school (Orenstein et al., 1990; Atkinson and Markowitz, 1991).

In 1990, there were large outbreaks of measles in Dallas, San Diego, and Los Angeles; each city reported more than 1,000 cases. In New York City, an outbreak that started in March 1990 continued through 1991, with more than 2,000 cases reported in the first five months of 1991. Epidemiologic data from the New York outbreak revealed that a majority of cases were among preschool-age black and Hispanic children who had not been immunized. Vaccination goals in this population were not being met (Centers for Disease Control, 1991d).

There have also been additional outbreaks among vaccinated school-age groups, indicating that in some cases the one-time vaccination was insufficient to prevent disease. In response, the American Academy of Family Physicians, the American Academy of Pediatrics, and the Immunization Practices Advisory Committee (ACIP; a committee of experts convened by the CDC) recommended, in 1989, that a second dose of measles vaccine (as part of the trivalent measles, mumps, and rubella vaccine) be given (Atkinson, 1991). In early 1991, the National Vaccine Advisory Committee issued recommendations to improve the availability of childhood vaccines and urged a two-dose schedule for the measles-mumps-rubella (MMR) immunization (National Vaccine Advisory Committee, 1991).

Available data for 1991 indicate that the trend of rising measles incidence is reversing itself. As of November 1991, there were 60 percent fewer cases than had been reported during the same period in 1990 (Cotton, 1991). Although efforts have been made over the past several years to reduce the number of people, particularly children, who have not been vaccinated against measles, the present decline in cases is too great to be attributable to better vaccine coverage alone (Cotton, 1991). At this time, however, a full explanation is not available.

War

When deployed outside of this country, U.S. military forces are at high risk of being exposed to a variety of infectious disease agents. In past conflicts, infectious diseases have produced higher hospital admission rates among U.S. troops and, until World War II, higher mortality rates, than battle injuries (Gordon, 1958; Reister, N.d.; Washington Headquarters Service Directorate for Information, Operations, and Reports, 1985). Table 2-8 shows the types of infectious diseases that have accounted for the greatest morbidity among American soldiers.

The relative importance to deployed forces of any particular infectious disease depends on a number of environmental factors and operational circumstances, including, principally, the geographic area of deployment, the time of year, the mission and composition of the force, and the intensity of the conflict. For example, military operations generally result in large numbers of susceptible individuals living in close proximity, circumstances that can facilitate the transmission of respiratory diseases. Under field conditions, food and water sanitation services may be rudimentary and subject to disruptions, opportunities to exercise good personal hygiene are diminished, and there may be exposure to the bites of infected arthropod vectors of both human and zoonotic diseases. In addition, warfare usually creates some degree of social disruption, which can produce refugee populations that are frequently subject to epidemics of infectious disease. Troops may be at added risk of infection to the extent that they become involved in the supervision and care of the refugees. Because troops are frequently living under relatively primitive field conditions, there is also the potential for accidental transmission of previously unknown zoonotic diseases. The return of

TABLE 2-8 Infectious Diseases Causing High Morbidity in U.S. Forces in Past Conflicts: World War II, Korea, Vietnam, and Operation Desert Storm

Disease Category	Conflict
Acute respiratory diseases and influenza	All
Acute diarrheal diseases	All
Malaria	WWII, Korea, Vietnam
Hepatitis	WWII, Korea, Vietnam
Sexually transmitted diseases	WWII, Korea, Vietnam
Arthropod-borne diseases[a]	WWII, Vietnam
Rickettsial diseases[b]	WWII, Vietnam
Leptospirosis	WWII, Vietnam
Leishmaniasis	WWII, Desert Storm
Schistosomiasis	WWII[c]

NOTE: WWII=World War II.

[a]Especially dengue fever, sandfly fever, hemorrhagic fevers, and encephalitides.

[b]Principally scrub typhus, whose distribution is limited to parts of Asia and northern Australia.

[c]Principally in engineer bridge-building units in Luzon, Philippines.

SOURCE: L. J. Legters, Department of Preventive Medicine, Division of Tropical Public Health, Uniformed Services University of the Health Sciences, Bethesda, Maryland.

U.S. troops from foreign soils offers a unique opportunity for the introduction or reintroduction of infectious diseases into the United States.

The following examples describe infectious diseases that have emerged in association with military operations, some of which involved U.S. troops.

• Epidemic typhus, caused by *Rickettsia prowazekii*, has been a frequent accompaniment of warfare in Europe, dating back to the siege of Naples by the French in 1528 (Zinsser, 1935). The disease, which is acquired by contact with the feces of infected body lice, was a major problem in World War II.

• Trench fever, caused by *Rochalimaea quintana* (*Rickettsia quintana*), which are transmitted by body lice, made its first appearance in troops during World War I (Fuller, 1964).

• Epidemic hemorrhagic fever, now known to be due to a zoonotic infection caused by Hantaan virus, was reported in Japanese and Soviet troops in Manchuria before the onset of World War II and was later (1951) recognized in United Nations troops in Korea (Benenson, 1990).

• Scrub typhus, caused by a rickettsia transmitted by the bite of an infected larval mite of the genus *Leptotrombidium*, was a major medical problem (surpassed only by malaria in some areas) in the Pacific Theater in both World War II (Philip, 1948) and the Vietnam conflict (Berman et al., 1973).

• A massive outbreak (involving 30,000 to 50,000 cases) of acute schistosomiasis, caused by *Schistosoma japonicum*, is reputed to have occurred in Chinese troops in 1950. The troops were being taught to swim in infected canals in southern China in preparation for what, because of the outbreak, became an aborted invasion of Taiwan in 1950 (Kiernan, 1959).

• Leptospirosis, caused by *Leptospira interrogans*, was first identified as an important military disease in British troops during jungle operations against Communist terrorists in what was then Malaya in the late 1950s (U.S. Army Medical Research Unit, Malaya, 1962).

• Leishmaniasis, due to *Leishmania tropica*, was known to be endemic in the Persian Gulf region before U.S. troops were committed in Operation Desert Shield. Known to cause cutaneous lesions, the capacity of *L. tropica* to "visceralize" (i.e., invade bone marrow, liver, and spleen) was not well documented before its discovery in returning U.S. troops. The apparently atypical visceral expression of the disease may not be unusual at all but merely a natural consequence of the exposure of more than 500,000 susceptible troops to infected sand fly vectors in an endemic area. A total of 26 cases of leishmaniasis in U.S. troops—17 cutaneous and 9 visceral—had been diagnosed as of April 1992 (M. Grogl, Chief, Leishmania Section, Division of Experimental Therapeutics, Walter Reed Army Institute of Research, Washington, D.C., personal communication, 1992).

3

Addressing the Threats

The process by which an infectious disease emerges and is recognized and responded to can be complex. Chapter 2 dealt with the many factors involved in emergence. This chapter addresses disease recognition and intervention and provides specific recommendations for improving the ability of the United States and the global community to respond to future microbial threats to health. The relationships between and among recognition activities and interventions are diagrammed in Figure 3-1.

Chapter 3 is divided into two sections. The first, on recognition, addresses domestic and international surveillance. The recommendations in this section, if implemented, would strengthen U.S. surveillance activities and encourage efforts to develop a global infectious disease surveillance network. The second section, on interventions, is divided into subsections that address the U.S. public health system, research and training, vaccine and drug development, vector control, and public education and behavioral change. Each subsection includes one or more recommendations directed at improving the current U.S. capability to respond to outbreaks of emerging infectious diseases.

RECOGNITION

The key to recognizing new or emerging infectious diseases, and to tracking the prevalence of more established infectious diseases, is surveillance. Surveillance and rapid response to identified disease threats are at the core of preventive medicine. A well-designed and well-implemented infectious disease surveillance program can provide a means to detect unusual clusters of disease, document the geographic and demographic spread of an out-

RECOGNITION ACTIVITIES

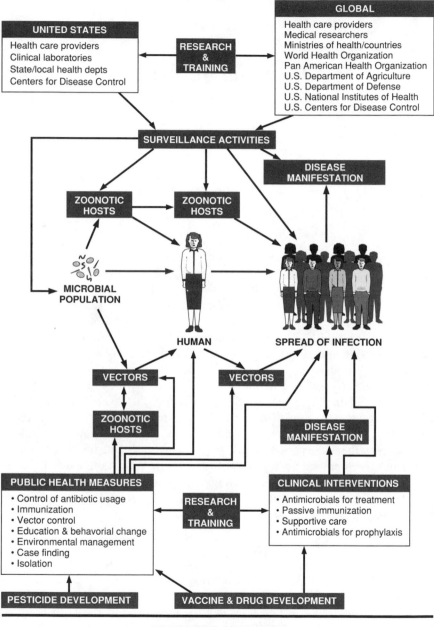

GLOBAL
Health care providers
Medical researchers
Ministries of health/countries
World Health Organization
Pan American Health Organization
U.S. Department of Agriculture
U.S. Department of Defense
U.S. National Institutes of Health
U.S. Centers for Disease Control

UNITED STATES
Health care providers
Clinical laboratories
State/local health depts
Centers for Disease Control

RESEARCH & TRAINING

SURVEILLANCE ACTIVITIES

DISEASE MANIFESTATION

ZOONOTIC HOSTS

ZOONOTIC HOSTS

MICROBIAL POPULATION

HUMAN

SPREAD OF INFECTION

VECTORS

VECTORS

ZOONOTIC HOSTS

DISEASE MANIFESTATION

PUBLIC HEALTH MEASURES
• Control of antibiotic usage
• Immunization
• Vector control
• Education & behavorial change
• Environmental management
• Case finding
• Isolation

RESEARCH & TRAINING

CLINICAL INTERVENTIONS
• Antimicrobials for treatment
• Passive immunization
• Supportive care
• Antimicrobials for prophylaxis

PESTICIDE DEVELOPMENT

VACCINE & DRUG DEVELOPMENT

RESPONSE ACTIVITIES

FIGURE 3-1 Recognition of and interventions for emerging infectious diseases.

break, estimate the magnitude of the problem, describe the natural history of the disease, identify factors responsible for emergence, facilitate laboratory and epidemiological research, and assess the success of specific intervention efforts.

Unfortunately, there is insufficient awareness of and appreciation for the value of comprehensive surveillance programs. Even among public health personnel, involvement in surveillance activities is often limited to collecting and transmitting disease-related data, a viewpoint that can mask the objectives and significance of the overall effort. Some health care and public health professionals are unfamiliar with surveillance methods, mainly because the topic is covered inadequately in medical schools and even in schools of public health (Thacker and Berkelman, 1988). The result is incomplete, underrepresentative, and untimely disease reporting. Poor surveillance leaves policymakers and practitioners without a basis for developing and implementing policies for controlling the spread of infectious diseases.

Surveillance can take many forms, from complex international networks involving sophisticated laboratory and epidemiological investigations, to small, community-based programs or a single astute clinician. Disease surveillance often is a passive process that is based on individual health care workers who report instances of unusual or particularly contagious human illnesses, usually to a government health agency. In other instances, more formal surveillance can take place, in which public health workers actively seek out cases of disease and report their findings regularly to a central data collection point.

The importance of surveillance to the detection and control of emerging microbial threats cannot be overemphasized. Active monitoring of such factors as population growth and migration, vector abundance, development projects that disturb the environment, and natural environmental factors (especially temperature and precipitation) is an essential component of surveillance and can influence the spread of emerging infectious diseases and the effectiveness of efforts to control them.

Surveillance is important to any disease control effort; it is absolutely essential if that effort's goal is eradication. Without the information obtained through disease surveillance, it is not possible to know how and where disease control efforts should be focused or to analyze the impact of ongoing efforts. The smallpox eradication program, discussed below, is an excellent example of the use of surveillance for case finding and program monitoring.

Surveillance in Action: The World Health Organization's Smallpox Eradication Program

An often overlooked but very significant contributor to the success of global smallpox eradication was disease surveillance. Of course, smallpox eradication would have been impossible had there not been an effective vaccine and a simple, inexpensive means of delivering it—the bifurcated needle. The fact that humans were the only known reservoir for the small-pox virus also simplified the task of eradication, since no insect vector or nonhuman animal hosts were involved in disease transmission.

Smallpox is transmitted by the respiratory route, by contact with pox lesions, or by infective material, such as bed linens, recently contaminated with discharge from lesions. A distinctive rash and skin lesions develop within 10 to 14 days in virtually all who are infected by the smallpox virus. Because those infected are contagious only from the time the rash appears to the time the resulting scabs fall off, and because subclinical cases play no role in disease spread, tracing the chain of transmission is fairly straight-forward. During the eradication period, when a case of disease was located, the affected individual was isolated and potential contacts were vaccinated. At the same time, an effort was made to find the person from whom the patient had presumably contracted the disease, and that individual's con-tacts were similarly vaccinated.

Perhaps the most difficult part of the eradication effort was the develop-ment of adequate national surveillance programs, since they were either nonexistent or nearly so in all participating countries when the program began. At the outset, it was evident that most smallpox cases were not being reported even though smallpox was, by international treaty, a reportable disease. It has been estimated that less than 1 percent of cases were being reported when the World Health Organization's (WHO) global smallpox eradication program got under way in 1967 (Henderson, 1976a,b).

Thus, one of the early steps in the eradication campaign was to establish disease reporting systems in countries that did not have them and to up-grade the quality of reporting systems in countries that did. It was a formi-dable task. In African countries and in Brazil, this was often done by as-signing teams of two to four persons to an administrative area that en-compassed a population of from 2 million to 5 million. The teams were charged with regularly visiting health centers and hospitals to encourage health personnel to report cases (or the absence of cases) each week, with investigating and containing outbreaks, and with distributing vaccine and vaccination supplies.

These teams played a vital role in the development and success of the reporting system. Not only did they discover unreported cases, but their prompt response to smallpox outbreaks also served to encourage case-reporting by health workers. As the incidence of the disease fell, periodic searches were conducted on a house-by-house basis. In some countries, such as India, Pakistan, and Bangladesh, rewards were offered for reporting cases.

Another key feature of the smallpox surveillance effort, and one that is common to all effective surveillance initiatives, was information dissemination. Those taking part directly in the eradication effort, as well as others with a "need to know," were regularly supplied with surveillance reports. The reports contained weekly tallies of cases from each reporting unit, comments, and other items of interest, such as specimen collection procedures or information about other smallpox programs.

In 1971, four years after the global campaign had begun, the number of countries reporting smallpox cases had fallen from 44 to 16 (Henderson, 1976a,b). By 1975, only one country, Ethiopia, remained endemic for the disease; two years later, the last known case of naturally occurring smallpox was diagnosed. Finally, in 1979, after long and careful review, the WHO certified the world free of smallpox.

LESSONS FROM THE SMALLPOX EXPERIENCE

Because every disease is different, in terms of how it is diagnosed, whom it affects, and where it occurs, surveillance efforts must be individually tailored. The experience with smallpox eradication was unique in several respects. Most important, eradication is not the goal of most public health activities that use surveillance. The fact that vaccination was the primary tool used to combat the disease also sets smallpox apart from most other situations in which surveillance plays a role. Nevertheless, the eradication campaign illustrated a number of important principles about surveillance that might be applied to other efforts to monitor and control the spread of infectious diseases.

One of the most fundamental is that a reduction in disease incidence is the ultimate measure of success in disease control. In the case of smallpox, for example, tallying the number of vaccinations performed in order to gauge the campaign's success would have been of little value because the immune response to the vaccine was not the same for all who were vaccinated. Not everyone to whom vaccine was administered was effectively vaccinated in terms of protection from contracting smallpox.[1] In addition, as the eradication campaign developed, it became clear that special efforts to vaccinate those at high risk, particularly contacts of infected individuals, were the most effective strategy. By focusing on disease incidence, it was possible to identify the epidemiological factors responsible for cases of disease that occurred despite ongoing efforts to prevent them. Once these

---

[1] Failures might be attributed to substandard vaccine (prior to 1970, when all vaccine used in the eradication program met international standards for potency and stability) or to poor (or absent) host immune response. Many other vaccines are likely to be somewhat less effective than smallpox vaccine (vaccinia); nevertheless, they may be important and useful tools for disease control.

factors had been identified, disease control efforts could be modified accordingly.

The importance of flexibility in surveillance activities was underscored early in the eradication campaign. The initial strategy had been to conduct mass vaccinations in every endemic country and at the same time improve surveillance capabilities. It was felt that once 80 percent of a country's population was immunized, any remaining foci of infection could be rapidly identified, contained, and eliminated.

Once the campaign was under way, however, it became clear that achieving the 80 percent immunization goal might not be necessary. A more targeted approach, called surveillance-containment, was tried. Infected individuals were located and isolated, and known or suspected contacts were vaccinated, thus preventing the disease from spreading to others. The new strategy worked because smallpox infection is never silent, because it spreads slowly compared with many other infectious diseases, and because vaccination could produce immunity within the incubation period for the disease.

Current U.S.-Supported Surveillance Efforts

Current U.S. surveillance efforts include both domestic and international components. Although the domestic program, in which a number of federal government agencies participate independently, is fairly comprehensive, U.S. international surveillance activities at this time are fragmented and inadequate to detect emerging infectious disease threats on a timely basis.

DOMESTIC EFFORTS

Surveillance of infectious diseases in the United States is a passive process. It relies on physicians, hospitals, and other health care providers to report cases to state and local organizations that are responsible for disease surveillance. The Centers for Disease Control (CDC) works in cooperation with the states in monitoring the domestic incidence of specific infectious diseases (such as measles, mumps, rubella, pertussis, diphtheria, and hepatitis B). Each state has its own regulations regarding the reporting of specific diseases. These "notifiable" diseases may duplicate or expand on the list of 49 diseases that are reportable to the CDC (see Table 3-1).

Notifiable Diseases Surveillance

The bulk of the federal reporting requirements are implemented through the National Notifiable Diseases Surveillance System (NNDSS), established in 1961. The list of nationally notifiable diseases is maintained and revised as needed by the Council of State and Territorial Epidemiologists in col-

TABLE 3-1 Diseases Currently Reportable to the Centers for Disease Control

Acquired immunodeficiency syndrome	Amebiasis
Anthrax	Aseptic meningitis
Botulism, food borne	Botulism, infant
Botulism, wound	Botulism, unspecified
Brucellosis	Chancroid
Cholera	Congenital rubella syndrome
Diphtheria	Encephalitis, post chickenpox
Encephalitis, post mumps	Encephalitis, post other
Encephalitis, primary	Gonorrhea
Granuloma inguinale	Hansen disease
Hepatitis A	Hepatitis B
Hepatitis, non-A, non-B	Hepatitis, unspecified
Legionellosis	Leptospirosis
Lyme disease	Lymphogranuloma venereum
Malaria	Measles
Meningococcal infections	Mumps
Pertussis	Plague
Poliomyelitis, paralytic	Psittacosis
Rabies, animal	Rabies, human
Rheumatic fever	Rocky Mountain spotted fever
Rubella	Salmonellosis
Shigellosis	Syphilis, all stages
Syphilis, primary and secondary	Syphilis, congenital
Tetanus	Toxic shock syndrome
Trichinosis	Tuberculosis
Tularemia	Typhoid fever
Yellow fever	

SOURCE: Wharton et al., 1990.

laboration with the CDC. Reporting of diseases on the list is voluntary, with the exception of the diseases that require quarantine: yellow fever, cholera, diphtheria, infectious tuberculosis, plague, suspected smallpox, and viral hemorrhagic fevers. Regulatory authority for disease surveillance in the United States is provided through state legislation.

Reportable disease data are provided to the CDC on a weekly basis by state health departments, New York City, the District of Columbia, Puerto Rico, the Virgin Islands, Guam, American Samoa, and the Commonwealth of the Northern Mariana Islands. Since 1984, disease reporting has been accomplished through a computer-based telecommunications system, the National Electronic Telecommunications System for Surveillance (NETSS). The CDC analyzes the data and disseminates it in its *Morbidity and Mortality Weekly Report*. As of June 1990, aggregate or case-specific data for a total of 49 infectious diseases were being reported to the CDC by all

U.S. states and territories. Individual states require reporting on more than 100 additional infectious diseases or infectious disease-related conditions (Centers for Disease Control, 1991k).

Data on disease incidence obtained through the NNDSS are important for public health decision making. Data supplied by private physicians and laboratories, the points of contact within the health care system for individuals who become ill, are critical elements in this process. In those instances in which a patient is diagnosed with a reportable disease, this information is supposed to be transmitted to the local or state health department. Unfortunately, this does not always happen. Laboratories may not have sufficient resources for reporting or may decide that reporting is unimportant. (Some states, however, require laboratories to report specific diseases.) Some physicians may be unaware of the requirement to report the occurrence of a specific disease or may not appreciate the importance of such a requirement.

Outbreaks of any disease that is not on CDC's current list of notifiable illnesses may go undetected altogether or may be detected only after an outbreak is well under way. In fact, except for food-borne and waterborne diseases, the United States has no comprehensive national system for detecting outbreaks of infectious disease. Emerging infectious diseases also are not usually detected and reported through established surveillance activities. Instead, private physicians who see small clusters of unusual cases may report them in the medical literature. What is needed is a way to bring these small clusters to the attention of the appropriate agencies in a timely manner.

The committee recommends the development and implementation of strategies that would strengthen state and federal efforts in U.S. surveillance. Strategy development could be a function of the Centers for Disease Control (CDC). Alternatively, the strategy development and coordination functions could be assigned to a federal coordinating body (e.g., a subcommittee of the Federal Coordinating Council for Science, Engineering, and Technology's [FCCSET] Committee on Life Sciences and Health,[2] specifically constituted to address this issue. Implementation of the strategies would be assigned to the appropriate federal agen-

---

[2]The FCCSET is a federally appointed body of experts that serve on seven standing committees and act as a mechanism for coordinating science, engineering, technology, and related activities of the federal government that involve more than one agency. In addition to conducting cross-cutting analyses of programs and budgets, the various committees and their subcommittees (interagency working groups) examine wide-ranging topics with the goal of reaching consensus on fundamental assumptions and procedures that can guide the actions of the participating agencies in achieving their mission objectives more effectively.

cies (e.g., CDC, National Institutes of Health, U.S. Department of Agriculture). **Approaches for consideration could include simplifying current reporting forms and procedures, establishing a telephone hotline by which physicians could report unusual syndromes, and using electronic patient data collected by insurance companies to assist in infectious disease surveillance.**

The committee believes that an excellent example of appropriate coordination of surveillance (and other) activities related to the emergence of a microbial threat to the U.S. population is the recent effort spearheaded by the CDC. Recognizing the seriousness of the emerging multidrug-resistant TB (MDRTB) epidemic, the CDC convened a federal task force in December 1991 at the request of James Mason, the Assistant Secretary for Health. This effort resulted in the *National Action Plan to Combat Multidrug-Resistant Tuberculosis* (National MDR-TB Task Force, 1992). The plan lays out a series of objectives, in the areas of epidemiology and surveillance, laboratory diagnosis, patient management, screening and preventive therapy, infection control, outbreak control, program evaluation, information dissemination/training and education, and research. These objectives are based on specific problems identified by the task force to meet these objectives. The plan specifies a series of activities, responsible organizations, and time frames for implementation. The committee feels that a similar task force could be convened to implement the above recommendation, as well as the one presented later in this chapter on U.S. international efforts in surveillance.

Nosocomial Infections Surveillance

A second major domestic disease surveillance effort is the National Nosocomial Infections Surveillance System (NNISS), which gathers data from approximately 120 sentinel hospitals. The NNISS is operated by the CDC's Hospital Infections Program (HIP); it is the nation's only database devoted to tracking nosocomial infections, which annually affect some 2 million hospitalized patients. The system allows estimates to be made about the incidence of nosocomial infections in the United States, and it provides data that help to detect changes in patterns of incidence, distribution, antibiotic drug resistance, sites of infection, outcomes of infection, and risk factors for nosocomial infections.

Each year, the HIP receives more than 5,000 inquiries about nosocomial infections, including a small number that involve the management of acute outbreaks. In the past 10 years, HIP staff have investigated approximately 120 hospital outbreaks of infectious disease (Centers for Disease Control, 1991b).

Hospitals must apply for membership in the NNISS, and their identity remains confidential. Membership is approved based on adequacy of personnel support for infection control, availability of a computer compatible with the NNISS software, and agreement of the hospital administration. The system has several limitations. For example, it cannot correct for differences among participating hospitals in diagnostic testing, intensity of surveillance, and provisions for post discharge surveillance. The requirement that NNISS member hospitals have at least 100 beds and the fact that a relatively small sample of hospitals is included in the system are potential sources of bias (Gaynes et al., 1991). Even so, the NNISS is the only national database for nosocomial infections, and it is a critical element in the CDC's program to monitor disease incidence.

The system is still evolving. Current plans call for improvements in the dissemination of NNISS data, the inclusion of a surveillance component for immunosuppressed patients, and the addition of more sentinel hospitals, among other efforts (Gaynes et al., 1991). These improvements should lead to better detection of outbreaks and widespread trends in the emergence of resistance among nosocomial pathogens. The limited participation of hospitals in the NNISS, however, remains a problem; as a result, little improvement will occur in nosocomial surveillance in the more than 6,000 hospitals that are not NNISS participants. Since hospital surveillance activities are not income generating, there is little financial motivation for hospitals to become involved. It is likely that accrediting agencies will have to mandate greater full-time-equivalents before the surveillance and control of these pathogens will improve in the majority of hospitals.

The committee recommends that additional resources be allocated to the Centers for Disease Control to enhance the National Nosocomial Infections Surveillance System (NNISS) in the following ways:

1. Include data on antiviral drug resistance.

2. Include information on morbidity and mortality from nosocomial infections.

3. Increase the number of NNISS member hospitals.

4. Strive to make NNISS member hospitals more representative of all U.S. hospitals.

5. Evaluate the sensitivity and specificity of nosocomial infection surveillance activities performed in NNISS member hospitals.

6. Determine the reliability of antimicrobial susceptibility testing performed in NNISS member hospitals.

Outbreak Surveillance

Since 1988, the CDC has participated with a number of states in a pilot project to develop a system for computerized surveillance of outbreaks of diseases that are not currently notifiable. For food-borne or waterborne outbreaks, reporting is required when two or more cases occur; for other outbreaks, the threshold for reporting is three cases. During a five-month period in 1990, nine participating states reported 233 outbreaks involving 6,241 individual cases of disease (Centers for Disease Control, 1991k). This initiative should also provide data to help identify factors that increase the risks of outbreaks and make it easier to assess the effectiveness of outbreak prevention and control measures.

Influenza Surveillance

To monitor influenza incidence and the prevalence of particular virus strains in this country, the CDC, in addition to participating in the WHO's global influenza surveillance network (see the later discussion), operates a domestic influenza surveillance program. Data for the program come from state and territorial health departments, U.S.-based WHO collaborating laboratories (see Figure 3-2), 121 key U.S. cities, and "sentinel" U.S. physicians. The epidemiological information these sources gather is analyzed and released to public health officials, physicians, the media, and the public.

Access to Surveillance Information

Considerable effort and resources are being expended on the various surveillance activities in which U.S. government agencies and the private sector participate. Much of this information, however, is not readily accessible. There is currently no single database from which a physician, researcher, health care worker, public health official, or other interested party can obtain information on disease incidence, antibiotic drug resistance, drug and vaccine availability, or other topics that might be relevant to infectious disease surveillance, prevention, treatment, and control. The need for such a database is strong; given the current communications capabilities of personal computers and the relative ease with which information on a multitude of topics can be accessed, a database is not only technologically feasible but could be a valuable addition to U.S. surveillance efforts.

The committee recommends that the U.S. Public Health Service develop a comprehensive, computerized infectious disease database. Such a da-

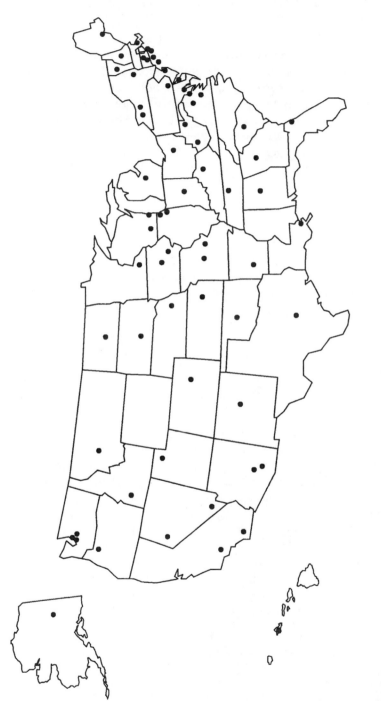

FIGURE 3-2 Location of World Health Organization influenza collaborating laboratories in the United States.
SOURCE: B. Mahy, Division of Viral and Rickettsial Diseases, National Center for Infectious Diseases, Centers for Disease Control.

tabase might consolidate information from more specialized sources, such as the National Nosocomial Infections Surveillance System (NNISS), the National Electronic Telecommunications System for Surveillance (NETSS), and the influenza surveillance system; it could also include additional information, such as vaccine and drug availability. As an alternative, expansion of currently available databases and provisions for easy access to these sources should be aggressively pursued. Also included in the implementation of such a program should be expanded efforts to inform physicians, public health workers, clinical laboratories, and other relevant target groups of the availability of this information.

INTERNATIONAL EFFORTS

U.S.-supported overseas infectious disease laboratories have played a historic role in the discovery and monitoring of infectious diseases. The United States and other nations first created these disease surveillance posts, many of them in tropical and subtropical countries, in an effort to protect the health of their citizens who were sent to settle or administer recently acquired territory. During and after World War II, there was a second blossoming of U.S. government-supported international disease research and surveillance activities. Several overseas laboratories staffed by Department of Defense (DoD) personnel were established. The Middle America and Pacific Research Units of the National Institutes of Health (NIH) were founded, and later terminated. The Gorgas Memorial Laboratory, in Panama, was until 1991, supported by the United States. Privately funded activities, like those of the Rockefeller Foundation Virus Program, were important contributors to surveillance efforts. Other private foundations and universities also played a role in surveillance overseas.

Over the past two decades, the number of such facilities has declined, largely as a result of shifts in program priorities. This trend is of concern to the committee, particularly in view of the many important achievements of the laboratories that have been closed. The loss of these facilities has left a major gap in U.S. overseas infectious disease surveillance, research, and training capabilities. Brief histories of some U.S.-supported overseas laboratories, several of which no longer operate, appear below. (See also the section on research and training later in this chapter.) Table 3-2 is a list of current U.S. government-supported overseas infectious disease laboratories.

Past Successes

The Gorgas Memorial Laboratory The Gorgas Memorial Laboratory (GML) in Panama, founded by the Gorgas Memorial Institute in 1928, was

TABLE 3-2 Sponsors and Locations of Current U.S. Government-Supported Overseas Infectious Disease Laboratories

Department of Defense
  Brazil
  Egypt
  Indonesia
  Kenya
  Peru
  South Korea
  Thailand
U.S. Public Health Service
  National Institute of Allergy and Infectious Diseases (NIAID), National Institutes of Health
    International Centers for Tropical Disease Research
      International Collaboration in Infectious Diseases Research (ICIDR)
            Brazil—with Cornell University
            Brazil—with Harvard University
            Brazil—with University of Virginia
            Brazil—with Vanderbilt University
            Israel—with Columbia University
            Sudan—with Brigham Young University
            Venezuela—with Albert Einstein College of Medicine
      Tropical Medicine Research Centers (TMRC)
            Colombia—at Centro Internacional de Entranamiento e Investigaciones
              Medicas
            Brazil—at Federal University of Bahia
            Philippines—at Research Institute for Tropical Medicine
    International Collaborations in AIDS Research (ICAR)
          Brazil—with Cornell University
          Malawi—with Johns Hopkins University
          Mexico—with Harvard University
          Senegal—with Harvard University
          Uganda—with Case Western Reserve University
          Zaire—with Tufts University
  Centers for Disease Control
    Côte d'Ivoire
    Guatemala
    Kenya
    Sierra Leone
    Thailand
    Zaire
U.S. Agency for International Development
  International Center for Diarrheal Disease Research—Bangladesh
  Ain Shams University—Egypt (administered by NIAID)
  Hebrew University—Israel (administered by NIAID)

throughout its existence funded directly by the U.S. Congress, although the Panamanian government donated the facilities in which the laboratory was housed. Named for General William C. Gorgas, a U.S. Army physician and engineer credited with controlling malaria and yellow fever during construction of the Panama Canal, the facility initially concentrated its research efforts on malaria, leishmaniasis, and yellow fever. Later, in fruitful collaboration with the Middle America Research Unit, an NIH field station (see below), the GML conducted studies of many arboviral infections indigenous to the American tropics. More recently, Gorgas scientists became known for their work on sexually transmitted diseases, human papillomavirus and cervical cancer, and hepatitis A.

In 1989, Congress decided that the money that historically had been given to the GML on a noncompetitive basis should be awarded through an open, national competition (*U.S. Medicine*, 1991). The laboratory was unable to enter the competition for funding, mainly because of its difficulty in retaining professional staff as a result of the political situation in Panama. The GML managed to survive through fiscal year 1990, while attempts were made to obtain funding through a cooperative U.S. Agency for International Development-Pan American Health Organization (USAID-PAHO) effort, or through the CDC. When these attempts failed, the Gorgas Memorial Institute relinquished the laboratory and its equipment to the Panamanian government and dismissed the staff. The Panamanian government has maintained the laboratory with a small cadre of scientists who survey dengue and leishmaniasis, and it is attempting to obtain funding from other sources to expand the laboratory's activities.

U.S. Army Medical Research Unit—Malaysia   Investigations into the efficacy of chloramphenicol for the treatment and prophylaxis of scrub typhus were initiated by American military scientists in Malaya in 1948. From the time it was formally established five years later, the U.S. Army Medical Research Unit in Kuala Lumpur not only investigated diseases of importance to the U.S. military but also frequently assisted the Malaysian government in the investigation of disease outbreaks of known and unknown etiology. Over more than four decades of scientific studies, the laboratory was involved in research on scrub typhus, typhoid fever, leptospirosis, malaria, and other tropical diseases (Oaks et al., 1983). Much of what is known about the vector of scrub typhus (the *Leptotrombidium* mite) was the result of collaborative efforts between the U.S. Army Unit and the Institute for Medical Research, Kuala Lumpur, in which the unit was housed (Ramanathan et al., 1976). Despite these achievements, this DoD laboratory, which had a strong research record (particularly in the area of vector-borne diseases), was closed in 1989 because of lack of funding.

Rockefeller Foundation Virus Program   The Rockefeller Foundation Virus Program was established in 1951 to investigate arthropod-borne viruses of vertebrates (Theiler and Downs, 1973). A number of foreign governments, including India, Brazil, Trinidad, South Africa, Colombia, and Nigeria, joined the effort. The program established a virus laboratory in each country in collaboration with a local university or government health agency. The costs of the research were split about equally between the foundation and the host country.

The program, through its surveillance of febrile and hemorrhagic diseases, was responsible for finding and characterizing scores of new infectious agents. In Belem, Brazil, for instance, more than 50 new tropical viruses were discovered, including eight in Groups C and Guama that were responsible for debilitating, nonfatal jungle fevers common in those living in the Amazon region. Kyasanur Forest disease was discovered at the Rockefeller laboratory in Puna, India. Crimean hemorrhagic fever in the former Union of Soviet Socialist Republics and Congo disease in East Africa were linked through studies by the Rockefeller arbovirus reference unit at Yale University (YARU). Several viruses related to rabies were discovered in Africa. Program scientists also searched for viruses in healthy wild animals and arthropods, an innovative approach to disease surveillance that identified a number of agents, such as the Oropouche virus in Trinidad and Brazil (Theiler and Downs, 1973). Oropouche virus in later years caused several major tropical epidemics (Pinheiro et al., 1981).

One of the deadliest of the agents identified by the program was Lassa virus, which was isolated in 1969 at YARU from the blood of a sick mission nurse who had been air-evacuated from Africa (Buckley and Casals, 1970). The discovery of this virus was the direct result of a surveillance program to find new agents that were infecting African missionaries.

The Rockefeller Foundation withdrew funding for the virus program in 1971, based on a policy decision of its board of trustees. During its two decades of operation, the program was an outstanding catalyst for international surveillance and research. YARU continues with support from the NIH, DoD, and WHO. Host country governments and international agencies assumed financial support for each of the field laboratories when Rockefeller withdrew its support. In most countries, these laboratories are now central national resources for disease surveillance and infectious disease research (R. Shope, Director, YARU, personal communication, 1992).

National Institutes of Health   In 1958, the NIH established the Middle America Research Unit (MARU) to study tropical infectious diseases, especially those of viral origin, in the U.S. Canal Zone. (A component of this effort was the U.S Army Medical Research Unit—Panama, which was charged with research on histoplasmosis and other fungal diseases of military importance.) Some of the MARU field studies were collaborations with the Gorgas Memorial Laboratory. MARU researchers conducted definitive studies on Bolivian hemorrhagic fever, Venezuelan equine encephalitis in Central America, and several viral infections that are transmitted by tropical sandflies. In the mid-1970s, as a harbinger of decreasing U.S. government commitment to international health research, MARU left the NIH to become part of the Gorgas Laboratory.

In 1960, the National Institute of Allergy and Infectious Diseases (NIAID) established the International Centers for Medical Research and Training (ICMRT) program to further support tropical disease research of benefit to U.S. citizens. In collaboration with foreign universities and government agencies, the program provided long-term overseas research training for U.S. scientists. ICMRT grants resulted in broadly productive research programs that studied a wide variety of infectious and noninfectious diseases. In 1979, as part of an overall plan to scale back its involvement in research training activities, the NIAID discontinued the ICMRT program.

Loss of Capacity

The establishment of a new laboratory (particularly on foreign soil), its staffing, and the development of a reputation for carefully conducted, rigorous scientific work are tasks that cannot be accomplished overnight. It is unfortunate that the U.S.-supported overseas laboratories discussed above were, for varying reasons, either discontinued or forced to scale back their efforts. Their achievements had a profound impact on the level of scientific knowledge of many previously known and newly recognized infectious diseases and their causative agents. A further loss is the many opportunities they provided for U.S. scientists to develop overseas field experience and to collaborate with foreign scientists and institutions, thereby acquiring infectious disease surveillance information of importance to U.S. monitoring activities.

Current Efforts

The purposes and entities discussed briefly below constitute current U.S. efforts in international infectious disease surveillance, most of which is conducted through passive monitoring.

• The NIAID's International Centers for Tropical Disease Research (ICTDR) program. Established as a means to provide more cohesion to existing and newly initiated programs in tropical infectious disease research, the ICTDR program laboratories, because of their geographic distribution (see Table 3-2 above), are well situated to conduct surveillance for new and emerging diseases. (This program and its subordinate elements are discussed in more detail in the research and training section later in this chapter.)

• The CDC's participation in the WHO global influenza surveillance network. Information obtained through the network allows the CDC to predict the potential impact of influenza on the United States in any given year. This information is crucial for influenza vaccine manufacturers, who need a minimum of six months' lead time to prepare and distribute adequate quantities of new vaccine.

As part of its international efforts, the CDC produces and sends (free of charge) WHO influenza virus detection and identification kits to 117 foreign national WHO collaborating laboratories and to 68 U.S. collaborating laboratories. These laboratories collect and identify influenza virus isolates and forward information about their findings, as well as actual virus samples, to the CDC on a weekly basis. The CDC also receives influenza virus isolates and information from about 50 foreign laboratories, provides the WHO with information collected from U.S. collaborating laboratories, and receives weekly reports from the WHO on the level of influenza activity in the other reporting countries.

Laboratories and research groups in several key areas of the world, such as the People's Republic of China, Hong Kong, Singapore, and the Pacific Basin, the areas in which most new strains originate, are also in regular contact with the CDC. Recently, the global influenza surveillance system improved its coverage of the Far East. In cooperation with the Chinese National Influenza Center in Beijing, the CDC has supported a national surveillance network in the People's Republic of China. This network has greatly increased the number and timeliness of influenza isolates that are available for analysis at the CDC from that country.

• The CDC's foreign field stations. Similar to the previously mentioned NIAID ICTDR program, the CDC overseas affiliates (see Table 3-2 above) provide passive surveillance information and expertise that is available to the host country for assistance in investigating outbreaks.

• Rockefeller Foundation's International Clinical Epidemiology Network. The network trains physicians from other nations in medical epidemiology, including infectious disease epidemiology. Through these efforts, a continuing interaction with U.S. universities is fostered, and collaborative activities aimed at infectious disease surveillance and response to emerging diseases are possible. (This program is discussed in greater detail in the research and training section later in this chapter.)

• USAID-supported International Center for Diarrheal Disease Research, Bangladesh (ICDDR,B). Of almost equal importance to its contributions in cholera epidemiology and treatment have been the pioneering efforts of this laboratory in the surveillance of diarrheal diseases throughout the Asian region. (This program is discussed in greater detail in the research and training section later in this chapter.)

• USAID's Program in Worldwide Control of Sexually Transmitted Diseases (STD)/HIV. This is a single-source contract to Family Health International, a non-profit organization committed to family planning; contraceptive safety, acceptability, effectiveness, and ease of use; maternal and child health; interventions to reduce the transmission of STDs; and other related issues.

Although the CDC appears to have a mandate for U.S. disease surveillance, other government agencies (e.g., the NIAID, U.S. Department of Agriculture [USDA], DoD, and USAID), private foundations, and universities may also independently play major or minor roles. Currently, there is little coordination among these agencies and organizations regarding infectious disease surveillance. The committee concludes that the effectiveness of their surveillance activities, particularly those pertaining to recognition of and response to emerging microbial threats, could be greatly improved by designating a central focus for such efforts.

The committee recommends that international infectious disease surveillance activities of U.S. government agencies be coordinated by the Centers for Disease Control (CDC). To provide the necessary link between U.S. domestic and international surveillance efforts, the body that is established for this purpose should be the same as that suggested earlier in the recommendation on domestic surveillance. Alternatively, a federal coordinating body (e.g., a subcommittee of the Federal Coordinating Council for Science, Engineering, and Technology's [FCCSET] Committee on Life Sciences and Health, specifically constituted to address this issue) could be assigned the coordinating function. Implementation of surveillance activities, however, should remain with the appropriate federal agencies (e.g., the CDC, Department of Defense, National Institutes of Health, U.S. Department of Agriculture).

Multilateral International Surveillance Efforts

The coordination efforts of multilateral international organizations, such as the WHO, are critical to infectious disease surveillance. Without these organizations, programs such as the successful worldwide eradication of smallpox and the interruption of polio transmission in the Americas would be little more than dreams. Any implementation of a global surveillance system for emerging infectious diseases must draw upon the capabilities of such organizations. Some of the ongoing and past programs of two of these bodies are discussed below.

WORLD HEALTH ORGANIZATION

The WHO is a focal point for surveillance data on global infectious diseases. Under the International Health Regulations, all countries (except Australia, Papua New Guinea, North Korea, and South Africa) must report to the WHO within 24 hours all cases of cholera, plague, and yellow fever (or any isolation of yellow fever virus from monkeys or mosquitoes). This information is published in the WHO's *Weekly Epidemiological Record.* Despite the requirement to do so, however, some countries are reluctant to release surveillance data. As a result, some outbreaks of these diseases are never discovered or are discovered only retrospectively after they have subsided.

The WHO also operates a number of networks, composed of selected laboratories worldwide (collaborating centers), that report and investigate outbreaks of specific diseases, such as influenza and HIV disease. The influenza surveillance network is designed to monitor newly emerging strains and subtypes of influenza virus. As noted earlier, the information it collects is used to determine the antigenic makeup of each year's influenza vaccines.

Among other activities, the HIV disease network is encouraging participating countries to do seroprevalence studies at sentinel sites (rather than just reporting numbers of cases) and to develop trend data on infection; it is also collecting geographically representative strains of HIV. More informally, the WHO gathers data about disease outbreaks through its contacts with tourist agencies and international companies, whose clients and employees often inadvertently act as sentinels for new or emerging diseases when they become infected while traveling in other countries.

As is true for many similar efforts, WHO disease surveillance activities are hindered by incomplete reporting and a frequent failure to obtain laboratory confirmation of reported cases of disease. Most cases of yellow fever, for example, are diagnosed on the basis of clinical symptoms alone and often occur in areas in which hepatitis or other tropical diseases with similar symptoms are prevalent. Although the WHO makes every attempt to obtain clinical specimens to allow a definitive diagnosis of reported cases, this is not always possible.

The WHO often is involved in early investigative efforts of newly emerging or reemerging infectious diseases, such as Ebola and Lassa fevers, yellow fever, and dengue fever. For example, when Ebola fever outbreaks occurred in Zaire and Sudan, the WHO provided rapid-response teams, composed of consultants from a number of countries, to help the governments of these nations determine the origin of the outbreaks and develop control strategies.

At one time, the WHO supported a series of serum banks, established in 1960 by John Paul, a physician-epidemiologist at Yale University who is considered the father of clinical and serological epidemiology; the banks contained thousands of well-documented serum samples from many areas of the world. The collections were located in the Department of Epidemiology and Public Health at Yale University; the Institute of Epidemiology and Microbiology, Prague, Czechoslovakia; the National Institute of Health, Tokyo, Japan; and the South African Institute for Medical Research, Johannesburg. The sera in these collections were useful for retrospective studies of specific disease agents. For example, using serum collected in Barbados, investigators were able to estimate vaccine coverage for childhood diseases and, recently, to document HTLV-I antibody. The WHO withdrew its support for these efforts in 1989, however, and in 1990, most of the sera from the Yale collection were transferred to the National Cancer Institute. The overseas serum banks apparently are receiving minimal support from their governments. Without the funding and coordination provided by an international organization like the WHO, it is doubtful whether the serum banks will continue to be maintained. Expansion of these collections at this time is uncertain at best (A. Evans, Professor of Epidemiology and Past Director, WHO Serum Reference Bank, Department of Epidemiology and Public Health, Yale University, personal communication, 1992).

Pan American Health Organization

In 1985, PAHO proposed a program to interrupt the transmission of poliomyelitis in the Americas by 1990. In 1986, the year prior to the actual start of the campaign, there were more than 900 confirmed cases of polio in the region. By the end of 1991, as a result of extensive immunization campaigns with oral polio vaccine, transmission appeared to be confined to only one country in the entire Western Hemisphere, Peru (De Quadros et al., 1991). In 1991, only eight isolates of wild poliovirus were detected in the Americas: six in Colombia (the last one in April 1991) and two in Peru (the last one in September 1991).

As with the smallpox eradication effort nearly 20 years earlier, surveillance has played a critical role in the PAHO polio eradication strategy. From the outset of the PAHO effort in September 1985, surveillance was a major component of the program. A number of important indicators were monitored by health facilities, including the proportion of sites reporting each week, the interval between diagnosis and the start of control measures, and the follow-up of cases (De Quadros et al., 1991). Reporting of cases of acute flaccid paralysis (including negative reports) was required in all countries, and by the end of 1991, there were nearly 20,000 health units involved in the reporting system, with approximately 80 percent of them reporting every week.

A cadre of epidemiologists was trained to do case investigation and follow-up to collect stool specimens and institute control measures. Eight diagnostic laboratories were identified and their personnel trained to conduct DNA-probe and polymerase chain reaction (PCR) assays for poliovirus identification and characterization. Between 1989 and 1991, a yearly average of 4,000 stool specimens were tested in this laboratory network. Twenty-four, 18, and 8 wild poliovirus isolates were identified in 1989, 1990, and 1991, respectively. This surveillance and laboratory network is being expanded to include one or two other vaccine-preventable diseases. The network has already proved to be of great assistance in the detection and follow-up of the cholera epidemic that recently struck the Western Hemisphere.

The Concept of Global Surveillance

Current U.S. and worldwide surveillance efforts are useful for detecting known infectious and noninfectious diseases. They fall short, however, in their ability to detect the emergence of infectious diseases. Although there are isolated examples of how such a system could work, there has been no effort to develop and implement a global program of surveillance for emerging diseases or disease agents (including agents with newly acquired drug resistance). Current surveillance efforts (even when adequate in specific areas for specific diseases) are not effectively linked; consequently, knowledge of small clusters of emerging diseases, even if detected, is not widely disseminated. Added to these factors is declining interest in studying, treating, and preventing infectious diseases as increasing attention has focused on chronic degenerative diseases.

To be effective, any global infectious disease surveillance network must be interactive and reciprocal. It is especially important that U.S.-funded laboratories engaged in infectious disease surveillance in foreign countries operate in partnership with host-country facilities. Developing countries, for their part, contribute surveillance data, but they must also be provided with a base of training and expertise, as well as with upgraded local surveillance, data acquisition, and analysis capabilities. The partnerships of U.S. and local facilities can work toward eliminating deficiencies in these areas. Global surveillance thus involves providing not only case numbers but the knowledge, skills, and tools necessary to improve disease surveillance and response within and among countries and regions. Such an effort, of necessity, will be multinational and will require regional and global coordination, advice, and resources from participating nations. These activities would not only benefit each participating country but, in the opinion of the committee, constitute the most economical means by far for developing and supporting a global surveillance network.

One of the biggest potential barriers to the implementation of a global surveillance network is the transfer of information from and to remote sites in many developing countries that have inadequate telecommunications capabilities. A new satellite technology is currently being tested that may help resolve this dilemma. The system uses a low-level communications satellite that has two-way communications with remote ground stations (each costing approximately $5,000). The requisite satellite, which is now in orbit, passes over every point on the globe at least twice each day. On each pass, it accepts information passed to it from files stored in a remote station's computer. The satellite stores the received information and then transfers it to the appropriate station on its next pass.

The system offers researchers and physicians in the developing world a simpler and less costly alternative for communicating with their peers and accessing information (e.g., scientific and medical journals). Tests of the system are ongoing in several East African sites, and licenses for additional testing sites are pending. Eventually, additional satellites will be placed in orbit to augment the system and provide more opportunities for data transfer each day (Pool, 1991; Clements, 1992). This technology may allow the earlier inclusion of many remote areas in a global infectious disease surveillance network.

A surveillance network must do more than detect cases of disease. It must also collect data on those cases, analyze them in some useful fashion, and disseminate the findings of the analyses to people who can use the information. Surveillance alone, however, is insufficient to address emerging infectious diseases adequately. A response mechanism is necessary as well. Thus, the committee believes that a global surveillance network for detecting emerging microbial threats should have four basic components:

1. a mechanism, based on clinical presentation, for detecting clusters of new or unusual diseases or syndromes (see Box 3-1);
2. laboratories capable of identifying and characterizing infectious agents;
3. an information system to record and analyze reportable occurrences and to disseminate summary data; and
4. a response mechanism to provide feedback to reporting agencies and individuals and, if necessary, to mobilize investigative and control efforts of local and international agencies.

Specific elements of a global infectious disease surveillance system are as follows:

• sustainability through continuity of funding;
• locally staffed surveillance centers to promote regional self-reliance and train local personnel;
• a research component with links to academic centers and other regional facilities involved in basic research;

**BOX 3-1   Clinical Circumstances That Require
High-Priority Surveillance Efforts**

- Acute respiratory disease
- Encephalitis and aseptic meningitis
- Hemorrhagic fever
- Acute diarrhea
- Febrile exanthems
- Other diseases with unusual clinical syndromes
- Unusual clusterings of disease or death
- Resistance to common treatment drugs

   • a network of laboratories/diagnostic facilities with people trained to examine specimens, identify isolates, search for clinical syndromes, prepare and distribute reagents, and develop physical and molecular markers for identification (these facilities should have discretionary capability to respond appropriately to emerging diseases by, for example, identifying causative agents and notifying appropriate national health authorities);
   • full clinical documentation of unsolved cases, with a system for archiving sera and pathological specimens;
   • a clinical arm for hospital-based surveillance and drug and vaccine trials;
   • a targeted disease approach with broad reporting criteria for maximum retrieval of data (e.g., "disease targeted: polio; reporting criterion: acute flaccid paralysis");
   • an effective specimen collection and transport system; and
   • an active system of data analysis and dissemination, with feedback to those providing data.

   The WHO's global influenza surveillance network and its collaborating centers for specific diseases, PAHO's polio eradication program, and previous efforts such as the WHO's smallpox eradication program and the Rockefeller Foundation's virus program, although all limited in scope, are nevertheless useful models to consider in the design of a global infectious disease surveillance system. The strengths and weaknesses of each component of these past and current programs should be carefully evaluated.
   In the case of current programs, when withdrawal of support threatens to close down a surveillance network, consideration should be given to preserving those components that prove to be of value. The infrastructure of a successful program can in some cases be continued and put to use in the cause of monitoring other diseases. The smallpox eradication surveillance

network is a good example. With appropriate planning and support, that network might have been shifted to surveillance for other diseases and now be useful as a basis for a global infectious disease surveillance system.

The committee recommends that the United States take the lead in promoting the development and implementation of a comprehensive global infectious disease surveillance system. Such an effort could be undertaken through the U.S. representatives to the World Health Assembly. The system should capitalize on the lessons from past successes and on the infrastructure, momentum, and accomplishments of existing international networks, expanding and diversifying surveillance efforts to include known diseases as well as newly recognized ones. This effort, of necessity, will be multinational and will require regional and global coordination, advice, and resources from participating nations.

INTERVENTION

The response to an emerging infectious agent or disease necessitates coordinated efforts by various individuals, organizations, and industries. The committee believes that the current U.S. capability for responding to microbial threats to health lacks organization and resources. This section addresses these deficiencies. It begins by discussing elements of response that actually precede intervention (the U.S. public health system and the research and training infrastructure), and it concludes with a discussion of and recommendations for specific interventions (in vaccine and drug development, vector control, and public education and behavioral change).

The U.S. Public Health System

Disease assessment, which includes the early recognition of emerging microbial threats, is the foundation on which knowledgeable public health policy decisions are based. In the United States, principal responsibility for protecting the public's health rests with the 50 state health departments, or their counterparts, and more than 3,000 local health departments. At the federal level, the national focus for disease assessment is the CDC.

A 1988 Institute of Medicine (IOM) report, *The Future of Public Health*, described the U.S. public health system as being in a state of disarray, which resulted in "a hodgepodge of fractionated interests and programs, organizational turmoil among new agencies, and well-intended but unbalanced appropriations—without coherent direction by well-qualified professionals." The report also cited several other problems.

• Many state and local facilities lack the capability for assessing health status.

• Policy at all levels often develops as a result of immediate and pressing needs rather than from analysis of carefully collected data.

• Unequal access to public health services means that certain populations, such as the poor, receive inadequate medical care.

• Public health leadership, particularly at the state and local levels, suffers from inadequate technical knowledge and rapid turnover, among other things.

It is the perception of this committee that there has been little positive change in the state of U.S. public health since the release of the 1988 IOM report. As partial evidence for this statement, the recent rapid increase in measles incidence (which is now beginning to subside) and the current upswing in cases of tuberculosis (TB) (including multidrug-resistant disease) can be offered. These emerging disease problems are largely the result of complacency—a misguided perception that the advanced U.S. health care system with its array of medical technologies is able to disarm almost any infectious disease.

In the case of measles, successful vaccination programs had diminished disease incidence to such a degree that the public, health care professionals, and public health organizations reduced their levels of vigilance and effort. The result was a resurgence in the disease that only last year reached a peak. Partly as a response, Congress appropriated an additional $40 million in 1992 (a 19 percent increase over 1991) to support the CDC immunization program. The money was targeted at children under the age of two living in communities in need, such as inner cities (National Foundation for Infectious Diseases, 1991).

As discussed earlier, the declines in incidence of TB since the early 1950s led to a belief held by many public health officials, beginning in the early 1980s, that the disease no longer posed a significant health problem. Research efforts waned, and in 1986, the CDC's surveillance program for tracking TB drug resistance trends was terminated. Increases in homelessness, poverty, substance abuse, HIV infection, and active TB among immigrants have now contributed to a resurgence in TB cases (Fox, 1992), which has been further complicated by outbreaks of multidrug-resistant TB (MDRTB) and poor availability or unavailability of some antituberculosis drugs. As recently as 1989, the Department of Health and Human Services developed a national plan to eliminate TB as a health problem in the United States, and at that time, the prospects appeared excellent for success. The plan was not implemented, however, because of both insufficient resources and a lack of conviction regarding the plan's effectiveness.

An aggressive response to the current TB/MDRTB crisis is now being pursued. A national coalition of more than 40 patient and provider organizations has been formed to address TB elimination issues (U.S. Department of Health and Human Services, 1992). Senior NIH and CDC officials are devoting more attention to the disease, in the form of research and public education. In April 1992, the Food and Drug Administration (FDA) arranged for a limited supply of streptomycin and para-aminosalicylic acid manufactured outside the United States to be available through the CDC under an investigational new drug agreement (Centers for Disease Control, 1992a). The FDA has also recently identified U.S. pharmaceutical companies that have agreed to manufacture these drugs and make them commercially available by late 1992 (Centers for Disease Control, 1992a). In addition, the FDA has promised to expedite the review process for TB-related products (Fox, 1992). Most recently, the CDC published a *National Action Plan to Combat Multidrug-Resistant Tuberculosis*. The plan lays out a series of specific activities (with organizational responsibility and time frames for action) that address nine objectives identified by the federal task force (National MDR-TB Task Force, 1992).

These responses, like those related to the resurgence of measles, are potentially of value in resolving the current problems with TB and MDRTB but they are reactive, not proactive. It is the committee's view that prevention of infectious diseases must be continually stressed if the U.S. public health system is to be maintained or, preferably, improved. Efforts directed at the recognition of and responses to emerging public health problems, particularly emerging infectious diseases, would help to achieve this goal. The country's recent episodes of measles and TB resurgence should reinforce the importance of upgrading and maintaining the U.S. public health system at all levels. Experience has taught that, in the long run, preventive action is generally more cost-effective than reactive response. For example, the current cholera epidemic, as of mid-1991, had cost Peru's economy an estimated $43 million in medical costs alone. Had that amount been spent over the past few years to provide clean water and adequate sanitation to the people of Peru, it is likely that the epidemic would not have progressed to its current state (Misch, 1991). Other examples of cost effectiveness include measles vaccination and the global eradication of smallpox. The benefit-cost ratio for measles prevention ranges from 11.9:1 to 14.4:1, depending on whether the vaccine administered is measles antigen alone or a combined vaccine (measles, mumps, and rubella) (Hinman et al., 1985). It has been estimated that, in 1967, global expenditures on smallpox annually were $1.35 billion. The 13-year (1967-1979) global smallpox eradication campaign totaled $299 million ($23 million per year), almost a 60-fold annual savings (Fenner et al., 1988).

Microbial disease assessment is a shared function. State and local health departments; the CDC; health care providers; private laboratories; schools of medicine, public health, and veterinary medicine; the FDA; the U.S. Department of Agriculture (USDA); and the NIH all contribute. The existing system for assessing microbial threats in the United States is based on a myriad of laws, practices, organizational structures, and shared responsibilities. Assessment capabilities, resources, and levels of commitment vary widely among the participants.

The nation's capacity for assessing microbial threats could be improved by strengthening the public health infrastructure to carry out assigned functions of disease assessment, policy development, and assurance of health with respect to microbial threats. Improving cooperation through the formation of consortia of schools of medicine, public health, and veterinary medicine, and departments of public health might also be an effective strategy, as would the availability of emergency funds to investigate, conduct research and surveillance on, and control major new or reemerging infectious diseases.

The quality of infectious disease surveillance varies according to the quality of disease reporting required by states from health care providers. Alert and capable clinical and, especially, laboratory staff are also crucial. In addition to surveillance, effective assessment of microbial threats requires epidemiological and laboratory research, and investigative capabilities at all levels of the health infrastructure. Without each of these, a public health system has little chance of succeeding.

The current U.S. economic climate has done little to help public health initiatives, which for years have lacked sufficient resources. Declining budgets have forced many local and state organizations to cut back on public health programs. Without strong local and state programs, the ability of federal agencies to promote the public health is greatly diminished. Diminishing resources have particularly threatened the state laboratories, which early in this century were major contributors to public health microbiology. The holes in the fabric of diagnostic, investigative, and research capabilities created by the dwindling activities of state laboratories are seldom repaired.

There is some indication that the United States' weakened public health infrastructure has become a concern to policymakers. Recently, the U.S. Public Health Service (PHS) published a plan designed to strengthen the U.S. public health infrastructure (Assistant Secretary for Health's Public Health Service Task Force to Strengthen Public Health in the United States, 1991). This document apparently comes as a response to *The Future of Public Health* (Institute of Medicine, 1988) and the national prevention objectives set out in *Healthy People 2000* (U.S. Department of Health and Human Services, 1990) and *Healthy Communities 2000* (American Public Health Association et al., 1991). The proposed PHS plan lays out strategies to improve surveillance, epidemiology, and communication, the three key areas identified in the 1988 IOM report. In reviewing these strategies, the committee found that a number of them were particularly applicable to emerging disease issues (see Box 3-2); moreover, if implemented, these

BOX 3-2 Extracts from Plan to Strengthen U.S. Public Health

Assessment strategy 1: Developing health information and health information systems that are useful to legislative and executive governmental bodies at the Federal, State, and local levels, and to other groups and organizations.
• CDC: Establish 10 regional centers for prevention and control of nosocomial infection linking about a thousand hospitals in a national surveillance network.
• CDC: Establish a county sentinel surveillance system for foodborne diseases.
• CDC: Establish mechanisms to collect the data through surveys and public health surveillance systems, and analyze and link data from existing data sets.

Assessment strategy 3: Building the capacity of States and local health departments and other relevant organizations to use health information systems to prevent disease, promote health, and increase access to services in their community.
• NIH: Support training grants and contracts that assist in developing health personnel, including training for epidemiologists, biostatisticians, and behavioral scientists.
• CDC: Develop State and local expertise, through training and personnel development, and provide assistance for the conduct of epidemiological investigations and studies designed to assess the health status of subject populations.

Policy development strategy 2: Developing strategies and programs to realize the goals.
• NIH: Support research to develop or improve vaccines against organisms causing such diseases as diarrhea (rotavirus), pertussis, influenza, and HIV infection and against cancer causing viruses.

Assurance strategy 1: Developing and maintaining the capacity of public health agencies at the State and local levels, and other organizations, to plan, implement, and assure the quality of the services that they provide or need to provide.
• FDA: Take a proactive approach to ease the entry of biotechnology-based products into the marketplace by facilitating and maintaining contact with manufacturers from the initial development stage of the approval process.
• CDC: Develop training programs for incorporating state-of-the-art information and techniques into prevention and control programs for infectious diseases.

continued on next page

Continued from previous page

Assurance strategy 3: Helping to ensure an adequate supply of appropriately trained health personnel.
   • NIH: Develop an active intramural training and education program for
scientists and assist in placing trainees in academic institutions and health
departments throughout the nation.
   • NIH: Support the PHS Epidemiology Fellowship Program to increase
the number of biomedical epidemiologists and attract them to PHS.
   • CDC: Establish a training program to assure the development of a
system to provide State and local health department personnel with state-
of-the-art skills in diagnostic evaluation and testing for infectious diseases.

Source: U.S. Department of Health and Human Services, 1991.

strategies will, in part, respond to recommendations made in this report.
Consequently, the committee supports the implementation of these strate-
gies (Assistant Secretary for Health's Public Health Service Task Force to
Strengthen Public Health in the United States, 1991).

Research and Training

Many of the factors that are responsible for, or that contribute to, emergence of infectious diseases are now known. However, our understanding of
these factors and of how they interact is incomplete. We are a considerable
way from being able to develop strategies to anticipate the emergence of
infectious diseases and prevent them from becoming significant threats to
health. Nevertheless, the committee sees the development of such strategies
as a desirable long-term goal and concludes that research to achieve it
should be strongly encouraged. Research of this kind will often be interdis-
ciplinary in nature and might include, for example, the development of
strategies to determine the potential for certain microorganisms to emerge
or of methods to assess the potential environmental and microbiological
consequences of development projects. Basic research in support of this
goal should also be encouraged.

Because emerging microbes are not limited by geographic boundaries,
research focusing on emerging infectious diseases must involve scientists
worldwide. Although this report focuses on U.S. public health, the importance of international research links and collaborations must not be forgot-
ten. Furthermore, the success of global surveillance for these microbes depends in part on an infrastructure that includes viable research programs in
nations on all continents. The United States could take a leading role, through
the WHO, to develop a program of international infectious disease research

and to enlist the participation of other nations and of foundations. This program could be targeted to research on specific emerging microbes, in addition to those already addressed by two extrabudgetary programs of the WHO: Special Programme for Research and Training in Tropical Diseases (TDR) and the Vaccine Development Programme (VDP). The TDR encompasses research on selected parasitic diseases and leprosy. The VDP supports research on vaccine development using molecular approaches. The international aspect of these efforts is one of their most prominent features. The funding is multinational, the review steering committees are composed of scientists from many countries, and scientists from any United Nations member nation may compete for funding under either program. These efforts may be useful models for a global infectious disease research program.

In July 1991, the NIAID convened a task force on microbiology and infectious diseases to identify promising research opportunities and to recommend research strategies for future NIAID programs. The report of the task force was released in January 1992 (U.S. Department of Health and Human Services, 1992). This committee has reviewed the report, believes that its and the work of the task force are complementary, and supports the conclusions and recommendations of the NIAID group. Following are 11 recommendations from the NIAID report that are particularly pertinent to dealing with emerging microbial threats to health:

1. Every effort should be made to continue and expand basic research on microbial pathogenesis. These studies, using state-of-the-art techniques, should provide a detailed knowledge of how microbes cause infection and disease.

2. More needs to be known about the insects that serve as vectors for infectious agents and about the interactions of microbes with their vectors.

3. Identify, through basic research on infectious agents, new molecular targets amenable for drug design, and improve methods for their cloning, expression, purification, and crystallization.

4. Establish a new mechanism to facilitate the production of experimental vaccines on a pilot-plant scale under conditions suitable for their subsequent use in clinical studies.

5. Fundamental studies should be aimed at providing ideal vaccines that would be entirely safe and would be as effective as current vaccines that are composed of infectious microbes.

6. Increase the research focus on prevention of infection.

7. Promote multifaceted approaches to disease control that cut across different disciplines.

8. Increase the research focus on insect and tick vectors of disease.

9. Research support for the surveillance of infectious diseases should be increased to enhance the detection of emerging infectious diseases in the United States.

10. New biomedical technology should be applied to the detection, identification, and control of emerging infectious pathogens.

11. There should be an increase in the support for international research units studying infectious disease outside the United States.

Much has been written about the present and projected future shortage of scientists, physicians, and others trained to conduct basic and applied research on infectious diseases. Previous reports from the National Research Council and the IOM, for example, have stressed that there are shortages of several kinds of crucial personnel: medical entomologists (National Research Council, 1983); clinical specialists trained in tropical disease diagnosis, prevention, and control; biomedical researchers (National Research Council and Institute of Medicine, 1987); and public health specialists (Institute of Medicine, 1988).

Although this committee was not charged with examining issues related to personnel, it considers it important to register its concern about these shortages. Particularly troubling is the personnel situation in very specific disciplines involving the study of uncommon organisms such as rickettsiae. In these instances, the committee is concerned that support for training and careers for interested students is insufficient to ensure that future research programs in these disciplines will be adequately staffed.

Recently, much infectious disease research has shifted toward an approach primarily based on molecular biology, a discipline that the committee believes is critical to the prevention and control of infectious diseases in general. As important, however, is that the nation maintain a core of generalists (who are well versed in molecular biology) to respond to emerging and other infectious disease problems. Therefore, the committee urges that future training in molecular biology be integrated with training in clinical infectious diseases, epidemiology, medical microbiology, entomology, tropical medicine, and public health.

There are a number of programs managed and supported by U.S. government agencies and U.S.-based foundations that conduct research related to, and train people in, the recognition, epidemiology, prevention, and control of emerging microbial threats. In addition to those programs that are discussed below, several others should be noted, all of which support international research and capacity building in epidemiology, health policy, and management. These include the National Epidemiology Boards (NEB), sponsored by the Rockfeller Foundation; the Community Epidemiology and Health Management Network (CEN), sponsored by the Ford Foundation; and the International Health Policy Program (IHPP), sponsored by the Pew Trusts and the Carnegie Foundation (Commission on Health Research for Development, 1990). Whether they involve U.S. or foreign scientists, have a broad or narrow focus, all of these programs contribute in some way to the international capability to recognize and respond to emerging microbial threats to health.

THE ROCKEFELLER FOUNDATION

In 1980, the Rockefeller Foundation established the International Clinical Epidemiology Network (INCLEN) to train junior medical school faculty from developing countries in the discipline of epidemiology. After receiving their training, these individuals return to their home countries where they become part of a medical school-based Clinical Epidemiology Unit (CEU) that helps evaluate the availability, effectiveness, and efficiency of health care in that nation. Faculty who complete a program at one of the five Clinical Epidemiology Resource and Training Centers (CERTC) receive a master's degree in one of several disciplines related to clinical epidemiology. The five CERTCs are located at McMaster University, Ontario, Canada; University of Newcastle, New South Wales, Australia; University of North Carolina at Chapel Hill; University of Pennsylvania in Philadelphia; and University of Toronto, Ontario, Canada (International Clinical Epidemiology Network, 1990).

The INCLEN program has resulted in the establishment of more than 25 CEUs in medical schools in Africa, Asia, India, and Latin America. The goal of each unit is to provide training to at least six epidemiologists, a biostatistician, a health economist, and a social scientist. CEU staff are to conduct research in areas that have a measurable impact on health or health care policy. In addition to supporting training at the CERTCs, the INCLEN program organizes annual scientific meetings and conducts site visits to evaluate progress at CEUs (International Clinical Epidemiology Network, 1990).

The hope is that selected CEUs will eventually become CERTCs, thus expanding the network. Closer links with other international training programs (e.g., the CDC's Field Epidemiology Training and International Health and Policy Programs) are being pursued (International Clinical Epidemiology Network, 1990).

NATIONAL INSTITUTES OF HEALTH

As part of its mandate, the NIH conducts research and training that covers a broad range of infectious and tropical infectious diseases. Both in-house and extramural programs contribute to this effort and are under the direction of the NIAID.

• In 1978, the agency established the International Collaboration in Infectious Disease Research (ICIDR) program. With both an international and a domestic component, ICIDR efforts focus on the study of tropical infectious diseases and are designed to promote collaboration and exchange of scientific knowledge between scientists from the United States and their overseas counterparts. The majority of the research under this program must take place in the country represented by the foreign collaborator, which allows U.S. scientists to develop overseas work experience, thereby increasing their understanding of endemic diseases in other countries and their value as a potential resource for investigating disease outbreaks.

• The Tropical Disease Research Units (TDRU) program, initiated in 1980, encourages research in tropical infectious diseases. A wholly domestic program, the grants allow investigators to use state-of-the-art technology in the study of tropical infectious diseases including the six diseases—filariasis, leishmaniasis, malaria, leprosy, schistosomiasis, and trypanosomiasis—designated by the WHO as major health problems in tropical countries.

• Recently, the NIAID initiated the International Centers for Tropical Disease Research (ICTDR) program, which is designed to coordinate the institute's efforts in tropical diseases and international health. It is anticipated that the program will create a forum to promote more efficient use of resources, provide a means to identify targets for further research, and streamline future planning. In addition to the ICIDR and TDRU programs, the ICTDR initiative will comprise the Tropical Medicine Research Centers (TMRC) and the Intramural NIAID Center for International Disease Research (INCIDR) programs established in 1991, as well as the AIDS Research Division and Office of Tropical Medicine of the NIAID. Table 3-2, in the earlier section on Recognition, showed overseas locations affiliated with the ICTDR program.

These NIH-supported programs do not specifically address the emergence of infectious diseases. Proposed research to investigate questions related to disease emergence currently is unlikely to receive a high priority for funding, an issue of concern to this committee. To deal with the problem, the committee suggests that the NIH and other funding organizations issue requests for proposals (RFP) that address specific issues related to infectious disease emergence, for example, those involving agent, host, vector, or environmental emergence factors.

The committee recommends the expansion and coordination of National Institutes of Health-supported research on the agent, host, vector, and environmental factors that lead to emergence of infectious diseases. Such research should include studies on the agents and their biology, pathogenesis, and evolution; vectors and their control; vaccines; and antimicrobial drugs. One approach might be to issue a request for proposals

(RFP) to address specific factors related to infectious disease emergence.

CENTERS FOR DISEASE CONTROL

The majority of research and training supported by the CDC in the area of infectious diseases is conducted by the National Center for Infectious Diseases (NCID). The CDC does not maintain formal overseas laboratories, but it does support a number of foreign field stations that carry out infectious disease research and training. These initiatives are collaborative efforts with the host country (see Table 3-2 in the earlier section on Recognition).

The CDC is home to more than 40 WHO collaborating centers, more than half of which are housed in the NCID. In addition, the CDC has nearly 50 employees stationed in foreign countries, many of whom are involved in activities related to infectious disease. In fiscal 1990, the agency mounted 25 international emergency responses, 10 of which were related to infectious disease outbreaks. Agency research personnel were sent to, among other locations, Brazil (Brazilian purpuric fever), Bolivia (yellow fever), Netherlands (filovirus in monkeys), and Uganda (meningitis). In fiscal 1991, CDC personnel were instrumental in investigations of the cholera epidemic in Latin America (ASM News, 1992).

From the mid-1960s to early-1970s, the CDC administered an extramural program that awarded grants to academia and other institutions for research in infectious disease prevention and control. This program, discontinued in 1973 by the CDC as a result of tight funding (the legislation for this program then lapsed), supported up to 102 separate research projects and varied from a high of approximately $3.9 million in fiscal year 1969 to a low of $1.7 million in its final year. Examples of areas in which support was provided included the evaluation of immunization techniques and the resulting effects on the immunity of populations, the development and evaluation of laboratory diagnostic tests, field studies on the epidemiology and control of specific diseases, and defining health hazards related to pesticide use. The committee concludes that the now defunct program filled a need for support in a critical area of research.

The committee recommends increased research on surveillance methods and applied control methods, on the costs and benefits of prevention, control, and treatment of infectious disease, and on the development and evaluation of diagnostic tests for infectious diseases. Reinstating and expanding (both in size and scope) the extramural grant program at the Centers for Disease Control, which ceased in 1973, would be one important step in this direction. Similarly, the FDA extramural grant

program should be expanded to put greater emphasis on the development of improved laboratory tests for detecting emerging pathogens in food.

The CDC's Epidemic Intelligence Service (EIS) provides health professionals with training and field experience in public health epidemiology. The two-year program graduated 70 EIS officers in 1991. EIS officers are assigned to CDC headquarters, one of CDC's seven domestic field stations, state and local health departments, or, on occasion, to other federal agencies such as the FDA or the NIH. Under the tutelage of an experienced epidemiologist, EIS officers carry out epidemiologic research and investigations. Over four decades, officers have participated in investigations of such problems as the Hong Kong influenza epidemics, Legionnaire's disease and toxic shock syndrome outbreaks, and the current HIV/AIDS pandemic (Thacker et al., 1990).

The EIS program is and will continue to be an important source of experienced public health epidemiologists. It is also the model for another evolving program, the joint CDC/WHO Field Epidemiology Training Program (FETP). Begun in 1980, FETP's first efforts were in Thailand. Other FETPs have followed in Indonesia, Mexico, Peru, the Philippines, Saudi Arabia, and Taiwan. The programs are funded by the host country and international organizations, such as the WHO. FETPs provide their host countries with field-oriented epidemiologists who can actively participate in the development and implementation of needed disease prevention and control programs (Music and Schultz, 1990).

The committee considers the EIS and FETP two of the nation's primary resources for the training of epidemiologists. Current and former EIS officers and FETP graduates are important sources of information on emerging diseases. Moreover, because these individuals form an informal global network, their participation in the implementation of a global surveillance system for infectious diseases could be particularly valuable. Currently, however, their distribution is geographically restricted because of the limited number of graduates each year.

The committee recommends the domestic and global expansion of the Center for Disease Control's (CDC) Epidemic Intelligence Service program and continued support for CDC's role in the Field Epidemiology Training Program.

DEPARTMENT OF DEFENSE

The seven overseas medical research laboratories maintained by the DoD are the most broadly based international infectious disease research laboratories supported by the United States. DoD has maintained overseas research activities since 1900, when the Yellow Fever Commission was established in Cuba. The U.S. Army supported laboratories in the Philippines from 1900 to 1934, and in Panama from 1936 to 1945. During World War II, the Navy established a tropical disease research laboratory on Guam, which was later designated the Naval Medical Research Unit No. 2 (NAMRU-2). This was followed by the establishment of additional laboratories in Burma and Egypt, the latter being the forerunner of the current NAMRU-3 laboratory in Cairo (Armed Forces Epidemiological Board, 1991).

Since that time, the DoD has supported a total of 20 strategically located overseas laboratories, research teams, and research units. At present, the department operates laboratories in Thailand, Indonesia, Egypt, Brazil, Kenya, Peru, and Korea; all of them cooperate with scientists of the host country and serve as focal points for basic and applied disease research, especially on diseases of military significance. In addition to being well situated to recognize and study emerging disease threats, the laboratories are valuable sites for testing new drugs and vaccines, since they are located in areas in which the targeted diseases are endemic. The laboratories are also a vital resource for recruiting and training medical personnel for the U.S. military (Armed Forces Epidemiological Board, 1991). The committee is concerned that some of these laboratories have been closed in the past, for reasons related both to insufficient funding and changes in mission priorities, and that further closings could jeopardize the United States' ability to detect and respond to emerging infectious disease threats.

The committee recommends continued support—at a minimum, at their current level of funding—of Department of Defense overseas infectious disease laboratories.

OTHER PROGRAMS

An excellent model of U.S. involvement in tropical infectious disease research is the USAID-supported International Center for Diarrheal Disease Research, Bangladesh (ICDDR,B), earlier known as the Cholera Research Laboratory. The ICDDR,B was founded in 1959 in Dhaka with funds from the International Cooperation Agency, the USAID predecessor. Much of our current understanding of cholera epidemiology and treatment is the result of studies conducted in Dhaka. The center's involvement in the development of oral rehydration therapy for cholera was a major contribution to international health. Over time, with additional support from numerous countries, the facility has evolved into a high-caliber multinational research organization.

Another potentially useful program model is the National Health Service Corps (NHSC). The NHSC was created in 1970 by Public Law 91-623 to improve the delivery of medical services in medically underserved areas of the United States. In 1972, the NHSC Scholarship Program was initiated. This program underwrites the costs of medical education and in return requires physicians trained with NHSC money to repay their debt by serving in areas in which health services are inadequate (Brown and Stone, 1990). The committee is unaware of any similar program directed toward those who wish to train for careers in public health and related disciplines, such as epidemiology, infectious disease, and medical entomology. Because more individuals with training in these disciplines are likely to be needed to fulfill the United States' commitments to the implementation of a global infectious disease surveillance network, the establishment of such a program, modeled after the NHSC, might help to attract individuals who otherwise would not consider public health careers.

The committee recommends that Congress consider legislation to fund a program, modeled on the National Health Service Corps, for training in public health and related disciplines, such as epidemiology, infectious diseases, and medical entomology.

Vaccine and Drug Development

Vaccines and antimicrobial drugs have led to dramatic improvements in public health in the United States and in much of the rest of the world during the latter half of this century. Despite this encouraging history, the committee is concerned that many of the vaccines and drugs available today have been used for decades. It believes that there is a need to review the present vaccine and drug armamentaria with a view toward improving availability and surge capacity (potential for emergency response), as well as safety and efficacy.

VACCINES

Vaccines are one of the most cost-effective means now available for preventing disease. The *Haemophilus influenza* type B (Hib) vaccine is a good example. With its newly approved use (the vaccine is given at 2 months of age instead of at 18 months) and assuming an effectiveness rate of 72 percent, the total cost savings for vaccinating a one-year cohort of infants is estimated to be more than $359 million. (Including the cost of providing and administering the vaccine, this works out to $106 million in vaccine costs versus $465.3 million in disease/morbidity/mortality costs [M. Rowe, Policy Analysis and Legislation Branch, NIAID, personal communication, 1992].)

In addition to protecting the individual who has been vaccinated, the effects of immunization can extend to unvaccinated persons through so-called herd immunity. Herd immunity protects nonimmune individuals by reducing the number of infected individuals in the community (either because of previous exposure/natural immunity or vaccination) below the critical level needed to sustain transmission. Within such a community, the likelihood of a susceptible individual coming into contact with someone who has the specific disease is thus reduced. Vaccines can also have significant secondary public health and economic benefits. For example, hepatitis B vaccination may prevent the development of hepatocellular carcinoma, and influenza vaccine may prevent secondary bacterial pneumonia.

In many countries, including the United States, the use of vaccines has reduced or eliminated death and illness from infectious diseases. There are now effective vaccines against a number of once common childhood illnesses, including diphtheria, pertussis, measles, mumps, rubella, and polio. The global eradication of smallpox was possible because of the availability of a vaccine; polio is on the verge of being eradicated from the Western Hemisphere for the same reason. Influenza vaccine reduces morbidity in the young and prevents fatal disease in the elderly. Newer vaccines, against *Hemophilus influenza* B, hepatitis A and B, and *Streptococcus pneumoniae*, when used to full advantage, will significantly reduce morbidity and mortality as well. Altogether, there are more than 20 infectious diseases that can be prevented through the use of vaccines; nevertheless, there are many diseases for which no vaccine is available. These facts constitute a strong argument for making vaccine development an important first consideration for controlling microbial threats to health.

The route by which vaccines move from the research laboratory into the doctor's office is quite complex; it involves many government agencies and private organizations, and is only very loosely coordinated. There are multiple steps in the process, each with different decision makers who respond to diverse political, social, and economic forces (see Table 3-3). Federal vaccine development efforts are the responsibility of the PHS's National Vaccine Program Office, but there is considerable autonomy for program direction within the principal agencies—the NIH, CDC, FDA, and DoD.

The foundation for developing new or improved vaccines is basic research in microbiology, immunology, and disease pathogenesis. This research is largely carried out at the NIH, DoD (understandably, DoD's efforts are oriented toward military needs), universities, and biotechnology firms; it is funded by federal grants, private foundations, and the biotechnology industry. The level of effort reflects the priority decisions of the funding organizations—principally, the NIAID and DoD.

Applied research, which leads directly to vaccine development, is also funded by the NIAID, often through contracts, and by DoD. There is also significant investment at this level by industry. The rate of progress in any

TABLE 3-3 The U.S. Domestic Vaccine Research, Development, and Utilization Process

RDU Activity	Major Support	Major Performers
Basic research	NIH, NSF	Academia
	Private foundations	NIH
Applied research	NIH, CDC, FDA	Academia
	Private foundations	NIH, CDC, FDA
	Industry	Industry
(Transition to development)	—	**FDA regulates**
Pilot manufacturing	Industry	Industry
Preclinical testing	Industry, NIH, FDA	Industry, NIH, FDA, CDC, academia
IND application	Industry	Industry
Phase 1-3 clinical and field testing	Industry, NIH	Academia, CDC, NIH
Large-scale manufacturing	Industry	Industry
(Licensing)	—	**FDA**
Postlicensure operational testing	CDC, industry, FDA	CDC, academia, industry
Postlicensure safety evaluation	CDC, industry, FDA	CDC, FDA, industry
Purchasing and utilization	CDC, states, private medicine	CDC, states, private medicine

RDU, research, development, and utilization; NIH, National Institutes of Health; NSF, National Science Foundation; CDC, Centers for Disease Control; FDA, Food and Drug Administration; IND, application for investigational new drug.

given field can be strongly influenced by the level of NIAID and DoD funding, as is the case with HIV vaccine research.

The decision to move a vaccine candidate from laboratory research to industrial development is in the hands of the private sector vaccine manufacturers. It is based on an assessment of technical feasibility, estimated development costs, and market analysis (including the potential for liability problems). In most cases, public policy only indirectly influences the decision to pursue vaccine development and thus has little effect on the character of the vaccines that eventually enter the marketplace.

During the course of vaccine development but before licensure, there is a requirement for a series of studies to prove clinical safety and efficacy. Government support for this phase of the development process is becoming increasingly common and varies in extent, depending on the priorities of NIH and the willingness of the vaccine's developers to cooperate with government agencies. Government support of these studies is an important subsidization of the vaccine development process.

On the demand side, the purchase, distribution, and administration of vaccines are carried out through a mixture of federal, state, and private sector activities. The FDA subserves the regulatory role in vaccine licensing; the CDC is a major buyer of vaccines for federal and state programs, purchasing more than half of the vaccines used for childhood immunizations in the United States. The cost to consumers of vaccines purchased by the CDC is much lower than the cost of vaccines sold by the private sector market. Policies for the use of vaccines are developed by the Immunization Practices Advisory Committee, a CDC advisory committee, within the licensed-use guidelines set by the FDA.

Many decisions influence the life cycle of a new vaccine. In the public sector, such decisions are made independently by a number of agencies or committees (e.g., the FDA, CDC, Immunization Practices Advisory Committee [ACIP]) and are loosely coordinated by the PHS through its National Vaccine Program Office. (This agency is a coordinating office for the PHS but has no directive authority.) Corporate decision making responds primarily to market forces. The relationship between the public and private sectors is defined mainly by FDA guidelines and federal purchasing regulations and, as a result, is as often confrontational as cooperative.

Advances in immunology, molecular biology, biochemistry, and drug delivery systems have stimulated major new initiatives in vaccine development. The generation of vaccines that will come into use in the next decade is likely to be different from previous generations of vaccines. Some will contain more than one highly purified antigen and will rely on new delivery methods. Programmed-release biodegradable microspheres offer the possibility of single-dose regimens for parenteral vaccines. New oral vaccination methods will improve our ability to protect against enteric and respiratory agents.

Extensive investigations are also centering on vaccines that use attenuated viruses and bacteria as vectors to introduce specific antigenic components of disease-causing microbes. For example, a fowlpox virus recombinant, which has had parts of the genome of rabies virus inserted into its DNA, has been tested in animals to determine its ability to induce immunity to rabies. In two of five vertebrate species examined in one study, inoculation of the fowlpox recombinant vaccine candidate resulted in the induction of an immune response that protected against subsequent challenge with live rabies virus (Taylor et al., 1988). Other attenuated organisms being considered for use as vaccine vectors are vaccinia virus, baculovirus, poliovirus, *Salmonella typhimurium*, and bacille Calmette-Guerin (BCG). A major advantage of the vectored vaccine concept is that the vector genome can accommodate genetic material from more than one agent (perhaps as many as six or more); thus, it might be possible to develop a single vaccine that would immunize a person against multiple agents. This area offers much promise for the future of vaccine development.

For all of their potential, however, vaccines should not be viewed as so-called magic bullets for defeating emerging microbial threats. The potential value of vaccination and the speed with which vaccines can be developed depend on many factors. Especially important are the existing scientific knowledge of the agent (or similar organisms), its molecular biology, rate of transmission, pathogenesis, how the human immune system responds to natural infection, and the nature of the protective immunity the vaccine induces.

Successful vaccines were first developed against organisms (such as smallpox and yellow fever viruses) that produce acute infections and generate a natural immune response that protects against reinfection. For such diseases, it was only necessary to induce an immune response through vaccination that was similar to that induced by the natural infection. Bacterial diseases like diphtheria and tetanus, whose clinical effects are the result of exotoxins, were good first targets for vaccine development because of the strong immune reaction stimulated by the toxins. For a number of viral diseases (such as polio), attenuated vaccines, which mimic the wild-type virus's ability to produce protective immunity, have been quite effective.

Vaccine development for other infectious diseases, particularly those caused by protozoans, helminths, and fungi, has proved to be quite difficult, often because the responsible pathogens are able to evade the body's normal immune defenses. In such cases, even natural infection does not always induce protective immunity. In malaria, for example, the protozoa that cause the disease go through a multistage life cycle. At each stage, the antigens exposed to the immune system are different; these changes effectively create a "moving target" that is difficult for the body, and for vaccine developers, to combat effectively. An additional problem in malaria is that the body is "tricked" into mounting an immune response against noncritical parts of the organism rather than against those parts that are capable of inducing effective antimalarial immunity (Institute of Medicine, 1991a).

Vaccine development may be impeded by economic factors as well as by inherent mechanisms in the pathogens under study. The development of vaccines requires an extensive, up-front investment in research that most vaccine manufacturers (and policymakers) are reluctant to make, since few vaccines are highly profitable and the very strict FDA requirements for proof of a vaccine's safety and efficacy make the risk of failure an important consideration. This reluctance of vaccine manufacturers to invest in research contrasts with the attitude of drug manufacturers, who invest considerable funds in research and development. One reason for the difference may be that, as a group, drugs have a much better record of profitability.

Vaccine developers must also take into account the extra costs that may arise from liability claims for injuries or deaths owing to vaccine administration. This concern has forced a number of U.S. vaccine manufacturers out of the market over the past decade. Whereas in 1985, there were 10 licensed manufacturers of human vaccines (seven commercial, two state laboratories, and a single university) (Institute of Medicine, 1985), today there are only five.

Industry currently lacks economic incentives to stimulate efforts at preventing infectious diseases with vaccines for which there is little or no foreseeable market. Nor does the public health sector (with specific exceptions) have a mechanism for setting development programs in motion. There are ways in which industry might be encouraged to assume a greater role in vaccine development. A comprehensive strategy is urgently needed.

One approach would be to establish public/private sector collaborations in vaccine research and development, a strategy exemplified by the National Cooperative Vaccine Development Groups (NCVDG), whose goal is to address the problem of HIV. The NCVDGs represent the core of the investigator-initiated HIV vaccine development effort sponsored by the Vaccine Research and Development Branch (VRDB) of NIAID's Division of AIDS. These collaborative research teams are composed of scientists from industry, academia, and government working to develop and test experimental HIV vaccines. Current vaccine strategies being evaluated in animal models include inactivated virus, recombinant proteins, live recombinant viruses, synthetic peptides, anti-idiotypic antibodies, and passive immunization (Marta Glass, Division of AIDS, NIAID, personal communication, 1992). An alternative approach would be to offer industry economic incentives to develop vaccines. These incentives could range from partial or complete "socialization" of responsibility (government cost sharing and involvement in development decisions) to long-term guaranteed purchases of minimum amounts of a vaccine at a price that would allow the manufacturer to recover the costs of development and production.

Another current study at the Institute of Medicine is exploring issues that are likely to influence the participation and cooperation of American private and public sector organizations in the international initiative to accelerate development of new, improved childhood vaccines. The IOM Committee on the Children's Vaccine Initiative is examining legal, regulatory, economic, and practical impediments to optimal application of available national resources to the International Children's Vaccine Initiative. The results of this study, which is due to be completed in 1993, may have implications for the development of vaccines for microbial diseases in both children and adults.

Emerging microbes offer a different challenge for vaccine development than that presented by a well-established pathogen, and there are potentially catastrophic consequences if the development process is left entirely to free enterprise (see Box 3-3). It is understandably difficult to promote private investment in vaccine development for diseases that may not materialize for 5, 10, or 20 years, if at all. If a company did stockpile vaccines for potentially emergent diseases, it would either lose its investment if the disease threat never materialized or be forced to charge extraordinary prices, when the need arose, to compensate for research (if applicable—vaccine research often is done by other than commercial manufacturers) and development costs and wasted inventory—a requirement that probably would not be tolerated by society.

The United States, with only five vaccine manufacturers, is in a precarious position should an infectious disease emergency occur. Although there are vaccine manufacturing facilities outside the United States, obtaining vaccines from these facilities in an emergency would be complicated and time-consuming. In addition, overseas regulations for licensure may differ from those of the United States, another factor that must be considered when attempting to import vaccines. New technologies and production facilities need to be developed in this country for rapid response capability.

BOX 3-3 Are We Prepared? A Hypothetical Case

Consider the city of New Orleans, with a population of about 500,000 people. Early in this century, in cities along the lower Mississippi River, deaths from yellow fever were as high as 50 percent of those infected. We know that the insect vector for yellow fever, the mosquito *Aedes aegypti*, is still in the area in abundance, as is a newly introduced potential vector, *Ae. albopictus*. An effective vaccine exists but is not manufactured in the United States; only small stocks are available in North America, from a Canadian manufacturer. Larger stocks are stored in Brazil but would take time to mobilize.

Were yellow fever to break out in New Orleans and a determination be made to vaccinate the city's population, the existing North American vaccine supply would be exhausted within several days. "Acceptable" pesticidal approaches effective for control of the vector are not available, and it would probably be necessary to undertake massive spraying and source reduction to stem the epidemic. If that approach proved to be unacceptable, because there are no effective drugs and because no U.S. manufacturer could produce sufficient vaccine in a timely fashion, we could project with some confidence that 100,000 people would become ill with yellow fever and that 10,000 would likely die within a 90-day period. In addition to the loss of life, monetary costs to the health care system and to the New Orleans economy can be predicted to be in the tens of millions of dollars.

BOX 3-4 Responding to the 1976 Influenza Outbreak

Timetable of Response (1976)

January 19	Virus isolated at Fort Dix, New Jersey
February 6	Virus received by the Centers for Disease Control, Atlanta, Georgia
February 10	Virus identified as swine influenza (presumed antigenic prototype of 1918)
February 17	Virus forwarded to academic laboratory for genetic reassortment
March 1	First reassortant strain sent to manufacturers
April 30	Second reassortant strain sent to manufacturers
April	Human vaccine trials
May-August	Political problems with vaccine liability
September 2	Vaccine released by the Food and Drug Administration
October-December	National Influenza Immunization Program—40 million of 115 million doses administered

Total elapsed time: Approximately one year

There is no infrastructure in place today that allows for anticipatory vaccine development in response to future pandemics. The current system barely suffices for vaccines that have a predictable, established demand. The FDA does not have primary responsibility for ensuring that needed innovations are promptly developed and marketed; instead, the innovations are expected to emerge as firms pursue their organizational goals. Vaccines against future (some would say speculative) threats are looked upon by manufacturers as offering little promise for recovery of the investment needed to drive the system.

The overall process of vaccine development, manufacturing, and use is fragmented. There is no direct connection between research and development on the one hand and the purchasing and use of vaccines on the other. The various decision makers do not work together; in fact, they respond to different pressures. This imperfect system for the development of new vaccines could easily fail to produce new products rapidly enough in the face of an emerging disease threat.

The example of influenza vaccines is instructive. The sequence of events that constituted the response to the 1976 influenza epidemic began with the initial recognition of the new virus and culminated in the production and use of a vaccine (see Box 3-4 above). It should be noted that the time intervals can vary, as a result of both technical and political factors, and that this is a class of viruses with which researchers and manufacturers have had previous experience. In cases in which the agent is unknown, the timetable would be extended. Also of note is that these actions would have blunted a winter epidemic but not an earlier one.

The basic technology for the production of influenza vaccine is 50 years old, and global surveillance for influenza viruses was initiated by the WHO in 1947. Since then, several new subtypes of influenza A virus have emerged or reemerged, each posing the threat of pandemic disease. The system in place for responding to these threats requires the combined and integrated efforts of the CDC, academic laboratories, private industry, and the FDA to recognize a new antigenic variant of influenza virus, fabricate (through genetic reassortment) an acceptable vaccine strain, distribute the strain to manufacturers, and monitor production lots. The system works reasonably well. But as with so many other vaccine programs, influenza vaccines are underused—only a fraction of those at increased risk of fatal outcome are vaccinated. Influenza thus remains essentially an uncontrolled disease.

To bring a new vaccine rapidly from the research laboratory into general use—a necessary criterion if one hopes to prevent or control an emerging infectious disease—will require an integrated national process that

- defines the need for a vaccine and its technical requirements;
- defines the target populations and delivery systems;
- ensures the purchase and use of the developed product, through purchase guarantees and targeted immunization programs;
- relies as much as possible on the capability of private industry to manage the vaccine development process, through the use of contracted production if necessary;
- utilizes the capacity of the NIAID to manage and support basic and applied research and to conduct clinical studies and field evaluations;
- utilizes the capacity of the CDC and academia to conduct field evaluations and develop implementation programs;
- is centrally coordinated to take maximal advantage of the capabilities of the public and private sectors and ensures the continued existence of a competitive, efficient, reliable vaccine manufacturing industry within the United States; and
- is prepared for the possible rapid emergence of novel disease threats, such as occurred in the 1918–1919 influenza pandemic.

The committee recommends that the United States develop a means for generating stockpiles of selected vaccines and a "surge" capacity for vaccine development and production that could be mobilized to respond quickly to future infectious disease emergencies. Securing this capabil-

ity would require development of an integrated national process, as described above. The committee offers two options for implementation of this recommendation:

1. Develop an integrated management structure within the federal government and provide purchase guarantees, analogous to farm commodity loans, to vaccine manufacturers that are willing to develop the needed capacity.

2. Build government-supported research and development and production facilities, analogous to the National Cancer Institute's program for cancer therapeutics and the federal space, energy, and defense laboratories. The assigned mission of these new facilities would be vaccine development for future infectious disease contingencies.

ANTIMICROBIAL DRUGS

Since the 1940s, antimicrobial agents have served to control many previously life-threatening infections. Antimicrobials have the unique ability to cure certain diseases, to provide prophylaxis for others, and to reduce sources of infection. The usefulness of these drugs must be protected by careful and responsible use, and by continuing to encourage the development of new antimicrobial drugs. The development of resistance by microorganisms (see Chapter 2), as well as the emergence of new organisms, will require replacement drugs to be in the pipeline even while existing drugs are still effective. Success depends on the alertness of the clinical community in identifying resistant organisms through surveillance and in reaching consensus on the need for new drugs. Data from the CDC's NNISS will be crucial to surveillance efforts and for developing guidelines for the rational use of antimicrobial drugs, as a means to delay the development of resistance. Should a global infectious disease surveillance system be put in place, such as the one suggested in this report, tracking antimicrobial resistance worldwide may be possible.

The development of public/private sector alliances, along the lines of the National Cooperative Drug Development Groups at the NIH (similar to the vaccine groups discussed above), may be desirable. There may also be circumstances similar to the current shortage of antituberculosis drugs in which the active involvement of the FDA may be necessary to encourage manufacturers to produce specific drugs or to pursue the development of drugs for a specific purpose.

The committee recommends that clinicians, the research and development community, and the U.S. government (Centers for Disease Control, Food and Drug Administration, U.S. Department of Agriculture,

and Department of Defense) introduce measures to ensure the availability and usefulness of antimicrobials and to prevent the emergence of resistance. These measures should include the education of health care personnel, veterinarians, and users in the agricultural sector regarding the importance of rational use of antimicrobials (to preclude their unwarranted use), a peer review process to monitor the use of antimicrobials, and surveillance of newly resistant organisms. Where required, there should be a commitment to publicly financed rapid development and expedited approval of new antimicrobials.

Vector Control

The United States and other developed countries have been able to free themselves to a remarkable degree from the burden of vector-borne diseases using a variety of methods of vector control. If that level of vigilance is maintained, there is a chance of minimizing new outbreaks of vector-borne disease. The potential for vector-borne disease to emerge in the United States still exists, however, because of the abundance of certain vectors, such as *Aedes albopictus* mosquitoes. And even in Lyme disease, a vector-borne illness with a known vector—the *Ixodes* tick—there is currently no agreement on intervention strategies.

Vector control generally includes the use of one or more measures to reduce vector abundance, vector longevity, and human-vector contact. Depending on the type of vector, common control measures include, but are not limited to, indoor and outdoor spraying of chemical pesticides, application of biological control agents, destruction or treatment of larval development sites, and personal protective measures, such as covering exposed areas of the body, application of repellents, sleeping under bednets, or reducing human contact with infective insects by remaining away from areas inhabited by the vectors. Innovative methods of vector control, such as genetic modification of vectors, the development of antivector vaccines, and the use of biological control techniques are currently being examined, particularly for use in the control of mosquito vectors of malaria (Institute of Medicine, 1991a).

The transovarial transmission (from infected female vectors through their eggs to succeeding generations) of pathogens, such as arboviruses, poses some unique problems for the development of control programs. A transovarially infected adult mosquito vector can transmit infection immediately after it emerges. In the case of the LaCrosse virus, for example, it is important to preclude adult emergence and/or reduce the abundance of adult vectors that emerge in the spring or early summer. Any reduction in vector-control efforts is likely to be followed by a resurgence of the vector population.

For a disease agent that is known or suspected to be transmitted by an arthropod vector, efforts to control the vector can be crucial in containing or halting an outbreak. This is true even for those vector-borne diseases, such as yellow fever or malaria, for which there is or may eventually be an effective vaccine. To be effective, a vaccine must have time—often several weeks—to elicit an immune response in recipients. Vector control may provide this opportunity (see Box 3-5).

BOX 3-5 Vector Control in Action

Venezuelan equine encephalomyelitis was introduced into Texas in 1971. This was not a new virus but a highly pathogenic (in both equines and people) strain that had emerged in Central America in 1969. The disease advanced from Guatemala through Mexico and into Texas, a distance of more than 4,000 kilometers, in two years. The virus produced high-titer viremias in equines and was isolated from many species of mosquitoes that fed on equines and people. Most of these mosquito species previously had been considered to be pests rather than vectors of disease (Sudia et al., 1975).

The initial approach to containing the epidemic was to immunize equine populations (horses, mules, donkeys, and burros) across extensive areas of Central America and Mexico. The objective was to create an immunological barrier to prevent further spread. Fortunately, a vaccine developed by U.S. Army researchers (Berge et al., 1961) had been stockpiled, and additional doses were rapidly prepared. Although more than 4 million equines were vaccinated in Mexico in a two-year period, the virus continued to spread. There were tens of thousands of equine cases and 8,000 to 10,000 equine deaths in Mexico alone. Almost 17,000 cases (but no deaths) were reported in humans (Sudia et al., 1975).

Once it was recognized that the disease had invaded Texas, a massive campaign to eliminate the virus was initiated (Pan American Health Organization, 1972). A total of 2.25 million equines were vaccinated over an 11-state area, and a quarantine was established to prevent movement of the equines out of infected areas. Malathion and dibrom pesticides were applied over 8 million acres in Texas and Louisiana to control mosquito populations. With completion of these activities in 1972 and the onset of winter, the pathogenic strain of the virus disappeared from Texas, Mexico, and Central America. The program's cost exceeded $30 million (Sudia et al., 1975).

The virus has not reappeared, and it must be assumed that the vaccinated equine population has, after 20 years, been replaced by susceptible animals. Thus, this region is now receptive to the reintroduction of a pathogenic virus from South America or to the reemergence of a virulent strain from the Venezuelan equine encephalomyelitis viruses endemic in Central America and Florida.

In temperate zones, epidemic onset of a newly emergent vector-borne disease occurs most often in the spring or summer, since both vector and pathogen depend on higher temperatures to maintain a rapid rate of reproduction. The spread of infection during the summer months may be rapid, particularly if humans are an effective source of vector infection or if the agent has become widespread in a nonhuman reservoir population. Thus, to be effective, vector control efforts must be launched shortly after the disease is first recognized or, ideally, before the disease is apparent.

For most vector-borne infectious diseases, the onset of winter dampens transmission or can even eliminate the vector or infectious agent. The exception is pathogens that can survive in humans for long periods and produce chronic infection (e.g., malaria and typhus). Vectors native to temperate areas, if introduced into new regions, may be able to survive at low temperatures, while those native to the tropics may not. In much of North America, cold weather is a second line of defense against most newly emerged or introduced pathogens that depend on vectors to be transmitted to humans. A sudden decrease in incidence of an unidentified disease at the start of winter may be the first epidemiological evidence that the disease is vectorborne.

VECTOR-CONTROL RESOURCES

North America has extensive vector-control resources. In fact, vector control is an essential part of environmental health programs in many communities. California's mosquito control, for example, covers most of the state and involves some 72 agencies with a 1991 budget of more than $48.9 million for an area with a population of more than 20 million (California Mosquito and Vector Control Association, Inc., 1991). Statewide surveillance for mosquito-borne encephalitis, plague, malaria, and Lyme disease is coordinated by the California Department of Health Services.

There are approximately 1,000 additional regional and community vector-control and vector-surveillance programs in the United States and Canada (American Mosquito Control Association, 1991). Most of these programs are geared to protecting local populations from indigenous vector-borne diseases and arthropod pests. They may also provide an early line of defense against newly introduced or resurgent vector-borne diseases. In the United States, responsibility for organizing surveillance data and investigating epidemics of emerging vector-borne diseases, such as encephalitis, plague, and Lyme disease, rests with the CDC's Division of Vector-Borne Infectious Diseases in Fort Collins, Colorado.

The control methods used in a particular region depend on the vectors that are present and on what is known about their biology and behavior. Chemical and biological agents and environmental modification can be used individually or together in an integrated control effort. Although many local and regional vector-control programs can effectively combat local and even regional outbreaks of vector-borne disease, they are not equipped to deal with outbreaks that are national in scope. For example, regional vector-control programs cannot declare a health emergency or bypass the many legal restrictions that now limit the use of certain pesticides that are potentially useful for vector-control efforts. That authority rests with health and environmental agencies at the state and federal levels.

PESTICIDES FOR VECTOR CONTROL

A growing problem in controlling vector-borne diseases is the diminishing supply of effective pesticides. Federal and state regulations increasingly restrict the use and supply of such chemicals, largely as a result of concerns over human health or environmental safety. All pesticides must be registered with the U.S. Environmental Protection Agency (EPA) before they can be offered for sale in the United States. A 1972 amendment to the Federal Insecticide, Fungicide, and Rodenticide Act (FIFRA), called for all pesticides to be re-registered by 1975 in order to meet new health and safety standards (Public Law No. 92-516). By 1986, only one of approximately 1,200 previously registered pesticides had met all of the re-registration requirements. A 1988 amendment to FIFRA moved the re-registration deadline to 1997, giving manufacturers additional time to locate or develop scientific data necessary for re-registration that were not in the original registration materials for their products. If adequate data are not submitted by the cut-off date, pesticide makers face the loss of registration (Moses, 1992).

Some manufacturers have chosen not to re-register their products because of the expense of gathering the required safety data. Partly as a result, many effective pesticides developed over the past 40 years to control agricultural pests and vectors of human disease are no longer available because their registrations have been canceled or suspended in the United States.

For example, malathion, a pesticide used worldwide for both agricultural and public health purposes, is currently registered in the United States but must be re-registered in accordance with the provisions of FIFRA. The manufacturer (American Cyanamid Corporation) has sold the rights to malathion to a Danish company, which may or may not apply for re-registration in the United States. Because malathion is an effective, relatively inexpensive broad-spectrum pesticide, a failure to re-register would be considerable cause for concern.

Pyrethrum, a plant product that has been used successfully to control adult vectors for many years, is currently being reviewed for its potential environmental and health hazards. This product is not produced in the

United States, and supply is often a problem. Nevertheless, its failure to be re-registered would be a serious loss to the vector-control armamentarium in this country.

In addition, the new registration frequently limits the circumstances under which products may be applied. In many instances, compounds that were once approved for pest-control applications are now restricted to certain narrow agricultural uses, such as for pest control in a single crop. The result is that many pesticides that might have been used to control emerging vector-borne diseases are either no longer registered or are not available in sufficient quantity.

In accordance with federal endangered species legislation, the EPA further restricts pesticide use through its Endangered Species Protection Plan. The plan prohibits the use of a wide range of pesticides within the habitat of any endangered species. Prohibitions extend in some cases to urban and suburban environments, in which outbreaks of vector-borne disease pose a particular threat. Efforts have been made to develop a workable, legal strategy for vector control in the event of a public health emergency. Specifically, EPA has developed an emergency exemption procedure in collaboration with the California Mosquito and Vector Control Association and the American Mosquito Control Association. The plan calls for specific steps to be followed when surveillance data suggest that the possibility of an outbreak of a vector-borne disease is great. After the local vector-control agency has determined a need to invoke the exemption, it must follow a 12-step procedure that includes review of the area for endangered species, consultation with the U.S. Fish and Wildlife Service (FWS), submission of a request for a public health exemption to the state public health agency or the CDC, a review and determination by the state agency or the CDC (which must be performed within 10 days if an emergency is anticipated or within 24 hours if the emergency is in progress), review and revision (if necessary) of the original plan and submission of a final plan to the state or the CDC, submission (within 15 days) by the CDC of a request to the EPA for an exemption, EPA consultation with the FWS, EPA approval or denial of the request (within 15 days), and, finally, implementation of the plan (B. Eldridge, Director, Mosquito Research Program, Department of Entomology, University of California at Davis, personal communication, 1992).

The committee recommends that the Environmental Protection Agency develop and implement alternative, expedited procedures for the licensing of pesticides for use in vector-borne infectious disease emergencies. These procedures would include a means for stockpiling designated pesticides for such use.

As with vaccines, there is little economic incentive for firms to develop new pesticides for public health use because such use makes up a very small part of the pesticide market. The committee feels strongly, however, that pesticide development in this area needs to be given some priority. Pesticide development is now driven mainly by the demands of agriculture. Moreover, as pesticide development has become ever more specialized, there are fewer compounds available that have both agricultural and public health uses.

Agricultural applications account for about 75 percent of pesticide use in the United States. Approximately 407,000 tons of pesticide were used in 1987, of which about 89,500 tons were insecticides. Public health use accounts for about 10 percent of all pesticides globally; the major public health uses are for control of malaria, filariasis, schistosomiasis, onchocerciasis, and trypanosomiasis (Moses, 1992).

Dichlorodiphenyl trichloroethane (DDT), one of the most effective and economical pesticides ever developed, was first marketed in 1942, three years after Swiss chemist Paul Mueller discovered that the compound had insecticidal properties. In 1972, all agricultural use of DDT in the United States was banned because of its adverse environmental effects. Its use is now restricted by the EPA to public health emergencies, as defined under FIFRA. DDT is still used in many developing countries for public health purposes, particularly malaria control. Currently, aldrin, benzene hexachloride, chlordane, chlordimeform, DBCP, diazinon, dieldrin, dinogeb, ethylene dibromide, andrin, EPN, heptachlor, lindane, mirox, nitrofen (TOK), 2,4,5-T/silvex, and toxaphene also are banned, suspended, or severely restricted in their use as pesticides within the United States (Moses, 1992).

The use of insect growth regulators (so-called biorational or third-generation pesticides) to control vector populations is being investigated. These compounds affect certain biological processes of insects, such as metamorphosis, that are not present in mammals and other vertebrates. Biological control agents (the use of one organism to control another) are also considered biorational pesticides. Once licensed, many such materials will be used to control the immature stages of a number of insect vectors. They are likely to be of limited value as adulticides, however, since compounds used to control adult insects usually must produce mortality quickly. So far, only conventional broad-spectrum pesticides possess this characteristic. Resistance to biorational pesticides has recently been demonstrated in laboratory settings, even in the case of microbial pesticides.

The lack of a sufficient stockpile of effective pesticides, which might be required in the event of a major epidemic, continues to be a serious problem. The public health community has played a minor role in the formulation of pesticide use policy, which is mainly influenced by agricultural and environmental lobbying efforts. Until there are adequate alternative means for controlling disease-carrying vectors, it is critical that public health requirements for pesticides be considered when pesticide policy is being debated. There may well be instances in which the limited application of pesticides, such as DDT, to deal with a public health emergency may be acceptable—as long as the overall burden on the environment is not excessive. The committee believes that the current EPA contingency plan that addresses this issue is ineffective: the approval process for emergency use of pesticides is so cumbersome that approval would likely come after the critical period in which application of the pesticide could avert the outbreak. Under emergency circumstances, a tradeoff must be made, so that the process can be more expedient.

Several arboviruses (St. Louis, western, and eastern equine encephalitis) are examples of diseases that could erupt suddenly into emergency proportions that might require pesticide use. These arboviruses are enzootic in North America and are maintained in a cycle of infection between wild birds and vector mosquitoes, with little or no transmission to humans. Periodically, however, excessive rain or snow, followed by high summer temperatures, favors the emergence of increased vector populations, which may lead to the rapid spread of infection to humans.

These events can occur in both urban and rural communities, and when they do, there is an immediate need to implement a control program. The primary goal at the onset of mosquito-borne disease epidemics is to eliminate the infective mosquitoes as quickly as possible. Transmission can only be stopped by the effective application of a pesticide that kills adult mosquitoes. A control program directed against the preadult aquatic and adult stages of the vector would not have an immediate effect on virus transmission but might be valuable for preventing a prolonged epidemic.

St. Louis encephalitis (SLE) exemplifies the above scenario. It has frequently reemerged as an epidemic infection in the United States (Monath, 1980), most recently in Florida and Texas in 1990 (Centers for Disease Control, 1990d). In 1966, an effort was made, in the middle of an epidemic in Dallas, Texas, to evaluate the effectiveness of controlling populations of adult mosquitoes that transmit this disease. There were 545 suspected and 145 confirmed cases of SLE in a period of a few weeks (Hopkins et al., 1975). In an eight-day period, 475,000 acres of the area were aerially sprayed with 12,000 gallons of malathion in an ultra-low-volume, high-concentration mist. Observations made before and after the application indicated that there was a significant reduction in the vector population and its infection rate. Few new cases were detected during the two to three weeks after the spraying. This is one of the few epidemics of a reemerging infection for which a study was conducted on its economic impact. It was estimated that the SLE outbreak cost the community $796,500, of which almost $200,000 was spent on vector control (Schwab, 1968). The economic and public health consequences would certainly have been greater had pesticides not been available.

Alternative strategies for the control of epidemics of SLE and western equine encephalitis are considered in detail elsewhere (Reeves and Milby, 1990). In the event of an epidemic caused by one of these enzootic viruses, the control of adult vectors is probably the best approach for stopping the spread of disease. To be successful, it has been estimated that pesticide application should achieve a 90 percent or greater reduction in the infected vector population (W. Reeves, Professor of Epidemiology Emeritus, School of Public Health, University of California at Berkeley, personal communication, 1992) .

As in the drug arena, resistance to pesticides can present serious problems to disease control. Mosquitoes, flies, and other disease-carrying insects have relatively short life cycles and produce many generations per year. This is a major factor in the development of pesticide resistance, and it is usually in these groups that resistance to a given chemical is seen. There are many strategies that can be used to delay or prevent pesticide resistance. So-called pesticide resistance management can include the rotation of chemicals, avoidance of sublethal doses, and the use of biodegradable materials. More research is needed, however, to hone the usefulness of these approaches.

The committee recommends that additional priority and funding be afforded efforts to develop pesticides (and effective modes of application) and other measures for public health use in suppressing vector-borne infectious diseases.

Public Education and Behavioral Change

The areas of public education and behavioral change in relation to emerging infectious diseases currently show visible activity; the media, for example, have been presenting information to the public about the control of Lyme disease and HIV transmission. The committee was not constituted to address these two issues; however, because the topics represent potentially important aspects of emerging infectious disease prevention and control, it was considered appropriate to address them briefly here.

Public policy discussions and scientific efforts sometimes focus on vaccine and drug development and fail to give appropriate consideration to education and behavioral change as means for preventing and controlling infectious diseases. This is unfortunate, since it is often only by changing patterns of human activity—from travel and personal hygiene to sexual behavior and drug abuse—that the spread of disease can be halted.

For many infectious disease problems, however, particularly those that result from emerging microbes, the use of vaccines and drugs is not practical. Often, for newly recognized diseases, the causative agent is unknown, making vaccine and drug development essentially impossible. Because of the long development process, vaccines and drugs can contribute little to disease control at the onset of an outbreak of a newly emergent disease. Only in a case in which an effective drug has already been developed for use against another organism and is found be efficacious against the newly discovered agent will drugs be of use in such circumstances.

HIV disease illustrates these problems quite clearly. It has been almost a decade since HIV was isolated, yet there is no vaccine and few drugs that have been shown to slow the disease process. Since the major modes of transmission of HIV are behaviorally based, the pandemic offered a unique opportunity to put public education and behavior modification to use. Initially, officials were highly reluctant to provide candid information to the public on how to prevent the spread of HIV. Recently, however, efforts at education on HIV and AIDS, much of it from nongovernmental organizations, have been more straightforward. Among the more visible of the federal government efforts were the mailing of an AIDS information pamphlet to every household in the country in 1988 and the current television spots that provide a toll-free number to call to learn more about HIV disease. The concern of the committee is that these efforts are targeted to a general audience rather than to specific risk groups, and do not use the terminology that is most understandable to these populations.

Nevertheless, despite a disappointing beginning, the experience with HIV demonstrates that human behavior can be modified in part through education. Condom use has increased and numbers of sexual partners have decreased in most male homosexual populations that have been studied (National Commission on Acquired Immune Deficiency Syndrome, 1991). Evidence for similar behavioral change among those using intravenous drugs or crack cocaine is less encouraging.

Even when scientists and public health officials rely on education and encourage behavioral change to prevent or limit the spread of infectious disease, the public may not be convinced. Although scientists may see emerging microbes as a very real threat to public health, the average citizen may be unaware of the potential danger or may consider those dangers to be less important than other health risks, for example heart disease or cancer. In such instances, carefully conceived media campaigns may have a beneficial effect on behavior in relation to disease transmission.

The committee recommends that the National Institutes of Health give increased priority to research on personal and community health practices relevant to disease transmission. Attention should also be focused on developing more effective ways to use education to enhance the health-promoting behavior of diverse target groups.

* * * *

It is the committee's hope that this report will be an important first step in highlighting the growing problem of emerging microbial threats to health and focus attention on ways in which the United States and the global community will attempt to address such threats, now and in the future. The major emphasis in the American health care system has always been on curing rather than prevention. The committee strongly believes that the best way to prepare for the future is by developing and implementing preventive strategies that can meet the challenges offered by emerging and reemerging microbes. It is infinitely less costly, in every dimension, to attack an emerging disease at an early stage and prevent its spread than to rely on treatment to control the disease.

In some instances, what this report proposes will require additional funds. The committee recognizes and has wrestled with the discomforts that such recommendations can bring—for example, the awareness that there are other compelling needs that also justify—and require—increased expenditures. But everyone must realize and understand the potential magnitude of future epidemics in terms of human lives and monetary costs.

The 1957 and 1968 influenza pandemics killed 90,000 people in the United States alone. The direct cost of medical care was $3.4 billion (more than three times the NIAID budget for fiscal year 1992), and the total economic burden was $26.8 billion[3]—almost three times the total NIH budget for fiscal year 1992 (Kavet, 1972). A more current example offers a similar lesson. The recent resurgence of TB (from 22,201 cases in 1985 to 26,283 cases in 1991, or 10.4 per 100,000 population) (Centers for Disease Control, 1992g), after a steady decline over the past several decades, will be costly. Every dollar spent on TB prevention and control in the United States produces an estimated $3 to $4 in savings; these savings increase dramatically when the cost of treating multidrug-resistant tuberculosis is factored in. We also have a recent example of what results when early prevention and control efforts are lacking. The costs of AIDS/HIV disease—in human lives as well as dollars—have been staggering, and the end is not yet in sight. The objective in the future should be earlier detection of such emerging diseases, coupled with a timely effort to inform the population about how to lower their risk of becoming infected.

Obviously, even with unlimited funds, no guarantees can be offered that an emerging microbe will not spread disease and cause devastation. Instead, this committee cautiously advocates increased funding and proposes some more effective ways for organizations—domestic and international, public and private—as well as individuals—both health professionals and the lay public—to work together and, in some cases, combine their resources. These efforts will help to ensure that we will be better prepared to respond to emerging infectious disease threats of the future.

---

[3]Study staff converted the figures in the original publication (Kavet, 1972) to 1992 dollars using the NIH Biomedical Research and Development Price Index (BRDPI).

References

Advisory Committee on Foreign Quarantine. 1966. Report to the Surgeon General of the Public Health Service by the Advisory Committee on Foreign Quarantine (June), Washington, D.C.

Afzelius, A. 1921. Erythema chronicum migrans. Acta Dermato-Venereologica 2:120-125.

Agency for Health Care Policy and Research. 1990. Large percentage of elders face nursing home use. Research Activities 134:6.

Allison, R., C. Thompson, and P. Ahlquist. 1990. Regeneration of a functional RNA virus genome by recombination between deletion mutants and requirement for cowpea chlorotic mottle virus 3a and coat genes for systemic infection. Proceedings of the National Academy of Sciences, USA 87:1820-1824.

Alter, M. J., S. C. Hadler, H. S. Margolis, W. J. Alexander, P. Y. Hu, F. N. Judson, A. Mares, J. K. Miller, and L. A. Moyer. 1990. The changing epidemiology of hepatitis B in the United States. Journal of the American Medical Association 263:1218-1222.

American Cancer Society. 1991. Cancer Facts and Figures—1991. Atlanta: American Cancer Society, p. 10.

American Mosquito Control Association. 1991. Directory of Mosquito Control Agencies in the United States and Canada. Baton Rouge, Louisiana: American Mosquito Control Association.

American Public Health Association, Association of State and Territorial Health Officials, National Association of County Health Officials, U.S. Conference of Local Health Officers, and Centers for Disease Control. 1991. Healthy Communities 2000: Model Standards, Guidelines for Community Attainment of Year 2000 National Health Objectives, 3rd ed. Washington, D.C.: American Public Health Association.

Ampel, N. M. 1991. Plagues—what's past is present: thoughts on the origin and history of new infectious diseases. Reviews of Infectious Diseases 13:658-665.

Anderson, C. 1991. Cholera epidemic traced to risk miscalculation. Nature 354:255.

Anderson, R. M., R. M. May, M. C. Boily, G. P. Garnett, and J. T. Rowley. 1991. The spread of HIV-1 in Africa: sexual contact patterns and the predicted demographic impact of AIDS. Nature 352:581-589.

Archer, D. L., and F. E. Young. 1988. Contemporary issues: diseases with a food vector. Clinical Microbiology Reviews 1:377-98.

Armed Forces Epidemiological Board. 1991. Department of Defense Overseas Infectious Diseases Research Program. Fort Detrick, Maryland: U.S. Army Medical Research and Development Command.

ASM News. 1992. Peru's cholera epidemic: health system's baptism by fire. Vol. 58, pp. 178-180.

Assistant Secretary for Health's Public Health Service Task Force to Strengthen Public Health in the United States. 1991. A plan to strengthen public health in the United States. Public Health Reports 106(Suppl. 1):1-86.

Atkinson, W. L. 1991. Measles returns. American Family Physician 43(1):104, 106.

Atkinson, W. L., and L. E. Markowitz. 1991. Measles and measles vaccine. Seminars in Pediatric Infectious Diseases 2:100-107.

Baek, L. J., R. Yanagihara, C. J. Gibbs, Jr., M. Miyazaki, and D. C. Gajdusek. 1988. Leakey virus: a new hantavirus isolated from *Mus musculus* in the United States. Journal of General Virology 69:3129-3132.

Bailey, T. M., and P. M. Schantz. 1990. Trends in the incidence and transmission patterns of trichinosis in humans in the United States: comparisons of the periods 1975–1981 and 1982–1986. Reviews of Infectious Diseases 12:5-11.

Bean, N. H., and P. M. Griffin. 1990. Foodborne disease outbreaks in the United States, 1973–1987: pathogens, vehicles, and trends. Journal of Food Protection 53:804-817.

Becker, R. L. 1983. Absence of induced radioactivity in irradiated foods. In: Recent Advances in Food Irradiation. P. W. Elias and A. J. Cohen (eds.). Amsterdam: Elsevier Biomedical Press.

Behbehani, A. M. 1991. The smallpox story: historical perspective. ASM News 57:571-576.

Benditt, E. P., T. Barrett, and J. K. McDougall. 1983. Viruses in the etiology of atherosclerosis. Proceedings of the National Academy of Sciences, USA 80: 6386 6389.

Benenson, A. S. (ed.). 1990. Control of Communicable Diseases in Man, 15th ed. Washington, D.C.: American Public Health Association.

Berge, T. O., I. S. Banks, and W. D. Tiggert. 1961. Attenuation of Venezuelan equine encephalomyelitis virus by in vitro cultivation in guinea-pig heart cells. American Journal of Hygiene 73:209-218.

Berman, S. J., G. S. Irving, W. D. Kundin, J.-J. Gunning, and R. H. Watten. 1973. Epidemiology of the acute fevers of unknown origin in South Vietnam: effect of laboratory support upon clinical diagnosis. American Journal of Tropical Medicine and Hygiene 22:796-801.

Bernier, R. 1991. Assessment of immunization coverage: a critical element in the strategy to reach 90 percent levels, In: Proceedings of the 25th National Immunization Conference, June 10–14, Washington, D.C. Atlanta: Centers for Disease Control.

172   EMERGING INFECTIONS

Berrang, M. E., R. E. Brackett, and L. R. Beuchat. 1989. Growth of *Listeria monocytogenes* on fresh vegetables stored under controlled atmosphere. Journal of Food Protection 52:702-705.

Blostein, J. 1991. Shigellosis from swimming in a park pond in Michigan. Public Health Reports 106:317-322.

Branati, R., R. F. Fritz, and A. C. Hollister. Jr. 1954. An outbreak of malaria in California. American Journal of Tropical Medicine and Hygiene 3:779-788.

Brazilian Purpuric Fever Study Group. 1987a. Brazilian purpuric fever: epidemic purpura fulminans associated with antecedent purulent conjunctivitis. Lancet 2:757-761.

Brazilian Purpuric Fever Study Group. 1987b. *Haemophilus aegyptius* bacteraemia in Brazilian purpuric fever. Lancet 2:761-763.

Brinton, L. A., W. C. Reeves, M. M. Brenes, R. Herrero, E. Gaitan, F. Tenorio, R. C. de Britton, M. Garcia, and W. E. Rawls. 1989. The male factor in the etiology of cervical cancer among sexually monogamous women. International Journal of Cancer 44:199-203.

Brown, J., and V. Stone. 1990. Decline in NHSC physicians threatens patient care. American Journal of Public Health 80(11):1395-1396.

Brummer-Korvenkontio, M., A. Vaheri, T. Hovi, C.-H. von Bonsdorff, J. Vuorimies, T. Manni, K. Penttinen, N. Oker-Blom, and J. Lahdevirta. 1980. Nephropathia epidemica: detection of antigen in bank voles and serologic diagnosis of human disease. Journal of Infectious Diseases 141:131-134.

Bryan, J. A., J. D. Lehmann, I. F. Setiady, and M. H. Hatch. 1974. An outbreak of hepatitis A associated with recreational lake water. American Journal of Epidemiology 99:145-154.

Buchanan, R. L., and S. A. Palumbo. 1985. *Aeromonas hydrophila* and *Aeromonas sobria* as potential food poisoning species: a review. Journal of Food Safety 7:15-29.

Buckley, S. M., and J. Casals. 1970. Lassa fever, a new virus disease of man from West Africa. II. Isolation and characterization of the virus. American Journal of Tropical Medicine and Hygiene 19:680-691.

Burk, R. D., A. S. Kadish, S. Calderin, and S. L. Romney. 1986. Human papillomavirus infection of the cervix detected by cervicovaginal lavage and molecular hybridization: correlation with biopsy results and Papanicolaou smear. American Journal of Obstetrics and Gynecology 154:982-989.

Caldwell, M. 1987. The Last Crusade: The War On Consumption, 1862–1954. New York: Atheneum.

California Mosquito and Vector Control Association (CMVCA), Inc. 1991. Yearbook of the California Mosquito and Vector Control Association, Inc. Sacramento, California: CMVCA, Inc.

Canfield, C. J. 1972. Malaria in U.S. military personnel, 1965–1971. Proceedings of the Helminthological Society of Washington 39:15-18.

Carey, D. E., G. E. Kemp, H. A. White, L. Pinneo, R. F. Addy, A. L. M. D. Fom, G. Stroh, J. Casals, and B. E. Henderson. 1972. Lassa fever: epidemiological aspects of the 1970 epidemic, Jos, Nigeria. Transactions of the Royal Society of Tropical Medicine and Hygiene 66:402-408.

Carman, W. F., M. R. Jacyna, S. Hadziyannis, P. Karayiannis, M. McGarvey,

A. Makris, and H. C. Thomas. 1989. Mutation preventing formation of e antigen in patients with chronic HBV infection. Lancet 2:588-591.

Carman, W. F., A. R. Zanetti, P. Karayiannis, J. Waters, G. Manzillo, E. Tanyi, A. J. Zuckerman, and H. C. Thomas. 1990. Vaccine-induced escape mutant of hepatitis B virus. Lancet 336:325-329.

Carman, W. F., E. A. Fagan, S. Hadziyannis, P. Karayiannis, N. C. Tassopoulos, R. Williams, and H. C. Thomas. 1991. Association of a precore genomic variant of hepatitis B virus with fulminant hepatitis. Hepatology 14:219-222.

Carnahan, A. M., and S. W. Joseph. 1991. Spotlight on *Aeromonas*—a human pathogen of aquatic origin. LabO 2:1-2.

Carnahan, A. M., M. A. Marii, G. R. Fanning, M. A. Pass, and S. W. Joseph. 1989. Characterization of *Aeromonas schubertii* strains recently isolated from traumatic wound infections. Journal of Clinical Microbiology 27:1826-1830.

Catteneo, R. A., A. Schmid, P. Spielhofer, K. Kaelin, K. Baczko, V. Ter Meulen, J. Pardowitz, S. Flanagan, B. K. Rima, S. Udem, and M. A. Billeter. 1989. Mutated and hypermutated genes of persistent measles viruses which caused lethal human brain diseases. Virology 173:415-425.

Centers for Disease Control. 1985. Preliminary report: epidemic fatal purpuric fever among children—Brazil. Morbidity and Mortality Weekly Report 34:217-219.

Centers for Disease Control. 1986. Brazilian purpuric fever: *Haemophilus aegyptius* bacteremia complicating purulent conjunctivitis. Morbidity and Mortality Weekly Report 35:553-554.

Centers for Disease Control. 1990a. Imported malaria associated with malariotherapy of Lyme disease—New Jersey. Morbidity and Mortality Weekly Report 39:873-875.

Centers for Disease Control. 1990b. Outbreak of multidrug-resistant tuberculosis—Texas, California, and Pennsylvania. Morbidity and Mortality Weekly Report 39:369-372.

Centers for Disease Control. 1990c. Transmission of *Plasmodium vivax* malaria in San Diego County, California, 1988 and 1989. Morbidity and Mortality Weekly Report 39:91-94.

Centers for Disease Control. 1990d. Update: St. Louis encephalitis—Florida and Texas, 1990. Morbidity and Mortality Weekly Report 39:756-759.

Centers for Disease Control. 1991a. The HIV/AIDS epidemic: the first ten years. Update: Acquired immunodeficiency syndrome—United States, 1981–1990. Morbidity and Mortality Weekly Report 40:357-369.

Centers for Disease Control. 1991b. Hospital Infections Program (pamphlet). Atlanta: National Center for Infectious Diseases, Centers for Disease Control. December.

Centers for Disease Control. 1991c. Imported dengue—United States, 1990. Morbidity and Mortality Weekly Report 40:519-520.

Centers for Disease Control. 1991d. Measles outbreak—New York City, 1990–1991. Morbidity and Mortality Weekly Report 40:305-306.

Centers for Disease Control. 1991e. Mortality attributable to HIV infection/AIDS— United States, 1981–1990. Morbidity and Mortality Weekly Report 40: 41-44.

Centers for Disease Control. 1991f. Mosquito-transmitted malaria—California and Florida, 1990. Morbidity and Mortality Weekly Report 40:106-108.

Centers for Disease Control. 1991g. Primary and secondary syphilis—United States 1981–1990. Morbidity and Mortality Weekly Report 40:314.

Centers for Disease Control. 1991h. Summary of notifiable diseases, United States: 1990. Morbidity and Mortality Weekly Report 39(53):30.

Centers for Disease Control. 1991i. Trichinosis surveillance—United States, 1987–1990. Morbidity and Mortality Weekly Report 40:36-41.

Centers for Disease Control. 1991j. Unavailability of streptomycin, para-aminosalicylic acid—United States. Morbidity and Mortality Weekly Report 40:715.

Centers for Disease Control. 1991k. Update: surveillance of outbreaks—United States, 1990. Morbidity and Mortality Weekly Report 40:173-175.

Centers for Disease Control. 1992a. Availability of streptomycin and para-aminosalicylic acid—United States. Morbidity and Mortality Weekly Report 41:243.

Centers for Disease Control. 1992b. Cases of selected notifiable diseases, United States, weeks ending December 28, 1991, and December 29, 1990 (52nd Week). Morbidity and Mortality Weekly Report 40(51/52):899-900.

Centers for Disease Control. 1992c. Cholera associated with an international airline flight, 1992. Morbidity and Mortality Weekly Report 41:134-135.

Centers for Disease Control. 1992d. Eastern equine encephalitis virus associated with *Aedes albopictus*—Florida, 1991. Morbidity and Mortality Weekly Report 41:115-121.

Centers for Disease Control. 1992e. HIV/AIDS Surveillance: Year-End Edition. (U.S. AIDS cases reported through December 1991; issued January 1992.) Atlanta: Centers for Disease Control.

Centers for Disease Control. 1992f. Syphilis cases, by 4-week period of report—United States, 1984–1991. Morbidity and Mortality Weekly Report 41:49.

Centers for Disease Control. 1992g. Tuberculosis morbidity—United States, 1991. Morbidity and Mortality Weekly Report 41:240.

Centers for Disease Control. 1992h. Update: foodborne listeriosis—United States, 1988–1990. Morbidity and Mortality Weekly Report 41:251, 257-258.

Childs, J. E., G. W. Korch, C. E. Glass, J. W. LeDuc, and K. V. Shah. 1987. Epizootiology of Hantavirus infections in Baltimore: isolation of a virus from Norway rats and characteristics of infected rat populations. American Journal of Epidemiology 126:55-68.

Clements, C. 1992. HealthNet connects Africa to vital medical data. Satellite Communications (Jan.):18-21.

Cohen, M. L., and R. V. Tauxe. 1986. Drug-resistant salmonella in the United States: an epidemiologic perspective. Science 234:964-969.

Commission on Health Research for Development. 1990. Health Research: Essential Link to Equity in Development. New York: Oxford University Press.

Cortes, E., R. Detels, D. Aboulafia, X. L. Li, T. A. Moudgil, M. C. Bonecker, A. Gonzaga, L. Oyafuso, M. Tondo, C. Boite, N. Hammershlak, C. Capitani, D. J. Slamon, and D. D. Ho. 1989. HIV-1, HIV-2, and HTLV-I infection in high-risk groups in Brazil. New England Journal of Medicine 320:953-958.

Cotton, P. 1991. Reported measles decline continues; research seeks to avert resurgence. Journal of the American Medical Association 266:2521-2522.

Council for Agricultural Science and Technology. 1986. Ionizing Energy in Food Processing and Pest Control: I. Wholesomeness of Food Treated with Ionizing Energy. Ames, Iowa: Council for Agricultural Science and Technology.

Cover, T. L., and R. C. Aber. 1989. *Yersinia enterocolitica*. New England Journal of Medicine 321:16-24.

Cox, M. F., C. A. Meanwell, N. J. Maitland, G. Blackledge, C. Scully, and J. A. Jordon. 1986. Human papillomavirus type 16 homologous DNA in normal human ectocervix (letter). Lancet 2:157-158.

Cronon, W. 1983. Changes in the Land: Indians, Colonists, and the Ecology of New England. New York: Hill and Wang.

Crosby, A. W., Jr. 1972. The Columbian Exchange. Westport, Connecticut: Greenwood Press.

Crosby, A. W., Jr. 1976. Epidemic and Peace, 1918. Westport, Connecticut: Greenwood Press.

Daily, O. P., S. W. Joseph, J. C. Coolbaugh, R. I. Walker, B. R. Merrell, D. M. Rollins, R. J. Seidler, R. R. Colwell, and C. R. Lissner. 1981. Association of *Aeromonas sobria* with human infection. Journal of Clinical Microbiology 13:769-777

Davis, R. M., E. D. Whitman, W. A. Orenstein, S. R. Preblud, L. E. Markowitz, and A. R. Hinman. 1987. A persistent outbreak of measles despite appropriate control measures. American Journal of Epidemiology 126:438-449.

Davis, W. A., J. G. Kane, and V. G. Garagusi. 1978. Human *Aeromonas* infections: a review of the literature and a case report of endocarditis. Medicine 57:267-277.

Dealer, S., and R. W. Lacey. 1990. Transmissible spongiform encephalopathies: the threat of BSE to man. Food Microbiology 7:253-279.

Dealer, S., and R. W. Lacey. 1991. Transmissible spongiform encephalopathies: the threat of BSE to man—a reply to K. C. Taylor. Food Microbiology 8:259-262.

DeFreitas, E., B. Hilliard, P. R. Cheney, D. S. Bell, E. Kiggundu, D. Sankey, Z. Wroblewska, M. Palladino, J. P. Woodward, and H. Koprowski. 1991. Retroviral sequences related to human T-lymphotropic virus type II in patients with chronic fatigue immune dysfunction syndrome. Proceedings of the National Academy of Sciences, USA 88:2922-2926.

Dentler, R. A. 1977. Urban Problems. Chicago: Rand McNally.

De Quadros, C. A., J. K. Andrus, J. M. Olive, C. M. Da Silviera, R. M. Eikhof, P. Carrasco, J. W. Fitzsimmons, and F. P. Pinheiro. 1991. Eradication of poliomyelitis: progress in the Americas. Pediatric Infectious Diseases Journal 10:222-229.

Desmyter, J., K. M. Johnson, C. Deckers, J. W. LeDuc, F. Brasseur, and C. Van Ypersele de Strihou. 1983. Laboratory rat associated outbreak of haemorrhagic fever with renal syndrome due to Hantaan-like virus in Belgium. Lancet 2:1445-1448.

deVilliers, E. M. 1989. Heterogeneity of the human papillomavirus group. Journal of Virology 63:4898-4903.

Diglisic, G., A. Gligic, R. Stojanovic, M. Obradovic, D. Volimirovic, V. Lukac, S. Y. Xiao, C. A. Rossi, and J. W. LeDuc. 1991. Outbreak of hemorrhagic fever with renal syndrome in Yugoslavia associated with domestic rats and mice. American Journal of Tropical Medicine and Hygiene 45(Suppl.):153.

Digoutte, J. P., and C. J. Peters. 1989. General aspects of the 1987 Rift Valley fever epidemic in Mauritania. Research in Virology 140:27-30.

Domingo, E., D. Sabo, T. Taniguchi, and C. Weissman. 1978. Nucleotide sequence heterogeneity of an RNA phage population. Cell 13:735-744.

Domingo, M., L. Ferrer, M. Pumarola, A. Marco, J. Plana, S. Kennedy, M. McAliskey, and B. K. Rima. 1990. Morbillivirus in dolphins (letter). Nature 348:21.

Dominguez, G., C. Y. Wang, and T. K. Frey. 1990. Sequence of the genome RNA of rubella virus: evidence for genetic rearrangement during togavirus evolution. Virology 177:225-238.

Dooley, C. P., P. L. Fitzgibbons, H. Cohen, M. D. Appleman, G. I. Perez-Perez, and M. J. Blaser. 1989. Prevalence of *Helicobacter pylori* infection and histologic gastritis in asymptomatic persons. New England Journal of Medicine 321:1562-1566.

Double Helix. 1990. Studies begin on opportunistic infections. Double Helix 15:2.

Dubos, R., and J. Dubos. 1987. The White Plague. New Brunswick, New Jersey: Rutgers University Press.

Duffy, J. 1990. The Sanitarians. Chicago: University of Illinois Press.

Fabricant, C. G., J. Fabricant, M. M. Litrenta, and C. R. Minick. 1978. Virus-induced atherosclerosis. Journal of Experimental Medicine 148:335-340.

Fabricant, C. G., J. Fabricant, C. R. Minick, and M. M. Litrenta. 1980. Herpesvirus-induced atherosclerosis. In: Viruses in Naturally Occurring Cancers. Cold Spring Harbor Conference on Cell Proliferation. Cold Spring Harbor, New York: Cold Spring Harbor Laboratory Press.

Fenner, F., D. A. Henderson, I. Arita, Z. Jezek, and I. D. Ladnyi. 1988. Lessons and benefits. In: Smallpox and Its Eradication. Geneva: World Health Organization, chap. 31.

Fleming, D. W., S. L. Cochi, K. L. MacDonald, J. Brondum, P. S. Hayes, B. D. Plikaytis, M. B. Holmes, A. Audurier, C. V. Broome, and A. L. Reingold. 1985. Pasteurized milk as a vehicle of infection in an outbreak of listeriosis. New England Journal of Medicine 312:404-407.

Fox, J. L. 1992. Coalition reacts to surge of drug-resistant TB. ASM News 58:135-139.

Frame, J. D., J. M. Baldwin, Jr., D. J. Gocke, and J. M. Troup. 1974. Lassa fever, a new virus disease of man from West Africa. I. Clinical description and pathological findings. American Journal of Tropical Medicine and Hygiene 19(4):670-676.

Fraser, D. W., C. C. Campbell, T. P. Monath, P. A. Goff, and M. B. Gregg. 1974. Lassa fever in the Eastern Province of Sierra Leone, 1970–1972, I. Epidemiologic studies. American Journal of Tropical Medicine and Hygiene 23:1131-1139.

Freeman, J., and J. E. McGowan. 1978. Risk factors for nosocomial infection. Journal of Infectious Diseases 138:811-819.

Friedman, C. T. H., A. S. Dover, R. R. Roberto, and O. A. Kearns. 1973. A malaria epidemic among heroin users. American Journal of Tropical Medicine and Hygiene 22:302-307.

Fuchs, P. C. 1979. Epidemiology of Hospital-Associated Infections. Chicago: American Society of Clinical Pathologists.

Fuller, H. S. 1964. Introduction. In: Communicable Diseases—Arthropodborne Diseases Other Than Malaria. J. B. Coates, Jr., E. C. Hoff, and P. M. Hoff (eds.). Washington, D.C.: Medical Department, United States Army.

Fuller, J. G. 1974. Fever! The Hunt for a New Killer Virus. New York: Reader's Digest Press.

Gao, F., L. Yue, A. T. White, P. G. Pappas, J. Barshue, A. P. Hanson, B. Greene, P. Sharp, G. M. Shaw, and B. H. Hahn. in press. Zoonotic infection by genetically diverse simian-related HIV-2 in West Africa. Nature.

Garry, R. F. 1990. Early case of AIDS in the USA. Nature 347:359.

Gasser, R. A., A. J. Magill, C. N. Oster, and E. C. Tramont. 1991. The threat of infectious disease in Americans returning from Operation Desert Storm. New England Journal of Medicine 324:859-864.

Gaynes, R. P., D. H. Culver, T. G. Emori, T. C. Horan, S. N. Banerjee, J. R. Edwards, W. R. Jarvis, J. S. Tolson, T. S. Henderson, J. B. Hughes, and W. J. Martone. 1991. The National Nosocomial Infections Surveillance (NNIS) System: Plans for the 1990s and beyond. American Journal of Medicine 91: 116S-120S.

Geisbert, T. W., and P. B. Jahrling. 1990. Use of immunoelectron microscopy to show Ebola virus during the 1989 United States epizootic. Journal of Clinical Pathology 43:813-816.

Georghiou, G. P. 1990. Resistance potential to biopesticides and consideration of counter measures, In: Pesticides and Alternatives: Innovative Chemical and Biological Approaches to Pest Control. J. E. Casida (ed.). New York: Elsevier Science Publishers Biomedical Division.

Gessain, A., F. Barin, and J. C. Vernant. 1985. Antibodies to human T-lymphotropic virus type-I in patients with tropical spastic paraparesis. Lancet 2:407-410.

Glass, G. E., J. E. Childs, A. J. Watson, and J. W. LeDuc. 1990. Association of chronic renal disease, hypertension, and infection with a rat-borne hantavirus. Archives of Virology (Supplement 1):69-80.

Glupczynski, Y., A. Burette, M. Labbe, M. Dereuck, and M. Deltenre. 1988. Campylobacter pylori-associated gastritis: a double blind, placebo-controlled trial with amoxicillin. American Journal of Gastroenterology 83:365-372.

Goldman, B. 1991. Growing number of "Jim Henson's" disease cases worries Ontario doctors. Canadian Medical Association Journal 144(6):760-764.

Goodstein, L. 1991. Study says drug-resistant TB on the rise. The Washington Post (Nov 20):A4.

Gordon, J. E. 1958. General considerations of modes of transmission. In: Communicable Diseases Transmitted Chiefly Through Respiratory and Alimentary Tracts. Coates, J. B., Jr., E. C. Hoff, and P. M. Hoff, eds., Washington, D.C.: Medical Department, United States Army.

Gorgas, M. D., and B. J. Hendrick. 1924. William Crawford Gorgas: His Life and Work. Philadelphia: Lea and Febiger.

Grachev, M. A., V. P. Kumarev, L. V. Mamaev, V. L. Zorin, L. V. Baranova, N. N. Denikina, S. I. Belikov, E. A. Petrov, V. S. Kolesnick, R. S. Kolesnick, V. M. Dorofeev, A. M. Beim, V. N. Kudelin, F. G. Nagieva, and V. N. Sidorov. 1989. Distemper virus in Baikal seals. Nature 338:209.

Gubler, D. J. 1991. Dengue haemorrhagic fever: a global update. Virus Information Exchange Newsletter 8:2-3.

Hahn, C. S., S. Lustig, E. G. Strauss, and J. H. Strauss. 1988. Western equine encephalitis is a recombinant virus. Proceedings of the National Academy of Sciences, USA 85:5997-6001.

Hallegraeff, G. M., and C. J. Bolch. 1991. Transport of toxic dinoflagellate cysts via ships' ballast water. Marine Pollution Bulletin 22:27-30.

Halstead, S. B. 1990. Global epidemiology of dengue hemorrhagic fever. Southeast Asian Journal of Tropical Medicine and Public Health 21:636-637.

Hamilton, W. D., R. Axelrod, and R. Tanese. 1990. Sexual reproduction as an adaptation to resist parasites: a review. Proceedings of the National Academy of Sciences, USA 87:3566-3573.

Hammon, W. McD., A. Rudnick, and G. E. Sather. 1960. Viruses associated with epidemic hemorrhagic fevers of the Philippines and Thailand. Science 131:1102.

Hanrahan, J. P., J. L. Benach, J. L. Coleman, E. M. Bosler, D. L. Morse, D. J. Cameron, R. Edelman, and R. Kaslow. 1984. Incidence and cumulative frequency of endemic Lyme disease in a community. Journal of Infectious Diseases 150:489-496.

Harding, G. K. M., L. E. Nicolle, A. R. Ronald, J. K. Preiksaitis, K. R. Forward, D. E. Low, and M. Cheang. 1991. How long should catheter-acquired urinary tract infection in women be treated? Annals of Internal Medicine 114:713-719.

Hardt-English, P., G. York, R. Stier, and P. Cocotas. 1990. Staphylococcal food poisoning outbreaks caused by canned mushrooms from China. Food Technology 44:74-77.

Hardy, J. L., E. J. Houk, L. D. Kramer, and W. C. Reeves. 1983. Intrinsic factors affecting vector competence of mosquitoes for arboviruses. Annual Reviews of Entomology 28:229-262.

Hart, C. D., G. C. Mead, and A. P. Norris. 1991. Effects of gaseous environment and temperature on the storage behavior of *Listeria monocytogenes* on chicken breast meat. Journal of Applied Bacteriology 70:40-46.

Hattori, T., A. Koito, K. Takatsuki, S. Ikematsu, J. Matsuda, H. Mori, M. Fujui, K. Akashi, and K. Matsumoto. 1989. Frequent infection with human T-cell lymphotropic virus type I in patients with AIDS but not in carriers of human immunodeficiency virus type I. Journal of Acquired Immune Deficiency Syndromes 2:272-276.

Hayden, F. G., and R. G. Douglas, Jr. 1990. Antiviral agents. In: Principles and Practice of Infectious Diseases, G. L. Mandell, R. G. Douglas, Jr., and J. E. Bennett (eds.). New York: Churchill Livingstone, chap. 34.

Hazen, T. C., C. B. Fleirmans, R. P. Hirch, and G. W. Esch. 1978. Prevalence and distribution of *Aeromonas hydrophila* in the United States. Applied Environmental Microbiology 33:114-122.

Henderson, D. A. 1976a. The eradication of smallpox. Scientific American 235:25-33.

Henderson, D. A. 1976b. Surveillance of smallpox. International Journal of Epidemiology 5:19-28.

Hendrix, M. G. R., P. H. J. Dormans, P. Kitslaar, F. Bosman, and C. A. Bruggeman. 1989. The presence of cytomegalovirus nucleic acids in arterial walls of atherosclerotic and nonatherosclerotic patients. American Journal of Pathology 134: 1151-1157.

Hendrix, M. G. R., M. M. M. Salimans, C. P. A. van Boven, and C. A. Bruggeman. 1990. High prevalence of latently present cytomegalovirus in arterial walls of patients suffering from grade III atherosclerosis. American Journal of Pathology 136:23-28.

Hess, A. D., C. E. Cherubin, and L. C. LaMotte. 1963. Relation of temperature to activity of western and St. Louis encephalitis viruses. American Journal of Tropical Medicine and Hygiene 12:657-667.

Hickman-Brenner, F. W., K. L. MacDonald, A. G. Steigerwalt, G. R. Fanning, D. J. Brenner, and J. J. Farmer III. 1987. *Aeromonas veronii*, a new ornithine decarboylase-positive species that may cause diarrhea. Journal of Clinical Microbiology 25:900-906.

Hickman-Brenner, F. W., F. W. Fanning, M. J. Arduino, D. J. Brenner, and J. J. Farmer III. 1988. *Aeromonas schubertii*, a new mannitol-negative species found in human clinical specimens. Journal of Clinical Microbiology 26:1561-1564.

Hildesheim, A., V. Mann, L. A. Brinton, M. Szklo, W. C. Reeves, and W. E. Rawls. 1991. Herpes simplex virus type 2: a possible interaction with human papillomavirus types 16/18 in the development of invasive cervical cancer. International Journal of Cancer 49:335-340.

Hillman, R., D. Tomlinson, D. Taylor-Brown, and J. R. W. Harris. 1989. Risks of AIDS among workers in the "sex industry." British Journal of Medicine 299: 622-623.

Hinman, A. R., K. J. Bart, and D. R. Hopkins 1985. Costs of not eradicating measles (letter). American Journal of Public Health 75(7):713-714.

Hintlian, C. B., and J. H. Hotchkiss. 1986. The safety of modified atmosphere packaging: a review. Food Technology 40:70-76.

Hintlian, C. B., and J. H. Hotchkiss. 1987. Comparative growth of spoilage and pathogenic organisms on modified atmosphere-packaged cooked beef. Journal of Food Protection 50:218-223.

Hirsch, A. 1885. Handbook of Geographical and Historical Pathology, Vol. 2. London: New Sydenham Society.

Hoehling, A. A. 1961. The Great Epidemic. Boston: Little, Brown and Company.

Holmberg, S. D., S. L. Solomon, and P. A. Blake. 1987. Health and economic impacts of antimicrobial resistance. Reviews of Infectious Diseases 9:1065-1078.

Holmes, G. P., J. B. McCormick, S. C. Trock, R. A. Chase, S. M. Lewis, C. A. Mason, P. A. Hall, L. S. Brammer, G. I. Perez-Oronoz, M. K. McDonnell, J. P. Paulissen, L. B. Schonberger, and S. P. Fisher-Hoch. 1990. Lassa fever in the United States: investigation of a new case and guidelines for management. New England Journal of Medicine 323:1120-1123.

Hopkins, C. C., F. B. Hollinger, R. F. Johnson, H. L. Dewlett, V. F. Newhouse, and R. W. Chamberlain. 1975. The epidemiology of St. Louis encephalitis in Dallas, Texas, 1966. American Journal of Epidemiology 102:1-15.

Ingham, S. C., J. M. Escude, and P. McCown. 1990. Comparative growth rates of *Listeria monocytogenes* and *Pseudomonas fragi* on cooked chicken loaf stored under air and two modified atmospheres. Journal of Food Protection 53:289-291.

Institute of Medicine. 1985. Vaccine Supply and Innovation. Washington, D.C.: National Academy Press.

Institute of Medicine. 1988. The Future of Public Health. Washington, D.C.: National Academy Press.

Institute of Medicine. 1989. Human Health Risks with the Subtherapeutic Use of Penicillin or Tetracyclines in Animal Feed. Washington, D.C.: National Academy Press.

Institute of Medicine. 1991a. Malaria: Obstacles and Opportunities. Washington, D.C.: National Academy Press.

Institute of Medicine. 1991b. Seafood Safety. Washington, D.C.: National Academy Press.

International Clinical Epidemiology Network. 1990. INCLEN: Design, Measurement, Evaluation (brochure). New York: Rockefeller Foundation.

Irino, K., I. M. L. Lee, M. Kaku, M. C. C. Brandelione, C. E. A. Melles, C. E. Levy, S. E. Berkley, D. W. Fleming, G. A. Silva, and L. H. Harrison. 1987. Fevre purpurica brasileira: resultados preliminares da investigacao etiologica. Reviews of the Institute of Tropical Medicine of São Paulo 29:147-177.

Jacoby, G. A. 1991. Emerging resistance to antimicrobial agents (paper prepared for the Committee on Emerging Microbial Threats to Health, Task Force on Bacteria, Rickettsia, and Chlamydia). April.

Jacoby, G. A., and G. L. Archer. 1991. New mechanisms of bacterial resistance to antimicrobial agents. New England Journal of Medicine 324:601-612.

Jaenson, T. G. T. 1991. The epidemiology of Lyme borreliosis. Parasitology Today 7:39-45.

Jahrling, P. B., T. W. Geisbert, S. W. Dalgard, E. D. Johnson, T. G. Ksiazek, W. C. Hall, and C. J. Peters. 1990. Preliminary report: isolation of Ebola virus from monkeys imported to USA. Lancet 1:502-505.

Janda, J. M., and P. S. Duffey. 1988. Mesophilic aeromonads in human disease: current taxonomy, laboratory identification, and infectious disease spectrum. Reviews of Infectious Diseases 10:980-997.

Johnston, J. 1991. New blood test for HIV-2 expected soon. Journal of NIH Research 3:29-30.

Joint Expert Committee on Food Irradiation. 1980. Wholesomeness of Irradiated Food: Summaries of Data Considered By the Joint FAO/IAEA/WHO Expert Committee. Geneva: World Health Organization.

Jones, M. M. 1991. Marine Organisms Transported in Ballast Water: A Review of the Australian Scientific Position. Canberra: Australian Government Publishing Service.

Jorgenson, N. 1971. A Guide to New England's Landscape. Barre, Massachusetts: Barre Publishers.

Joseph, S. W., A. M. Carnahan, P. R. Brayton, G. R. Fanning, R. Almazan, C. Drabick, E. W. Trudo, Jr., and R. R. Colwell. 1991. *Aeromonas jandaei* and *Aeromonas veronii* dual infection of a human wound following aquatic exposure. Journal of Clinical Microbiology 29:565-569.

Jouan, A., B. LeGuenno, J. P. Digoutte, B. Philippe, O. Riou, and F. Adam. 1988. A RVF epidemic in southern Mauritania. Annales de l'Institut Pasteur, Virology 139:307-308.

Kalyanaraman, V. S., M. G. Sarngadharan, M. Robert-Guroff, I. Miyoshi, D. Blayney,

D. Golde, and R. C. Gallo. 1982. A new subtype of human T-cell leukemia virus (HTLV-II) associated with a T-cell variant of hairy cell leukemia. Science 218:571-573.

Kannel, W. B., J. T. Doyle, A. M. Ostfield, C. D. Jenkins, L. Kuller, R. N. Podell, and J. Stamler. 1984. Optimal resources for primary prevention of atherosclerotic diseases. Circulation 70:157A-205A.

Kaplan, J. E., M. Osame, and H. Kubota. 1990. The risk of developing HTLV-I associated myelopathy/tropical spastic paraparesis (HAM/TSP) among persons infected with HTLV-I. Journal of Acquired Immune Deficiency Syndromes 3:1096-1101.

Karabatsos, N. (ed.). 1985. International Catalogue of Arboviruses, 3rd ed. San Antonio, Texas: American Society of Tropical Medicine and Hygiene.

Kautter, D. A., T. Lilly, Jr., and R. Lynt. 1978. Evaluation of the botulism hazard in fresh mushrooms wrapped in commercial polyvinylchloride film. Journal of Food Protection 41:120-121.

Kavet, J. 1972. Influenza and public health. Master's thesis, Harvard School of Public Health.

Kawaoka, Y., and R. G. Webster. 1988. Molecular mechanism of acquisition of virulence in influenza in nature. Microbial Pathogenesis 5:311-318.

Kennedy, S., J. A. Smyth, S. J. McCullough, G. M. Allan, F. McNeilly, and S. McQuaid. 1988. Confirmation of cause of recent seal deaths (letter). Nature 335:404.

Kew, O. M., and B. K. Nottay. 1984. Evolution of the oral polio vaccine strains in humans occurs by both mutations and intra-molecular recombination. In: Modern Approaches to Vaccines. R. M. Chanock and R. A. Lerner (eds.). Cold Spring Harbor, New York: Cold Spring Harbor Laboratory.

Kiernan, F. A., Jr. 1959. The blood fluke that saved Formosa. Harpers Magazine (April):45-47.

Kilbourne, E. D. 1987. Influenza. New York: Plenum Medical Book Company.

Kilbourne, E. D. 1991. New viruses and new disease: mutation, evolution, and ecology. Current Opinion in Immunology 3:518-524.

Klugman, K. P. 1990. Pneumococcal resistance to antibiotics. Clinical Microbiology Reviews 3:171-196.

Koch, H. W., and E. H. Eisenhower. 1967. Radioactivity criteria for radiation processing of foods. In: Radiation Processing of Foods, Advances in Chemistry, Series No. 65. Washington, D.C.: American Chemical Society.

Koop, C. E. 1991. AIDS. In: Koop: The Memoirs of America's Family Doctor. New York: Random House.

Kuefler, P. R., and P. A. Bunn, Jr. 1986. Adult T-cell leukemia/lymphoma. Clinical Haematology 15:695-726.

Laga, M., J. P. Icenogle, R. Marsella, R. W. Ryder, S. Vermund, W. Heyward, A. Nelson, and W. C. Reeves. 1992. Genital papillomavirus infection and cervical dysplasia—opportunistic complications of HIV infection. International Journal of Cancer 50:45-48.

Langone, J. 1990. Emerging viruses. Discover 11:63-68.

Last, J. M., and R. B. Wallace (eds.) 1992. Maxcy-Rosenau-Last Public Health and Preventive Medicine, 13th ed. Norwalk, Connecticut: Appleton & Lange.

Lastavica, C. C., M. L. Wilson, V. P. Barardi, A. Spielman, and R. D. Deblinger. 1989. Rapid emergence of a focal epidemic of Lyme disease in coastal Massachusetts. New England Journal of Medicine 320:133-137.

Laughlin, C. A., R. J. Black, J. Feinberg, D. J. Freeman, J. Ramsey, M. A. Ussery, and R. J. Whitley. 1991. Resistance to antiviral drugs. ASM News 57:514-517.

Lawson, H. W., M. M. Braun, R. I. M. Glass, S. E. Stine, S. S. Monroe, H. K. Atrash, L. E. Lee, and S. J. Englender. 1991. Waterborne outbreak of Norwalk virus gastroenteritis at a southwest U.S. resort: role of geological formations in contamination of well water. Lancet 337:1200-1204.

LeDuc, J. W. 1987. Epidemiology of Hantaan and related viruses. Laboratory Animal Science 37:413-418.

LeDuc, J. W., G. A. Smith, and K. M. Johnson. 1984. Hantaan-like viruses from domestic rats captured in the United States. American Journal of Tropical Medicine and Hygiene 33:993-998.

LeDuc, J. W., G. A. Smith, M. Macy, and R. J. Hay. 1985. Certified cell lines of rat origin appear free of infection with hantavirus. Journal of Infectious Diseases 152:1082-1083.

LeDuc, J. W., G. A. Smith, J. E. Childs, F. P. Pinheiro, J. I. Maiztegui, B. Niklasson, A. Antoniadis, D. M. Robinson, M. Khin, K. F. Shortridge, M. T. Wooster, M. R. Elwell, P. L. T. Ilbery, D. Koech, E. S. T. Roas, and L. Rosen. 1986. Global survey of antibody to Hantaan-related viruses among peridomestic rodents. Bulletin of the World Health Organization 64:139-144.

Lee, H. H., P. Swanson, J. D. Rosenblatt, I. S. Y. Chen, W. C. Sherwood, D. E. Smith, G. E. Tegtmeier, L. P. Fernando, C. T. Fang, M. Osame, and S. H. Kleinman. 1991. Relative prevalence and risk factors of HTLV-I and HTLV-II infection in US blood donors. Lancet 337:1435-1439.

Lee, H. W., P. W. Lee, and K. M. Johnson. 1978. Isolation of the etiologic agent of Korean hemorrhagic fever. Journal of Infectious Diseases 137:298-308.

Lee, H. W., L. J. Baek, and K. M. Johnson. 1982. Isolation of Hantaan virus, the etiologic agent of Korean hemorrhagic fever, from wild urban rodents. Journal of Infectious Diseases 146:638-644.

Lepes, T. 1981. Technical problems related to biological characteristics of malaria, as encountered in malaria control/eradication. Unpublished World Health Organization document WHO/MAL/81.934. Geneva.

Levi, R. I., and J. Moskovitz. 1982. Cardiovascular research: decades of progress, a decade of promise. Science 217:121-129.

Liang, T. J., K. Hasegawa, N. Rimon, J. R. Wands, and E. Ben-Porath. 1991. A hepatitis B virus mutant associated with an epidemic of fulminant hepatitis. New England Journal of Medicine 324:1705-1709.

Linnan, M. J., L. Mascola, D. L. Xiao, V. Goulet, S. May, A. Salmidurier, B. D. Plikaytis, S. L. Fannin, A. Kleks, and C. V. Broome. 1988. Epidemic listeriosis associated with Mexican-style cheese. New England Journal of Medicine 319:823-828.

Lloyd, G., E. T. W. Bowen, N. Jones, and A. Pendry. 1984. HFRS outbreak associated with laboratory rats in UK. Lancet 1:1175-1176.

Logan, R. P. H., P. A. Gummett, R. J. Polson, M. M. Walker, J. H. Baron, and J. Misiewicz. 1990. The recurrence of *H. pylori* in relation to duodenal ulcer.

Revista Española De Las Enfermedades Del Aparato Digestivo (Madrid) 78:S72-S73.

Lorber, B. 1988. Changing patterns of infectious diseases. American Journal of Medicine 84:569-578.

Maldonado, Y. A., B. L. Nahlen, R. R. Roberto, M. Ginsberg, E. Orelana, M. Mizrahi, K. McBarron, H. O. Lobel, and C. C. Campbell. 1990. Transmission of *Plasmodium vivax* malaria in San Diego County, California, 1986. American Journal of Tropical Medicine and Hygiene 42:3-9.

Maloney, J., D. Rimland, D. S. Stephens, P. Terry, and A. M. Whitney. 1989. Analysis of amikacin-resistant *Pseudomonas aeruginosa* developing in patients receiving amikacin. Archives of Internal Medicine 149:630-634.

Mandell, G. L., R. G. Douglas, Jr., and J. E. Bennett (eds.). 1990. Principles and Practice of Infectious Disease, 3rd ed. New York: Churchill Livingstone.

Marks, G., and W. K. Beatty. 1976. Epidemics. New York: Charles Scribner's Sons.

Marshall, E. 1991. Sullivan overrules NIH on sex survey. Science 253:502.

Martini, G. A. 1969. Marburg agent disease in man. Transactions of the Royal Society of Tropical Medicine and Hygiene 63:295-302.

Marton, A., M. Gulyas, R. Munoz, and A. Tomasz. 1991. Extremely high incidence of antibiotic resistance in clinical isolates of *Streptococcus pneumoniae* in Hungary. Journal of Infectious Diseases 163:542-548.

Martone, W. J. 1990. Hospital infections often preventable. U.S. Medicine 26(15/16):17-18.

Marwick, C. 1992. Do worldwide outbreaks mean tuberculosis again becomes "captain of all men of death"? Journal of the American Medical Association 267:1174-1175.

Matuschka, F. R., and A. Spielman. 1989. Lyme Krankheit durch Zechen: der verhaengisvolle Biss. Bild der Wissenschaft 8:54-64.

McAulcy, J. B. , M. K. Michelson, and P. M. Schantz. 1991. Trichinella infection in travelers. Journal of Infectious Diseases 164(5):1013-1016.

McEvedy, C. 1988. The bubonic plague. Scientific American 258:118-123.

McIntyre, P., G. Wheaton, J. Erlich, and D. Hansman. 1987. Brasilian purpuric fever in central Australia. Lancet 2:112.

McKerrow, J. H., Sakanari, J., and T. L. Deardorff. 1988. Revenge of the sushi parasite. New England Journal of Medicine 319:1228-1229.

McNeill, W. H. 1976. Plagues and Peoples. Garden City, New York: Anchor Press/Doubleday.

Meegan, J. M., and R. E. Shope. 1981. Emerging concepts on Rift Valley Fever. In: Perspectives in Virology. M. Pollard (ed.). New York: Alan R. Liss, Inc.

Mekalanos, J. J. 1983. Duplication and amplification of toxin genes on *Vibrio cholerae*. Cell 35:253-263.

Melnick, J. L., E. Adam, and M. E. DeBakey. 1990. Possible role of cytomegalovirus in atherogenesis. Journal of the American Medical Association 263:2204-2207.

Minick, C. R., C. G. Fabricant, J. Fabricant, and M. M. Litrenta. 1979. Atherosclerosis induced by infection with a herpesvirus. American Journal of Pathology 96:673-706.

Misch, A. 1991. Sanitation in the time of cholera. World Watch (Jul./Aug.):37-38.

Molloy, D. P. 1990. Progress in the biological control of black flies with *Bacillus thuringiensis israelensis*, with emphasis on temperate climates. In: Bacterial Control of Mosquitoes and Blackflies. de Barjac, H., and D. J. Sutherland, eds. New Brunswick, New Jersey: Rutgers University Press.

Monath, T. P. 1980. St. Louis Encephalitis. Washington, D.C.: American Public Health Association.

Monath, T. P., P. E. Mertens, R. Patton, C. R. Moser, J. J. Baum, L. Pinneo, G. W. Gary, and R. E. Kissling. 1973. A hospital epidemic of Lassa fever in Zorzor, Liberia, March–April 1972. American Journal of Tropical Medicine and Hygiene 22:773-779.

Morgan, D., W. Kraft, M. Bender, and A. Pearson. 1988. Nitrofurans in the treatment of gastritis associated with *Campylobacter pylori*. Gastroenterology 95:1178-1184.

Morris, A., and G. Nicholson. 1989. Experimental and accidental *C. pylori* infection of humans. In: *Campylobacter pylori* in Gastric and Peptic Ulcer Disease. M. J. Blaser (ed.). New York: Igaku Shoin Medical Publishers.

Morse, S. S. 1990. Regulating viral traffic. Issues in Science and Technology (Fall):81-84.

Moses, M. 1992. Pesticides. In: Maxcy-Rosenau-Last Public Health and Preventive Medicine. 13th ed., J. M. Last and R. B. Wallace (eds.). Norwalk, Connecticut: Appleton and Lange, chap. 24.

Murphy, E. L., B. Hanchard, and J. P. Figueroa. 1989. Modeling the risk of adult T-cell leukemia/lymphoma in persons infected with human T-lymphotropic virus type I. International Journal of Cancer 43:250-253.

Murray, C., K. Styblo, and A. Rouillon. In press. Tuberculosis. In: Disease Control Priorities in Developing Countries. D. T. Jamison and W. H. Mosley (eds.). New York: Oxford University Press.

Music, S. I., and M. G. Schultz. 1990. Field epidemiology training programs. Journal of the American Medical Association 263:3309-3311.

Musser, J. M., A. R. Hauser, M. H. Kim, P. M. Schlievert, K. Nelson, and R. K. Selander. 1991. *Streptococcus pyogenes* causing toxic-shock-like syndrome and other invasive diseases—clonal diversity and pyrogenic exotoxin expression. Proceedings of the National Academy of Sciences, USA 88:2668-2672.

Nair, G. B., R. K. Bhadra, T. Ramamurthy, A. Ramesh, and S. C. Pal. 1991. *Vibrio cholerae* and other vibrios associated with paddy field cultured prawns. Food Microbiology 8:203-208.

National Commission on Acquired Immune Deficiency Syndrome. 1991. America Living with AIDS. Washington, D.C.: National Commission on AIDS.

National Foundation for Infectious Diseases. 1991. President Bush increases immunization budget for FY '92 by $40 million. Double Helix 16(4):2.

National Institute of Allergy and Infectious Diseases. 1991a. Report of the Task Force on Microbiology and Infectious Diseases. Washington, D.C.: U.S. Department of Health and Human Services.

National Institute of Allergy and Infectious Diseases. 1991b. Research on AIDS and Opportunistic Infections. Bethesda, Maryland: National Institutes of Health.

National MDR-TB Task Force. 1992. National Action Plan to Combat Multidrug-Resistant Tuberculosis. Atlanta: Centers for Disease Control.

National Research Council. 1983. Manpower Needs and Career Opportunities in the Field Aspects of Vector Biology. Washington, D.C.: National Academy Press.

National Research Council. 1992. Global Environmental Change: Understanding the Human Dimensions. Washington, D.C.: National Academy Press.

National Research Council and Institute of Medicine. 1987. The U.S. Capacity to Address Tropical Infectious Disease Problems. Washington, D.C.: National Academy Press.

National Vaccine Advisory Committee. 1991. The measles epidemic: the problems, barriers, and recommendations. Journal of the American Medical Association 266:1547-1552.

Neurath, A. R., and S. B. H. Kent. 1988. The pre-S region of hepadnavirus envelope proteins. In: Advances in Virus Research. K. Maramorosch, F. A. Murphy, and A. J. Shatkin (eds.). San Diego: Academic Press.

Neustadt, R. E., and H. V. Fineberg. 1978. The Swine Flu Affair. Washington, D.C.: U.S. Department of Health, Education, and Welfare.

Nomura, A., G. N. Stemmerman, P.-H. Chyou, I. Kato, G. I. Perez-Perez, and M. J. Blaser. 1991. *Helicobacter pylori* infection and gastric carcinoma among Japanese Americans in Hawaii. New England Journal of Medicine 325:1132-1136.

Oaks, S. C., Jr., R. L. Ridgway, A. Shirai, and J. C. Twartz. 1983. Scrub Typhus. Bulletin No. 21. Kuala Lumpur, Malaysia: Institute for Medical Research.

O'Connor, H. J., Axon, A. T., and M. F. Dixon. 1984. *Campylobacter*-like organisms unusual in type A gastritis. Lancet 2:1091.

Office of Federal Public Health, Switzerland. 1988. Listeriosis in Switzerland. Bulletin of the Office of Federal Public Health 3:28-29.

Ognibene, A. J., and O. Barrett (eds.). 1982. Internal Medicine in Vietnam. Washington, D.C.: Office of the Surgeon General and Center for Military History, U.S. Army.

Omata, M., T. Ehata, O. Yokosuka, K. Hosoda, and M. Ohto. 1991. Mutations in the precore region of hepatitis B virus DNA in patients with fulminant and severe hepatitis. New England Journal of Medicine 324:1699-1704.

Orenstein, W. A., W. Atkinson, D. Mason, and R. H. Bernier. 1990. Barriers to vaccinating preschool children. Journal of Health Care for the Poor and Underserved 1:315-330.

Osame, M., K. Usuku, and S. Izumo. 1986. HTLV-I associated myelopathy, a new clinical entity (letter). Lancet 1:1031-1032.

Osame, M., A. Igata, and M. Matsumoto. 1990. HTLV-I associated myelopathy (HAM), treatment trials, retrospective survey, and clinical and laboratory findings. Hematology Reviews 3:271-284.

Osborn, J. E. (ed.). 1977. History, Science, and Politics: Influenza in America, 1918–1976. New York: Prodist.

Oshima, T. 1987. Anisakiasis—is the sushi bar guilty? Parasitology Today 3:44-48.

Pan American Health Organization. 1972. Venezuelan equine encephalitis. In: Workshop-Symposium on Venezuelan Encephalitis Virus, Washington, D.C.,

September 1971. Scientific Publication No. 243. Washington, D.C.: Pan American Health Organization.

Pan American Health Organization. 1991. Cholera situation in the Americas. An update. Epidemiological Bulletin 12:11-13.

Parsonnet, J., G. Friedman, D. P. Vandersteen, Y. Chang, J. H. Vogelman, N. Orentreich, and R. K. Sibley. 1991. *Helicobacter pylori* infection and the risk of gastric carcinoma. New England Journal of Medicine 325:1127-1131.

Pattyn, S. R. (ed.). 1978. Ebola Haemorrhagic Fever. North Holland: Elsevier Biomedical Press.

Pereira, B. J., E. L. Milford, R. L. Kirkman, and A. S. Levey. 1991. Transmission of hepatitis C virus by organ transplantation. New England Journal of Medicine 325:507-509.

Peters, W. 1987. Chemotherapy and Drug Resistance in Malaria, 2nd ed. London: Academic Press.

Peters, W. 1990. *Plasmodium*: resistance to antimalarial drugs. Annales de Parasitologie et Humaine Compare 65(Suppl. I):103-106.

Phelps, C. E. 1989. Bug/drug resistance. Medical Care 27:194-203.

Philip, C. B. 1948. Tsutsugamushi disease (scrub typhus) in World War II. Journal of Parasitology 34:169-191.

Phillips, R. E., S. Rowland-Jones, D. F. Nixon, F. M. Gotch, J. P. Edwards, A. O. Ogunlesi, J. G. Elvin, J. A. Rothbard, C. R. Bangham, and C. R. Rizzi. 1991. Human immunodeficiency virus genetic variation that can escape cytotoxic T cell recognition. Nature 354:433-434.

Pinheiro, F. P., A. P. A. Travassos da Rosa, J. F. S. Travassos da Rosa, R. Ishak, R. B. Freitas, M. L. C. Gomes, J. W. LeDuc, and O. F. P. Oliva. 1981. Oropouche virus. I. A review of clinical, epidemiological, and ecological findings. American Journal of Tropical Medicine and Hygiene 30:149-160.

Plumb, J. A. 1975. An 11-year summary of fish disease cases at the Southern Cooperative Fish Disease Laboratory. Proceedings of the Annual Conference of the Southeast Association of Game Fish Commissioners 29:254-260.

Poiesz, B. J., F. W. Ruscetti, and A. F. Gazdar. 1980. Detection and isolation of type C retrovirus particles from fresh and cultured lymphocytes of a patient with cutaneous T-cell lymphoma. Proceedings of the National Academy of Sciences, USA 77:7415-7419.

Pool, R. 1991. Opening up communications. Nature 353:293.

Post, L. S., D. Lee, M. Solberg, D. Furgang, J. Specchio, and C. Graham. 1985. Development of botulinal toxin and sensory deterioration during storage of vacuum- and modified atmosphere-packaged fish fillets. Journal of Food Science 50:990-996.

Prucha, R. J. 1991. Imported Canadian product: further implementation of the United States-Canada free-trade agreement. Federal Register 56:52218.

Quinn, T. C., J. M. Mann, J. W. Curran, and P. Piot. 1986. AIDS in Africa: an epidemiologic paradigm. Science 234:955-963.

Ramanathan, K., W. C. Cheah, and T. J. Dondero, Jr. (eds.). 1976. Seventy-Five Years of Medical Research in Malaysia, rev. ed. Petaling Jaya: Institute for Medical Research, Malaysia.

Rauws, E. A. J., W. Langenberg, H. J. Houthoff, H. C. Zanen, and G. N. J. Tytgat.

1988. *Campylobacter pyloris*-associated chronic active antral gastritis. Gastroenterology 94:33-40.

Reeves, W. C., and M. M. Milby. 1990. Strategies and concepts for vector control. In: Epidemiology and Control of Mosquito-Borne Arboviruses in California, 1943–1987. Sacramento: California Mosquito and Vector Control Association.

Reeves, W. C., D. Caussy, L. A. Brinton, M. M. Brenes, P. Montalvan, B. Gomez, R. C. deBritton, E. Morice, E. Gaitan, S. Loo de Lao, and W. E. Rawls. 1987. Case-control study of human papillomaviruses and cervical cancer in Latin America. International Journal of Cancer 40:450-454.

Reeves, W. C., W. E. Rawls, and L. A. Brinton. 1989. Epidemiology of genital papillomaviruses and cervical cancer. Reviews of Infectious Diseases 11:426-439.

Reister, F. A. N.d. Battle Casualties and Medical Statistics—U.S. Army Experience in the Korean War. Washington, D.C.: Surgeon General, Department of the Army.

Reyes, G. R., M. A. Purdy, J. P. Kim, K.-C. Luk, L. M. Young, K. E. Fry, and D. W. Bradley. 1990. Isolation of a cDNA from the virus responsible for enterically transmitted non-A, non-B hepatitis. Science 247:1335-1339.

Rich, A. R. 1944. The Pathogenesis of Tuberculosis. Baltimore, Maryland: Charles C. Thomas.

Rieckmann, K. H., D. R. Davis, and D. C. Hutton. 1989. *Plasmodium vivax* resistance to chloroquine? Lancet 2:1183-1184.

Robillard, N. J., and A. L. Scarpa. 1988. Genetic and physiological characterization of ciprofloxacin resistance in *Pseudomonas aeruginosa*. Antimicrobial Agents and Chemotherapy 32:535-539.

Rodcharoen, J., and M. S. Mulla. In press. Development of resistance in *Culex quinquefasciatus* (Diptera: Culicidae) to the microbial agent *Bacillus sphaericus*. Journal of Economic Entomology.

Ross, V. 1990. Nosocomial infections during the age of AIDS. ASM News 56:575-578.

Russell, C. 1991. Bled dry: nation's blood supply suffers chronic shortages. Washington Post (Oct. 15):11-12.

Saikku, P., M. Leinonen, L. Tenkanen, E. Linnanmaki, Marja-R. Ekman, V. Manninen, M. Manttari, M. H. Frick, and J. K. Huttunen. 1992. Chronic *Chlamydia pneumoniae* infection as a risk factor for coronary heart disease in the Helsinki Heart Study. Annals of Internal Medicine 116:273-278.

Salas, R., N. De Manzione, R. B. Tesh, R. Rico-Hesse, R. E. Shope, A. Betancourt, O. Godoy, R. Bruzual, M. E. Pacheco, B. Ramos, M. E. Taibo, J. G. Tamayo, E. Jaimes, C. Vasquez, F. Araoz, and J. Querales. 1991. Venezuelan haemorrhagic fever. Lancet 338:1033-1036.

Schaberg, D. R., D. H. Culver, and R. P. Gaynes. 1991. Major Trends in the Microbial Etiology of Nosocomial Infection. Atlanta: Hospital Infections Program, Center for Infectious Diseases, Centers for Disease Control.

Schaechter, M., G. Medoff, and D. Schlessinger (eds.). 1989. Mechanisms of Microbial Disease, 1st ed. Baltimore, Maryland: Williams and Wilkins.

Schlech, W. F., P. M. Lavigne, R. A. Bortolusse, A. C. Allen, E. V. Haldane, A. J. Wort, A. W. Hightower, S. E. Johnson, S. H. King, E. S. Nicholis, and C. V.

Broome. 1983. Epidemic listeriosis—evidence for transmission by food. New England Journal of Medicine 308:203-206.

Scholtissek, C., and E. Naylor. 1988. Fish farming and influenza pandemics. Nature 331:215.

Scholtissek, C., W. Rohde, V. Von Hoyningen, and R. Rott. 1978. On the origin of the human influenza virus subtypes H2N2 and H3N2. Virology 87:13-20.

Schwab, P. M. 1968. Economic cost of St. Louis encephalitis epidemic in Dallas, Texas, 1966. Public Health Reports 83:860-866.

Schwartz, I. K., E. M. Lackritz, and L. C. Patchen. 1991. Chloroquine-resistant *Plasmodium vivax* from Indonesia. New England Journal of Medicine 324:927.

Scrimenti, R. J. 1970. Erythema chronicum migrans. Archives of Dermatology 102:104-105.

Seideman, S. C., and P. R. Durland. 1984. The utilization of modified gas atmosphere packaging for fresh meat: a review. Journal of Food Quality 6:239-252.

Selander, R. K., and J. M. Musser. 1990. The population genetics of bacterial pathogenesis. In: Molecular Basis of Pathogenesis, B. H. Iglewski and V. L. Clark (eds.). New York: Academic Press.

Shapiro, M., T. R. Townsend, B. Rosner, and E. H. Kass. 1979. Use of antimicrobial drugs in general hospitals: patterns of prophylaxis. New England Journal of Medicine 301:351-355.

Shlaes, D., S. Levy, and G. Archer. 1991. Antimicrobial resistance: new directions. ASM News 57:455-458.

Smith, A. W., and P. M. Boyt. 1990. Caliciviruses of ocean origin: a review. Journal of Zoo and Wildlife Medicine 21:3-23.

Snider, D. E., and W. L. Roper. 1992. The new tuberculosis. New England Journal of Medicine 326:703-705.

Sonti, R. V., and J. R. Roth. 1989. Role of gene duplications in the adaptation of *Salmonella typhimurium* to growth on limiting carbon sources. Genetics 123: 19-28.

Soper, F. L., D. B. Wilson, S. Lima, and W. S. Antunes. 1943. The Organization of Permanent Nationwide Anti-*Aedes aegypti* Measures in Brazil. New York: The Rockefeller Foundation.

Southeastern Cooperative Wildlife Diseases Study. 1982–1988. White-Tailed Deer Populations—Maps. Washington, D.C.: Bureau of the Census, U.S. Department of Commerce.

Spielman, A. 1988. Lyme disease and human babesiosis: evidence incriminating vector and reservoir hosts. In: The Biology of Parasitism. P. T. Englund and A. Sher (eds.). New York: Alan R. Liss, Inc.

Spielman, A., M. L. Wilson, J. F. Levine, and J. Piesman. 1985. Ecology of *Ixodes dammini*-borne human babesiosis and Lyme disease. Annual Review of Entomology 30:439-460.

Spika, J. S., R. R. Facklam, B. D. Plikaytis, M. J. Oxtoby, and the Pneumococcal Surveillance Working Group. 1991. Antimicrobial resistance of *Streptococcus pneumoniae* in the United States, 1979–1987. Journal of Infectious Diseases 163: 1273-1278.

Steere, A. C., S. E. Malawista, D. E. Snydman, R. E. Shope, W. A. Andiman, M. R. Ross, and F. M. Steele. 1977. Lyme arthritis: an epidemic of oligoarticular arthritis in children and adults in three Connecticut communities. Arthrology and Rheumatology 20:7-17.

Steere, A. C., E. Taylor, M. L. Wilson, J. F. Levine, and A. Spielman. 1986. Longitudinal assessment of the clinical and epidemiological features of Lyme disease in a defined population. Journal of Infectious Diseases 154:295-300.

Stevens, D. L., M. H. Tanner, J. Winship, R. Swarts, K. M. Ries, P. M. Schlievert, and E. Kaplan. 1989. Severe group A streptococcal infections associated with a toxic shock-like syndrome and scarlet fever toxin A. New England Journal of Medicine 321:1-7.

Sudia, W. D., V. F. Newhouse, L. D. Beadle, D. I. Miller, J. G. Johnston, R. Young, C. H. Calisher, and K. Maness. 1975. Epidemic Venezuelan equine encephalitis in North America in 1971: vector studies. American Journal of Epidemiology 101:17-35.

Sugiyama, S., and K. H. Yang. 1975. Growth potential of *Clostridium botulinum* in fresh mushrooms packaged in semipermeable plastic film. Applied Microbiology 30:964-969.

Tabbara, S., A. D. M. Saleh, W. A. Andersen, S. R. Barber, P. T. Taylor, and C. P. Crum. 1992. The Bethesda classification for squamous intraepithelial lesions: histologic, cytologic, and viral correlates. Obstetrics and Gynecology 79:338-346.

Taylor, J., R. Weinberg, B. Languet, P. Desmettre, and E. Paoletti. 1988. Fowlpox virus based recombinant vaccines. In: Technological Advances in Vaccine Development, L. Lasky (ed.). New York: Alan R. Liss, Inc.

Taylor, K. C. 1991. Transmissible spongiform encephalopathies: the threat of BSE to man. Food Microbiology 8:257-258.

Terzaghi, E., and M. O'Hara. 1990. Microbial plasticity—the relevance to microbial ecology (review). Advances in Microbial Ecology 11:431-460.

Thacker, S. B., and R. L. Berkelman. 1988. Public health surveillance in the United States. Epidemiologic Reviews 10:164-190.

Thacker, S. B., R. A. Goodman, and R. C. Dicker. 1990. Training and service in public health practice, 1951–1990—CDC's Epidemic Intelligence Service. Public Health Reports 105:599-603.

Thayer, D. W. 1990. Food irradiation: benefits and concerns. Journal of Food Quality 13:147-169.

Theiler, M., and W. G. Downs. 1973. The Arthropod-Borne Viruses of Vertebrates (An Account of The Rockefeller Foundation Virus Program, 1951–1970). London: Yale University Press.

Thomson, B. F. 1977. The Changing Face of New England. Boston: Houghton Mifflin.

Tibayrenc, M., F. Kjellberg, J. Arnaud, B. Oury, S. F. Breniere, M. L. Darde, and F. J. Ayala. 1991a. Are eukaryotic microorganisms clonal or sexual—a population genetics vantage. Proceedings of the National Academy of Sciences, USA 88:5129-5133.

Tibayrenc, M., F. Kjellberg, and F. J. Ayala. 1991b. The clonal theory of parasitic protozoa—a taxonomic proposal applicable to other clonal organisms. BioScience 41:767-774.

Tirrell, S., R. Shope, J. Meegan, and C. Peters. 1985. Rift Valley fever diagnosis, surveillance, and control. Fourth International Conference on the Impact of Viral Diseases on the Development of African and Middle East Countries, Rabat, Morocco, April 14–19.

Toorn, P. G., J. R. Arrand, L. P. Wilson, and D. S. Sharp. 1986. Human papillomavirus infection of the uterine cervix of women without cytological signs of neoplasia. British Medical Journal 293:1261-1264.

Trias, J., and H. Nikaido. 1990. Outer membrane protein D2 catalyzes facilitated diffusion of carbapenems and penems through the outer membrane of *Pseudomonas aeruginosa*. Antimicrobial Agents and Chemotherapy 34:52-57.

Uchiyama, T., J. Yodoi, and D. Sagawa. 1977. Adult T-cell leukemia: clinical and hematologic features of 16 cases. Blood 50:481-491.

Umenai, T., H. W. Lee, P. W. Lee, T. Saito, T. Toyodat, M. Hongo, K. Yoshinaga, T. Nobunaga, T. Horiuchi, and N. Ishida. 1979. Korean hemorrhagic fever in staff in an animal laboratory. Lancet 1:1314-1316.

United Nations. 1985. United Nations Demographic Yearbook 1983. New York: Statistical Office, Department of International Economic and Social Affairs, United Nations.

U.S. Army Medical Research Unit, Malaya. 1962. Annual Progress Report, 1 July 1961–30 June 1962. Kuala Lumpur, Malaya: Institute for Medical Research.

U.S. Department of Health and Human Services. 1990. Healthy People 2000: National Health Promotion and Disease Prevention Objectives. DHHS Publication No. (PHS) 91-50212. Washington, D.C.: Public Health Service.

U.S. Department of Health and Human Services. 1991. A plan to strengthen public health in the United States. Public Health Reports 106(Supplement 1):1-86.

U.S. Department of Health and Human Services. 1992. Tuberculosis: an update. HHS Issue Profile 14:1-2.

U.S. Medicine. 1991. Panama health ministry will retain some operations at Gorgas Lab. U.S. Medicine (Feb.):16.

Usuku, K., S. Sonoda, and M. Osame. 1988. HLA haplotype-linked high immune responsiveness against HTLV-I in HTLV-I associated myelopathy: comparison with adult T-cell leukemia/lymphoma. Annals of Neurology 23:S143-S150.

Vartanian, J. P., A. Meyerhans, B. Asjo, and S. Wain-Hobson. 1991. Selection, recombination, and G: a hypermutation of human immunodeficiency virus type 1 genomes. Journal of Virology 65:1779-1788.

Waksman, S. A. 1964. The Conquest of Tuberculosis. London: Robert Hale, Ltd.

Ward, D. R. 1989. Microbiology of aquaculture products. Food Technology 43:82-86.

Warren, J. R., and B. Marshall. 1983. Unidentified curved bacilli on gastric epithelium in active chronic gastritis. Lancet 2:1273-1275.

Washington Headquarters Service Directorate for Information, Operations, and Reports, Department of Defense. 1985. U.S. Casualties in Southeast Asia— Statistics as of April 30, 1985. Washington, D.C.: U.S. Government Printing Office.

Watanabe, M., S. Iyobe, M. Inoue, and S. Mitsuhashi. 1991. Transferable imipenem resistance in *Pseudomonas aeruginosa*. Antimicrobial Agents and Chemotherapy 35:147-151.

Webster, R. G., J. Geraci, G. Petursson, and K. Skirnisson. 1981. Conjunctivitis in human beings caused by influenza A virus of seals. New England Journal of Medicine 304:911.

Weiss, R. 1992. On the track of "killer" TB. Science 255:148-150.

Wenzel, R. P. 1987. Towards a global perspective of nosocomial infections. European Journal of Clinical Microbiology 6:341-342.

Wenzel, R. P. 1988. The mortality of hospital-acquired bloodstream infections: need for a new vital statistic? International Journal of Epidemiology 17:225-226.

Wenzel, R. P., M. D. Nettleman, R. N. Jones, and M. A. Pfaller. 1991. Methicillin-resistant *Staphylococcus aureus*: implications for the 1990s and effective control measures. American Journal of Medicine 91(Suppl. 3B):221S-227S.

Wharton, M., T. L. Chorba, R. L. Vogt, D. L. Morse, and J. W. Buehler. 1990. Case definitions for public health surveillance. Morbidity and Mortality Weekly Report 39:1-43.

Williams, R. C. 1951. On guard against disease from without. In: The United States Public Health Service, 1798–1950. Washington, D.C.: Commissioned Officers Association of the United States Public Health Service, chap. 2.

Wilson, M. E. 1991. A World Guide to Infections: Diseases, Distribution, Diagnosis. New York: Oxford University Press.

Wimpfheimer, L., N. S. Altman, and J. H. Hotchkiss. 1990. Growth of *Listeria monocytogenes* Scott A, serotype 4 and competitive spoilage organisms in raw chicken packaged under modified atmospheres and in air. International Journal of Food Microbiology 11:205-214.

World Health Organization. 1991. In Point of Fact. Geneva: World Health Organization.

World Health Organization. 1992. Global Health Situations and Projections, Estimates 1992. Geneva: World Health Organization.

World Resources Institute. 1986. World Resources 1986: An Assessment of the Resource Base That Supports the Global Economy. New York: World Resources Institute, International Institute for Environment and Development, Basic Books.

Yamanishi, K., J. R. Dantas, M. Takahishi, T. Yamanouchi, K. Domae, J. Kawamata, and T. Kurata. 1983. Isolation of hemorrhagic fever with renal syndrome (HFRS) virus from a tumor specimen in a rat. Biken Journal 26:155-160.

Yamashiroya, H. M., L. Ghosh, R. Yang, and A. L. Robertson, Jr. 1988. Herpesviridae in the coronary arteries and aorta of young trauma victims. American Journal of Pathology 130:71-79.

Young, M. D., and D. V. Moore. 1961. Chloroquine resistance in *Plasmodium falciparum*. American Journal of Tropical Medicine and Hygiene 10:317-320.

Zinsser, H. 1935. Rats, Lice, and History. Boston: Little, Brown and Company.

Appendixes

A

Task Forces

At its first meeting, the Committee on Emerging Microbial Threats to Health decided to form four task forces to obtain input from the scientific community at large. Each task force (with the exception of Task Force 4) was composed of both committee and noncommittee members and a rapporteur. Task Forces 1 through 3 dealt with specific categories of organisms; Task Force 4 examined policy options that the committee might wish to consider in developing its recommendations. It was later decided to establish a fifth task force to refine the recommendations drafted by the full committee at its third meeting in January 1992. In the lists below, committee members are designated by an asterisk.

TASK FORCE 1

Bacteria, Rickettsiae, and Chlamydiae

Task Force 1 met in Washington, D.C. on May 20-21, 1991, with the following participants:

BARRY R. BLOOM,* Department of Microbiology and Immunology and Howard Hughes Medical Institute, Albert Einstein College of Medicine, Yeshiva University

ROBERT L. BUCHANAN,* Microbial Food Safety Research Unit, Agricultural Research Service, U.S. Department of Agriculture, Eastern Regional Research Center

J. THOMAS GRAYSTON, Department of Epidemiology, University of Washington

GEORGE A. JACOBY, JR., Infectious Disease Unit, Massachusetts General Hospital

GERALD L. MANDELL, (*Chair*),* Division of Infectious Diseases, Department of Internal Medicine, University of Virginia

WILLIAM A. PETRI, JR. (*Rapporteur*), Medicine and Microbiology, Divisions of Infectious Diseases and Geographic Medicine, University of Virginia Health Sciences Center

P. FREDERICK SPARLING,* Department of Medicine, University of North Carolina School of Medicine

ANDREW SPIELMAN,* Department of Tropical Public Health, Harvard School of Public Health

DAVID H. WALKER, Department of Pathology, University of Texas Medical Branch

RICHARD P. WENZEL, Department of Clinical Epidemiology, University of Iowa Hospital

TASK FORCE 2

Viruses

Task Force 2 met in Washington, D.C., on May 16-17, 1991, with the following participants:

BRUCE F. ELDRIDGE, University of California Mosquito Research Program, Department of Entomology, University of California at Davis

PATRICIA N. FULTZ,* Department of Microbiology, University of Alabama at Birmingham

DUANE J. GUBLER, Vector-Borne Infectious Diseases Division, National Center for Infectious Diseases, Centers for Disease Control

JAMES L. HARDY, School of Public Health, University of California at Berkeley

FREDERICK G. HAYDEN, Department of Internal Medicine, University of Virginia Hospital

JOHN J. HOLLAND,* Department of Biology and Institute for Molecular Biology, University of California at San Diego

RICHARD T. JOHNSON, Department of Neurology, Microbiology, and Neuroscience, Johns Hopkins University School of Medicine

EDWIN D. KILBOURNE,* Department of Microbiology, Mount Sinai School of Medicine

STEPHEN S. MORSE (*Chair*),* Rockefeller University

FREDERICK A. MURPHY, School of Veterinary Medicine, University of
California at Davis
THOMAS W. SCOTT (*Rapporteur*), Department of Entomology, University
of Maryland at College Park
ALEXIS SHELOKOV,* Salk Institute, Government Services Division

TASK FORCE 3

Protozoans, Helminths, and Fungi

Task Force 3 met in Washington, D.C., on May 8, 1991, with the following participants:

RONALD E. BLANTON (*Rapporteur*), Division of Geographic Medicine,
Department of Medicine, Case Western Reserve University, School
of Medicine
CARLOS C. CAMPBELL, Malaria Branch, Parasitic Diseases Division,
National Center for Infectious Diseases, Centers for Disease Control
WILLIAM E. DISMUKES, Department of Medicine, Division of Infectious
Disease, University of Alabama School of Medicine
ADEL A. F. MAHMOUD (*Chair*),* Department of Medicine, Case Western
Reserve University, University Hospitals of Cleveland
ROSEMARY SOAVE, Division of Infectious Diseases, Cornell Medical
Center, New York Hospital
ANDREW SPIELMAN,* Department of Tropical Public Health, Harvard
School of Public Health
ROBERT B. TESH, Yale Arbovirus Research Unit, Department of
Epidemiology and Public Health, Yale University School of Medicine

TASK FORCE 4

Policy Options

Task Force 4 met in Washington, D.C., on May 13-14, 1991, with the
following participants:

BARRY R. BLOOM,* Department of Microbiology and Immunology,
Howard Hughes Medical Institute, Albert Einstein College of Medicine,
Yeshiva University
CIRO A. DE QUADROS, Expanded Programme on Immunization, Pan
American Health Organization
WALTER R. DOWDLE, Centers for Disease Control

DEAN T. JAMISON,* Department of Community Health Sciences and
  Department of Education, University of California at Los Angeles
ADETOKUNBO LUCAS, Department of Population Sciences, Harvard
  School of Public Health
HARRY M. MEYER, JR., Medical Research Division, American
  Cyanamid Company
PHILIP K. RUSSELL, (*Chair*),* School of Hygiene and Public Health,
  Johns Hopkins University
ROBERT E. SHOPE,* Yale Arbovirus Research Unit, Yale University
  School of Medicine

TASK FORCE 5

Recommendations

Task Force 5 met in Washington, D.C., on February 17, 1992, with the
following participants:

JOSHUA LEDERBERG,* Rockefeller University
ADEL A. F. MAHMOUD,* Department of Medicine, Case Western Reserve
  University, University Hospitals of Cleveland
GERALD L. MANDELL, Division of Infectious Diseases, Department of
  Internal Medicine, University of Virginia
STEPHEN S. MORSE,* Rockefeller University
PHILIP K. RUSSELL,* School of Hygiene and Public Health, Johns
  Hopkins University
ROBERT E. SHOPE, (*Chair*),* Yale Arbovirus Research Unit,
  Yale University School of Medicine

B

Catalog of Emerging
Infectious Disease Agents

The material in this appendix is provided for those who are interested in more detail on each of the agents considered by this committee to be emerging or reemerging and listed earlier in the report (see Table 2-1). It is a brief summary of information compiled from three sources, listed below, as well as additional data provided by committee and task force members, and other experts. The individual summaries are separated into three sections, corresponding to the categorizations of the earlier charts.

Benenson, Abram S. (ed.) 1990. Control of Communicable Diseases in Man, 15th edition. Washington, D.C.: American Public Health Association.

Mandell, Gerald L.; Douglas, R. Gordon, Jr.; and Bennett, John E. (eds.) 1990. Principles and Practice of Infectious Disease, 3rd edition. New York: Churchill Livingstone.

Wilson, Mary E. 1991. A World Guide to Infections: Diseases, Distribution, Diagnosis. New York: Oxford University Press.

EMERGENT BACTERIA, RICKETTSIAE, AND CHLAMYDIAE

Aeromonas

DISEASE(S) AND SYMPTOMS

Aeromonad gastroenteritis
—acute diarrhea lasting several days, abdominal pain
—vomiting, fever, and bloody stools may be present

Cellulitis, wound infection, and septicemia
—septicemia occurs most often in predisposed patients

DIAGNOSIS

— identification of the organism in patient's feces or in wound secretions

INFECTIOUS AGENT

— *Aeromonas hydrophila*, *A. veronii* (biovariant *sobria*), *A. caviae*
— other species of *Aeromonas* (*A. jandaei*, *A. trota*, *A. schubertii*, and *A. veronii* biovariant *veronii*) have also been associated with human disease
— the natural habitats of *Aeromonas* bacteria are water and soil

MODE OF TRANSMISSION

— ingestion of contaminated water
— entry of organism through a break in the skin

DISTRIBUTION

— presence of organism in clinical specimens has been documented in the Americas, Africa, Asia, Australia, and Europe
— distribution is worldwide

INCUBATION PERIOD

— undefined; probably 12 hours to several days
— organism may persist for weeks to months in gastrointestinal tract

TREATMENT

— antibiotics: trimethoprim-sulfamethoxazole, the quinolones, aminoglycosides, and tetracyclines
— organisms tend to be resistant to penicillins and cephalosporins

PREVENTION AND CONTROL

— proper treatment of drinking water and monitoring of well water
— predisposed individuals should avoid aquatic environments

FACTORS FACILITATING EMERGENCE

— predisposition (e.g., immunosuppression)
— improved technology for detection and differentiation
— increased awareness

Borrelia burgdorferi

DISEASE(S) AND SYMPTOMS

Lyme disease
— distinctive skin lesion (erythema migrans) at site of tick bite that

appears as a red papule and expands in an annular fashion to at least 5 cm. in diameter
— fatigue, headache, stiffness, myalgia, lymphadenopathy
— neurologic (10 to 15% of patients) and cardiac (6 to 10% of patients) abnormalities may develop weeks to months after lesion
— months to years after onset, swelling and pain in large joints may develop and persist for years ("Lyme arthritis")

DIAGNOSIS

— currently based on clinical findings and serologic tests
— tests are poorly standardized and are insensitive during the first several weeks of infection

INFECTIOUS AGENT

— *Borrelia burgdorferi*, a spirochete bacterium

MODE OF TRANSMISSION

— bite of an *Ixodes* tick; transmission does not occur until tick has fed for several hours
— wild rodents (especially the white-footed mouse) and white-tailed deer maintain transmission cycle; tick depends on deer to reproduce and feeds on mice to become infected
— no evidence for person-to-person transmission
— transplacental transmission has been documented

DISTRIBUTION

— in the United States: Atlantic coastal states from Maine to Georgia; upper midwestern states (concentrated in Minnesota and Wisconsin); California and Oregon
— abroad: Europe, Canada, Japan, Australia, China, and the Commonwealth of Independent States

INCUBATION PERIOD

— erythema migrans appears 3 to 32 days after tick exposure

TREATMENT

— oral antibiotics (tetracycline, doxycycline, amoxicillin, erythromycin) for 10 to 30 days
— high-dose intravenous penicillin or ceftriaxone is used if neurologic abnormalities develop
— novel drug regimens are undergoing evaluation

PREVENTION AND CONTROL

— avoidance of tick-infested areas; securing of clothing at entry points (ankles, cuffs, etc.); application of tick repellent to outer clothing
— host (mice and deer) reduction

FACTORS FACILITATING EMERGENCE

— reforestation and consequent proliferation of deer
— housing development in wooded areas

Campylobacter jejuni

DISEASE(S) AND SYMPTOMS

Campylobacteriosis, campylobacter enteritis
— abdominal pain, diarrhea, fever
— illness typically lasts two to five days
— prolonged illness and relapses may occur
— infection is asymptomatic in many cases

DIAGNOSIS

— detection of organism in the stool

INFECTIOUS AGENT

— *Campylobacter jejuni*, a bacterium
— other species within the genus *Campylobacter* have been associated with similar disease

MODE OF TRANSMISSION

— ingestion of contaminated food, water, or milk
— fecal-oral spread from infected person or animal

DISTRIBUTION

— worldwide
— organism has a vast reservoir in animals

INCUBATION PERIOD AND COMMUNICABILITY

— incubation period is 2 to 5 days
— disease is communicable throughout the course of infection

TREATMENT

— rehydration and replacement of electrolytes
— antibiotic therapy is used in some cases, though it rarely shortens duration of symptoms

PREVENTION AND CONTROL

— chlorination of water
— proper cooking of foods (particularly poultry) and pasteurization of milk
— handwashing after animal contact

FACTORS FACILITATING EMERGENCE

— improved recognition of the organism
— an increase in poultry consumption in recent years

Chlamydia pneumoniae (TWAR Strain)

DISEASE(S) AND SYMPTOMS

TWAR infection, TWAR pneumonia
— fever, myalgias, cough, sore throat, sinusitis
— illness is usually mild, but recovery is slow; cough tends to last for more than two weeks

DIAGNOSIS

— isolation of organism from throat or sputum

INFECTIOUS AGENT

— *Chlamydia pneumoniae* (TWAR), a chlamydia
— strain name is derived from designation of first two isolates, TW-183 from Taiwan and AR-39 (acute respiratory)

MODE OF TRANSMISSION

— person to person; thought to be acquired by inhalation of infective organisms
— possibly by direct contact with secretions of an infected person

DISTRIBUTION

— probably worldwide
— the majority of cases have occurred in North America, Asia, and Europe

INCUBATION PERIOD AND COMMUNICABILITY

— 1 to 4 weeks
— period of communicability is unknown but presumed to be long, based on duration of documented outbreaks

TREATMENT

   — antibiotics: tetracycline or erythromycin

PREVENTION AND CONTROL

   — avoidance of overcrowding in living and sleeping quarters

FACTORS FACILITATING EMERGENCE

   — increased recognition

Chlamydia trachomatis

DISEASE(S) AND SYMPTOMS

  Genital chlamydia
   — urethritis in males, mucopurulent cervicitis in females (opaque discharge, itching, burning upon urination)
   — asymptomatic infection can occur
   — in women, infertility and ectopic pregnancy can result from chronic infection

DIAGNOSIS

   — identification of organism on intraurethral or endocervical swab material

INFECTIOUS AGENT

   — *Chlamydia trachomatis*, a bacterium

MODE OF TRANSMISSION

   — sexual intercourse

DISTRIBUTION

   — worldwide; recognition has increased in the United States, Canada, Europe, and Australia over the past two decades

INCUBATION PERIOD AND COMMUNICABILITY

   — incubation period is poorly defined, probably 7 to 14 days or longer
   — period of communicability is unknown

TREATMENT

   — oral antibiotics: tetracycline, doxycycline, or quinolone

PREVENTION AND CONTROL

   — condom use during sexual intercourse
   — prophylactic treatment of sexual partners

Factors Facilitating Emergence

— probably increased sexual activity

Clostridium difficile

Disease(s) and Symptoms

Clostridium difficile colitis
— antibiotic-associated colitis
— pseudomembranous colitis
— watery diarrhea, bloody diarrhea, abdominal pain

Diagnosis

— detection of *C. difficile* toxin in the stool
— visualization of characteristic pseudomembranes during endoscopy of colon

Infectious Agent

— *Clostridium difficile*, a toxin-producing bacterium

Mode of Transmission

— fecal-oral transmission
— acquisition of organism from the environment

Distribution

— worldwide
— an estimated 3 percent of healthy adults carry the organism in the gut

Incubation Period and Communicability

— colitis typically begins during, or shortly after, antibiotic administration (changes in gastrointestinal tract flora due to antibiotic use allow proliferation of the organism and its production of toxins)

Treatment

— discontinuation of aggravating antibiotic treatment if possible
— antibacterial agents: metronidazole, vancomycin, bacitracin

Prevention and Control

— avoidance of unnecessary antibiotic administration

Factors Facilitating Emergence

— immunosuppression
— increased recognition

Ehrlichia chaffeensis

DISEASE(S) AND SYMPTOMS

Ehrlichiosis
— fever, malaise, headache, lymphadenopathy, anorexia
— fever usually lasts 2 weeks
— meningitis is occasionally reported

DIAGNOSIS

— poor; few laboratories have antigen for immunoflourescence
  serology by surrogate *E. canis* antigen

INFECTIOUS AGENT

— *Ehrlichia chaffeensis*, a rickettsia
— reservoir is unknown

MODE OF TRANSMISSION

— an undetermined tick transmits the agent (possibly the widely
  distributed species, *Amblyomma americanum*)
— no evidence of person-to-person transmission
— although other types of Ehrlichia are transmitted to dogs by the
  brown dog tick, dogs have not been found to be reservoirs of human
  disease

DISTRIBUTION

— Southern and mid-Atlantic United States

INCUBATION PERIOD

— unknown; possibly 1 to 3 weeks

TREATMENT

— oral antibiotics: tetracycline

PREVENTION AND CONTROL

— avoidance of tick-infested areas; securing of clothing at entry points
  (ankles, cuffs, etc.); application of tick repellent to outer clothing

FACTORS FACILITATING EMERGENCE

— organism is probably newly recognized
— possible increase in reservoir and vector populations

Escherichia coli O157:H7

DISEASE(S) AND SYMPTOMS

— Hemorrhagic colitis; hemolytic uremic syndrome

DIAGNOSIS

— identification of antibodies to O157:H7 serotype

INFECTIOUS AGENT

— *Escherichia coli* O157:H7, a bacterium
— one of several "EHEC" (enterohemorrhagic *E. coli*) strains
— EHEC bacteria produce potent cytotoxins, called Shiga-like toxins 1 and 2
— cattle are believed to be the reservoirs of EHECs

MODE OF TRANSMISSION

— ingestion of contaminated food, typically poorly cooked beef and raw milk
— transmission by direct contact may occur in high-risk populations

DISTRIBUTION

— probably worldwide
— most cases have occurred in North America and Europe

INCUBATION PERIOD

— 12 to 60 hours

TREATMENT

— oral replacement of fluids and electrolytes (intravenous if necessary)

PREVENTION AND CONTROL

— proper cooking of meat
— hand washing
— proper sewage and water treatment

FACTORS FACILITATING EMERGENCE

— probably spread of a bacterial virus carrying the gene for Shiga-like toxin production into the otherwise unremarkable host, *E. coli* O157:H7

Haemophilus influenzae **biogroup** *aegyptius*

Disease(s) and Symptoms

Brazilian purpuric fever
— irritation of the conjunctivae of the eyes, followed by edema of the eyelids, photophobia, and mucopurulent discharge
— high fever appears 3 to 15 days after conjunctivitis, along with vomiting and purpura
— case fatality rate is 70 percent, with death occurring shortly after onset of systemic symptoms
— disease was first recognized in 1984

Diagnosis

— microscopic examination of bacterial culture of conjunctival discharge
— detection of organism in the blood

Infectious Agent

— *Haemophilus influenzae* biogroup *aegyptius*, a bacterium

Mode of Transmission

— contact with the conjunctival or respiratory discharges of infected persons
— eye flies are suspected mechanical vectors

Distribution

— nearly all reported cases of Brazilian purpuric fever have occurred in southern Brazil (most cases have been in young children)
— one case was reported from Australia

Incubation Period and Communicability

— incubation period is unknown
— disease is communicable for the duration of active infection

Treatment

— high-dose intravenous antibiotics: ampicillin, chloramphenicol

Prevention and Control

— prompt treatment of patients and close contacts
— avoidance of exposure to eye flies
— possibly vector control

Factors Facilitating Emergence

— possibly an increase in bacterial virulence due to mutation

Helicobacter pylori

DISEASE(S) AND SYMPTOMS

— dyspepsia, abdominal pain
— chronic infection may result in peptic ulcer, gastric cancer

DIAGNOSIS

— detection of antibodies in blood by ELISA
— biopsy and culture

INFECTIOUS AGENT

— *Helicobacter pylori*, a bacterium (formerly known as *Campylobacter pylori*)

MODE OF TRANSMISSION

— unknown; some studies suggest a zoonotic origin

DISTRIBUTION

— worldwide

INCUBATION PERIOD AND COMMUNICABILITY

— unknown

TREATMENT

— antibiotics: metronidazole, ampicillin, tetracycline
— bismuth

PREVENTION AND CONTROL

— none

FACTORS FACILITATING EMERGENCE

— increased recognition

Legionella pneumophila

DISEASE(S) AND SYMPTOMS

Legionnaires' disease, Pontiac fever
— initial symptoms include malaise, headache, myalgias, fever, chills, and cough
— fever rises rapidly within 1 day, and may precede the development of pulmonary symptoms

— changes in mental status occur in 25 to 75 percent of patients
— complications include renal failure, lung abscesses, and extrapulmonary infection
— Pontiac fever may represent a reaction to inhaled antigen rather than bacterial invasion; patients recover in 2 to 5 days without treatment

DIAGNOSIS

— isolation of the organism on special media
— demonstration of organism by direct immunofluorescence stain of involved tissue or respiratory secretions

INFECTIOUS AGENT

— *Legionella pneumophila*, a bacterium

MODE OF TRANSMISSION

— aerosol transmission via aerosol-producing devices (especially air cooling systems)
— person-to-person transmission has not been documented

DISTRIBUTION

— documented as an important cause of pneumonia in North America, Europe, Asia, and Australia
— also identified in South America and Africa

INCUBATION PERIOD

— 2 to 10 days for Legionnaires' disease
— 5 to 66 hours for Pontiac fever

TREATMENT

— for Legionnaires' disease, antibiotics: erythromycin and rifampin

PREVENTION AND CONTROL

— drainage of cooling towers when not in use
— hyperchlorination and elevation of hot water temperature have been partially successful in interrupting waterborne outbreaks

FACTORS FACILITATING EMERGENCE

— recognition in an epidemic situation

Listeria monocytogenes

DISEASE(S) AND SYMPTOMS

Listeriosis
— typically manifested as meningoencephalitis and/or septicemia (preceded by fever, headache, and vomiting)
— delirium, shock, and coma may occur
— disease is particularly dangerous to pregnant women, whose infants may be stillborn if infected
— immunosuppressive conditions facilitate infection
— fetuses and newborn infants are especially susceptible to infection

DIAGNOSIS

— isolation of organism from the blood or cerebrospinal fluid

INFECTIOUS AGENT

— *Listeria monocytogenes*, a bacterium

MODE OF TRANSMISSION

— ingestion of contaminated foods (particularly nonreheated hotdogs, undercooked chicken, various soft cheeses, and food purchased from store delicatessen counters[1])
— direct contact with organism or with soil contaminated with infected animal feces
— transmission can also occur by inhalation of the organism

DISTRIBUTION

— worldwide

INCUBATION PERIOD AND COMMUNICABILITY

— incubation period is extremely variable (from 3 to 70 days)
— disease is communicable for duration of infection

TREATMENT

— antibiotics: penicillin, ampicillin, cotrimoxazole

---

[1] Centers for Disease Control, 1992h.

PREVENTION AND CONTROL
- for pregnant women, avoidance of certain foods (see above) is recommended
- proper food-handling practices
- pasteurization of dairy products

FACTORS FACILITATING EMERGENCE
- increased awareness, recognition, and reporting

Mycobacterium tuberculosis

DISEASE(S) AND SYMPTOMS

Tuberculosis
- cough, weight loss, night sweats, and low-grade fever
- hemoptysis and chest pain are common
- extrapulmonary tuberculosis can cause symptoms involving any organ system including kidneys, liver, and central nervous system

DIAGNOSIS
- identification of tubercle bacteria in patient's sputum
- characteristic changes visible in chest x-ray

INFECTIOUS AGENT
- *Mycobacterium tuberculosis*, a mycobacterium

MODE OF TRANSMISSION
- inhalation of droplet nuclei containing the bacteria (droplet nuclei can remain suspended in the air for up to 2 hours)

DISTRIBUTION
- worldwide
- annually, 8 million people develop clinical tuberculosis and 3 million people die of tuberculosis
- it is estimated that up to 50 percent of the world's population (2 billion people) are infected, clinically or subclinically, with tuberculosis

INCUBATION PERIOD AND COMMUNICABILITY
- 4 to 12 weeks
- disease is communicable as long as viable bacteria remain in the sputum

TREATMENT

— chemotherapy involving a combination of antibiotics (esp. isoniazid and rifampin) for a period of 6 to 12 months

PREVENTION AND CONTROL

— treatment of patients with active infection to prevent spread
— strict respiratory isolation for patients with active pulmonary infection
— preventive antibiotic treatment of contacts

FACTORS FACILITATING EMERGENCE

— an increase in immunosuppressed populations

Staphylococcus aureus (and Toxic Shock Syndrome)

DISEASE(S) AND SYMPTOMS

Toxic shock syndrome
— although symptoms of infection with *S. aureus* can range from a single pustule to septicemia to death, "toxic shock syndrome," a newly emerged disease caused by *S. aureus* is the focus of this summary
— symptoms of toxic shock syndrome (TSS) include sudden onset of high fever, vomiting, profuse diarrhea, myalgia, hypotension, and, in severe cases, shock
— a sunburn-like rash is present in the acute phase of the disease, often accompanied by desquamation of the palms and soles
— disorientation and alterations in consciousness may be present

DIAGNOSIS

— isolation of the bacteria from the vagina or from abscess

INFECTIOUS AGENT

— *Staphylococcus aureus*, a bacterium

MODE OF TRANSMISSION

— TSS has been associated with use of super-absorbent tampons, prolonged use of diaphragms, and cesarean section deliveries
— reported cases of TSS in males have been linked to local *S. aureus* infections such as abscesses and postsurgical infections
— not directly transmitted from person to person

DISTRIBUTION

— sporadic cases throughout the world
— TSS epidemic in the United States occurred 1980-1981

INCUBATION PERIOD

— unknown

TREATMENT

— initial treatment involves replacement of lost fluids/electrolytes
— intravenous antibiotics

PREVENTION AND CONTROL

— avoidance/minimal use of highly absorbent tampons
— a better understanding of factors associated with nonmenstrual cases is needed

FACTORS FACILITATING EMERGENCE

— use of super-absorbent tampons

Streptococcus pyogenes (Group A)

DISEASE(S) AND SYMPTOMS

— the most common conditions caused by group A streptococcal bacteria are sore throat and skin infection
— other conditions caused by the bacteria include scarlet fever, rheumatic fever, puerperal fever, septicemia, wound infections, and pneumonia
— rarely, group A bacteria cause sepsis and streptococcal toxic shock syndrome (which can be fatal)

DIAGNOSIS

— identification of group A streptococcal antigen in pharyngeal secretions

INFECTIOUS AGENT

— *Streptococcus pyogenes* (group A), a bacterium

MODE OF TRANSMISSION

— direct or intimate contact with infected persons/carriers of the organism
— outbreaks of streptococcal sore throat have been linked to contaminated food

DISTRIBUTION

— worldwide

INCUBATION PERIOD AND COMMUNICABILITY

— 1 to 3 days
— with antibiotic therapy, period of communicability is as short as 1 to 2 days
— untreated cases, especially those involving purulent discharges, can be communicable for weeks to months

TREATMENT

— antibiotics: penicillin

PREVENTION AND CONTROL

— in some cases, prophylactic treatment of close contacts with penicillin
— people with respiratory infections or skin infections should not directly handle food

FACTORS FACILITATING EMERGENCE

— probably a change in the virulence of some streptococci in this group has been responsible for deadly infections

Vibrio cholerae

DISEASE(S) AND SYMPTOMS

Cholera
— sudden onset of profuse, watery diarrhea followed by profound dehydration
— can progress to shock within 4 to 12 hours
— in severe untreated cases, death can occur within hours

DIAGNOSIS

— isolation of organism from stool or rectal swab

INFECTIOUS AGENT

— *Vibrio cholerae* serogroup O1, biotypes *cholerae* and El Tor (bacteria)

MODE OF TRANSMISSION

— ingestion of water contaminated with the feces of infected persons (organism is easily killed with chlorination but can survive in ice cubes, salt water, and mineral water)
— ingestion of food washed with contaminated water

DISTRIBUTION

— epidemics are sporadic, the most recent being in South America in 1991
— disease is endemic in southern Asia

INCUBATION PERIOD AND COMMUNICABILITY

— from a few hours to 5 days; usually 2 to 3 days
— direct, person-to-person transmission is of minor importance in areas with good sanitary facilities

TREATMENT

— replacement of fluids and electrolytes (oral rehydration therapy [ORT])
— antibiotics eradicate organisms and shorten duration of illness, but are secondary in importance to rehydration

PREVENTION AND CONTROL

— currently available vaccine provides only partial protection (50%) of short duration (3 to 6 months) and thus is of no practical value in epidemic control
— avoidance of contaminated food and water, as well as raw and undercooked crabs and shellfish harvested from potentially contaminated water

FACTORS FACILITATING EMERGENCE

— breakdown of sanitation measures protecting water supplies
— in Peru, miscalculation of risks involved in chlorine use (and consequent lack of chlorine use)

Vibrio vulnificus

DISEASE(S) AND SYMPTOMS

— varies from cellulitis to fatal bacteremia associated with chronic cutaneous ulcers
— soft tissue infection and septicemia can occur if organism enters body percutaneously
— organism has occasionally been associated with diarrheal illness

DIAGNOSIS

— isolation of the organism from blood or cutaneous lesions in bacteremic cases

INFECTIOUS AGENT

— *Vibrio vulnificus*, a bacterium

MODE OF TRANSMISSION
- contact of superficial wounds with seawater or seafood containing the organism
- ingestion of contaminated water or food (usually raw or undercooked seafood) by immunocompromised persons, especially those with hepatic cirrhosis
- not transmitted person to person

DISTRIBUTION
- organism is most commonly found in the Gulf states of the United States and is probably part of the normal marine flora in warmer climates

INCUBATION PERIOD
- incubation period is 10 to 20 hours

TREATMENT
- antibiotic therapy
- surgical drainage may be necessary with soft tissue infections
- supportive treatment for diarrheal illness (e.g., oral fluid replacement)

PREVENTION AND CONTROL
- avoidance of exposure of open skin wounds to seawater
- careful handling of raw or undercooked seafood by persons with superficial wounds
- avoidance of raw or undercooked seafood, particularly by immunocompromised persons

FACTORS FACILITATING EMERGENCE
- increased recognition

EMERGENT VIRUSES

Bovine Spongiform Encephalopathy Agent

DISEASE(S) AND SYMPTOMS

Bovine spongiform encephalopathy (BSE) in cattle
- progressive neurological disease, staggering
- BSE agent has *not* caused any cases of human disease

DIAGNOSIS
- histology of brain tissue
- epidemiological characteristics
- no serological tests are currently available

INFECTIOUS AGENT

— BSE agent, a virus-like agent similar to scrapie prion in sheep

MODE OF TRANSMISSION

— probably ingestion by cattle of poorly disinfected sheep offal

DISTRIBUTION

— epidemic in England in 1990; cases in France and Switzerland

INCUBATION PERIOD AND COMMUNICABILITY

— unknown

TREATMENT

— none

PREVENTION AND CONTROL

— destruction of infected animals to prevent spread
— control measures instituted during 1990 epidemic: restrictions on use
of cattle serum and cells for pharmaceutical (including vaccines)
manufacturing in Europe
— changes in the rendering process (a return to batch processing and
solvent use) will probably provide effective control

FACTORS FACILITATING EMERGENCE

— changes in the rendering process: continuous processing and
elimination of solvents

California Serogroup Viruses
(LaCrosse, Jamestown Canyon, California Encephalitis)

DISEASE(S) AND SYMPTOMS

— acute, inflammatory viral diseases of short duration involving parts
of the brain, spinal cord, and meninges
— many infections are asymptomatic; severe infections involve acute
onset, headache, high fever, stupor, disorientation, tremors,
spasticity, and coma
— case fatality rate is 0.5 percent

DIAGNOSIS

— demonstration of antibodies in blood or cerebrospinal fluid

INFECTIOUS AGENT

— California serogroup viruses: LaCrosse, Jamestown Canyon, California encephalitis, and snowshoe hare virus

MODE OF TRANSMISSION

— bite of an infective mosquito
— not directly transmitted from person to person

DISTRIBUTION

— United States, Canada, and Commonwealth of Independent States
— cases typically occur in temperate latitudes in summer and early fall

INCUBATION PERIOD

— usually 5 to 15 days

TREATMENT

— supportive only

PREVENTION AND CONTROL

— avoidance of exposure to mosquitoes during hours of biting (dusk to dawn)
— mosquito control (elimination of breeding sites)

FACTORS FACILITATING EMERGENCE

— reforestation
— poor vector control
— increasing interface between human activity and endemic areas
— discarded tires as a source of mosquito breeding sites

Chikungunya Virus

DISEASE(S) AND SYMPTOMS

Chikungunya fever
— abrupt onset of fever, headache, myalgias
— joint pain, arthritis, hemorrhagic fever
— disease is usually acute and self-limited

DIAGNOSIS

— isolation of the virus from patient's blood

INFECTIOUS AGENT

— Chikungunya virus, a single-stranded RNA virus

MODE OF TRANSMISSION

— bite of an infective *Aedes* mosquito
— not directly transmitted from person to person

DISTRIBUTION

— primarily Africa, South Asia, and the Philippines

INCUBATION PERIOD

— 3 to 12 days

TREATMENT

— supportive only

PREVENTION AND CONTROL

— mosquito control in endemic areas
— a live, attenuated vaccine is being tested

FACTORS FACILITATING EMERGENCE

— unknown

Crimean-Congo Hemorrhagic Fever Virus

DISEASE(S) AND SYMPTOMS

Crimean-Congo hemorrhagic fever
— abrupt onset of fever, headache, chills, photophobia, myalgia, and abdominal pain
— nausea, vomiting, and diarrhea may be present; rash is common
— infection to death ratio is estimated at 25:1
— in pregnant women, infection is severe and often results in death

DIAGNOSIS

— isolation of the virus from cerebrospinal fluid, blood, or other tissues

INFECTIOUS AGENT

— Crimean-Congo virus, an RNA virus

MODE OF TRANSMISSION

— bite of an infective tick
— contact with blood or secretions/excretions of an infected person or animal
— virus has also spread by aerosolization

DISTRIBUTION

— Eastern Europe, central and western Asia, Middle East, Sub-Saharan and southern Africa

INCUBATION PERIOD AND COMMUNICABILITY

— 3 to 6 days
— blood of an infected person has high concentration of virus for 8 to 10 days

TREATMENT

— supportive
— ribavirin may be helpful

PREVENTION AND CONTROL

— strict isolation of infected patients
— avoidance of contact with ticks and infected persons and animals
— in the Commonwealth of Independent States, a killed vaccine is used in high-risk populations, with uncertain efficacy

FACTORS FACILITATING EMERGENCE

— lack of effective tick control
— lack of effective animal quarantine

Dengue Virus

DISEASE(S) AND SYMPTOMS

Dengue/dengue hemorrhagic fever (DHF)/dengue shock syndrome (DSS)
— sudden onset of fever, headache, joint and muscle pain
— nausea, vomiting, abdominal pain, and rash may be present
— fever typically lasts 3 to 7 days; convalescence may be prolonged
— initial phase of DHF/DSS may be similar to the above, but is followed by hemorrhagic phenomena, bleeding from multiple sites, and vascular collapse

DIAGNOSIS

— isolation of virus from blood
— serologic studies (ELISA, etc.)

INFECTIOUS AGENT

— dengue viruses, serotypes 1-4 (all four types can cause dengue hemorrhagic fever)

MODE OF TRANSMISSION

— bite of an infective *Aedes aegypti* or *Aedes albopictus* mosquito
— not directly transmitted from person to person

Distribution

— epidemic and endemic in tropical and subtropical areas of Africa, the Americas, Asia, Oceania, and Australia
— widespread in the Caribbean basin

INCUBATION PERIOD AND COMMUNICABILITY

— 3 to 14 days, average 7 to 10 days
— while disease is not transmitted from person to person, patients can be infective for mosquitoes from the day before to the end of the febrile period (5 to 7 days)

TREATMENT

— supportive only

PREVENTION AND CONTROL

— control of mosquitoes
— vaccine is not yet available

FACTORS FACILITATING EMERGENCE

— lack of effective mosquito control
— increased urbanization in the tropics
— increased air travel

Filoviruses (Marburg, Ebola)

DISEASE(S) AND SYMPTOMS

— sudden onset of fever, headache, joint and muscle pain, followed by sore throat, diarrhea, abdominal pain, vomiting, and rash

— after 3 to 5 days of fever, hemorrhagic manifestations begin
— case fatality rate for Marburg virus infection is 25 percent
— case fatality rates for Ebola infection have ranged from 50 to 90 percent

DIAGNOSIS

— isolation of virus from blood, other tissues, or body fluids
— serological detection of antibodies

INFECTIOUS AGENT

— Ebola virus
— Marburg virus

MODE OF TRANSMISSION

— close contact with infected persons or infected blood, tissues, secretions, or excretions
— transplacental and venereal transmission have occurred
— possibly contact with infected animal vectors (primates)

DISTRIBUTION

— Ebola: epidemics have taken place in Sudan and Zaire; virus may be endemic in other parts of Africa; monkeys infected with an Ebola like virus were imported to the United States from the Philippines in 1989 (no human illness resulted)
— Marburg: scattered human cases have occurred in central, eastern, and southern Africa; cases reported in Germany were a result of handling material from infected African green monkeys imported from Uganda

INCUBATION PERIOD AND COMMUNICABILITY

— for both virus infections, 5 to 10 days
— both viruses can persist in humans for at least 2 months

TREATMENT

— supportive only

PREVENTION AND CONTROL

— avoidance of contact with infected persons and their blood, other tissues, and body fluids
— strict isolation of infected persons

FACTORS FACILITATING EMERGENCE

— virus-infected monkeys shipped from developing countries via air

Hantaviruses (Hantaan, Puumala, and Seoul)

DISEASE(S) AND SYMPTOMS

Hemorrhagic fever with renal syndrome
— abrupt onset of fever, headache, and myalgias; abdominal pain, vomiting, and diarrhea
— the appearance of petechiae (reddish purple, blood-filled spots) on the palate
— in the severe form of the disease, initial febrile period may be followed by hypotension and hemorrhage from multiple sites
— most survivors regain normal renal function
— the most severe disease is caused by the Hantaan virus

DIAGNOSIS

— demonstration of specific antibodies using IFA or ELISA

INFECTIOUS AGENT

— hantaviruses, a group of RNA viruses
— several different subtypes exist, each associated with a single rodent reservoir species (Hantaan—*Apodemus* field mouse; Puumala—*Clethrionomys* bank vole; Seoul—rats)

MODE OF TRANSMISSION

— contact with infective material (feces, urine, saliva, tissue, etc.) of rodents
— contact is usually by aerosol
— transplacental transmission has been documented; other person-to-person spread has not been reported

DISTRIBUTION

— hantaviruses are found on all continents
— endemic and epidemic disease in China, Korea, and the Commonwealth of Independent States
— Hantaan virus is widely distributed in eastern Asia
— Puumala virus is common to Scandinavia and western Europe

INCUBATION PERIOD

— 4 to 42 days; average is 12 to 16 days

TREATMENT

— supportive only
— recent studies show that ribavirin may shorten illness and reduce mortality

PREVENTION AND CONTROL

— rodent control

FACTORS FACILITATING EMERGENCE

— human invasion of virus ecologic niche

Hepatitis B Virus

DISEASE(S) AND SYMPTOMS

Hepatitis B
— insidious onset of anorexia, abdominal pain
— sometimes arthralgias and rash, often progressing to jaundice
— chronic infection leads to cirrhosis of the liver

DIAGNOSIS

— elevated levels of certain liver enzymes
— serological antibody tests (RIA, ELISA)

INFECTIOUS AGENT

— Hepatitis B virus, a double-stranded DNA virus

MODE OF TRANSMISSION

— virus enters body through a break in the skin or through mucous membranes
— transmission via contaminated needles, transfusions of blood or blood products, sexual contact
— transplacental transmission

DISTRIBUTION

— worldwide

INCUBATION PERIOD AND COMMUNICABILITY

— 45 to 180 days, average 60 to 90 days
— blood containing the virus has been shown to be infective many weeks before the onset of first symptoms and to remain infective during the acute clinical course of the disease
— chronic carriers are infectious

TREATMENT

— supportive only

PREVENTION AND CONTROL

— immunization with Hepatitis B vaccine
— testing of donor blood

FACTORS FACILITATING EMERGENCE

— possibly increased sexual activity and intravenous drug abuse

Hepatitis C Virus

DISEASE(S) AND SYMPTOMS

Classic non-A, non-B hepatitis
— onset is insidious and accompanied by anorexia, nausea, vomiting, and jaundice
— course is similar to hepatitis B, but more prolonged
— strong tendency to progress to chronic hepatitis and liver disease, which can be asymptomatic
— the most common form of posttransfusion hepatitis

DIAGNOSIS

— diagnosed by exclusion of hepatitis A, B, and delta viruses and other causes of liver injury
— blood tests are now available for clinical use

INFECTIOUS AGENT

— exact viral agent is unknown
— agent appears to be a flavivirus

MODE OF TRANSMISSION

— percutaneous exposure to contaminated blood and plasma derivatives
— the role of sexual activity in transmission is not well defined

DISTRIBUTION

— worldwide
— common among dialysis patients, hemophiliacs, health care workers, and drug addicts

INCUBATION PERIOD AND COMMUNICABILITY

—20 to 90 days (mean: 50)
— period of communicability extends from one week after exposure into chronic stage

TREATMENT

- existing antivirals have little effect
- interferon may be helpful to chronic carriers

PREVENTION AND CONTROL

- no vaccine is available
- monitoring of blood supply for anti-HCV and elevated liver enzyme levels
- pasteurization of clotting factor concentrates

FACTORS FACILITATING EMERGENCE

- application of molecular virology techniques to identify etiologic agent
- an old disease syndrome newly documented

Hepatitis E Agent

DISEASE(S) AND SYMPTOMS

Hepatitis E

- also known as epidemic non-A, non-B hepatitis; waterborne non-A, non-B hepatitis; enterically transmitted non-A, non-B hepatitis
- sudden onset of fever, malaise, nausea, and anorexia
- disease varies in severity from a mild illness lasting 7 to 14 days, to a severely disabling disease lasting several months (rare)
- jaundice can be present
- no evidence of a chronic form

DIAGNOSIS

- liver function tests
- exclusion of other etiologies of hepatitis (especially hepatitis A) by serologic tests

INFECTIOUS AGENT

- virus is not yet fully characterized
- virus-like particles have been detected in the feces of infected patients

MODE OF TRANSMISSION

- ingestion of contaminated water (most outbreaks have been linked to fecal contamination of water)
- fecal-oral transmission

DISTRIBUTION

— may be widespread
— majority of outbreaks have been reported from Asia, Africa, the Commonwealth of Independent States, and Mexico

INCUBATION PERIOD AND COMMUNICABILITY

— 30 to 40 days
— period of communicability is unknown; may be similar to hepatitis A

TREATMENT

— supportive only

PREVENTION AND CONTROL

— educational programs stressing importance of sanitary disposal of feces, careful hand washing after defecation and before handling food

FACTORS FACILITATING EMERGENCE

— agent and disease are newly recognized

Human Herpesvirus-6

DISEASE(S) AND SYMPTOMS

— sudden onset of fever (fever lasts 3 to 5 days)
— maculopapular rash (*exanthem subitum/roseola infantum*) that appears on the trunk and spreads to rest of body
— febrile seizures have been reported in very few cases

DIAGNOSIS

— serology
— ELISA is now available experimentally

INFECTIOUS AGENT

— Human herpesvirus-6

MODE OF TRANSMISSION

— unknown

DISTRIBUTION

— appears ubiquitous in United States and Japan (antibody prevalence as high as 90 percent)

— disease usually occurs in children under 4 years of age
— incidence is highest in the spring

INCUBATION PERIOD AND COMMUNICABILITY

— incubation period is 10 days

TREATMENT

— supportive only

PREVENTION AND CONTROL

— none

FACTORS FACILITATING EMERGENCE

— newly recognized

Human Immunodeficiency Virus (HIV), Types 1 and 2

DISEASE(S) AND SYMPTOMS

HIV disease; acquired immunodeficiency syndrome (AIDS); AIDS-related complex (ARC)
— clinical features of infection are correlated with degree of immune dysfunction and range from asymptomatic to progressive and lethal
— manifestations can involve any organ system of the body
— initially: fever, weight loss, diarrhea, fatigue, cough, lymphadenopathy, oral thrush, and skin lesions (AIDS-related complex)
— several opportunistic infections and cancers are very common and are considered specific indicators of HIV infection, including tuberculosis and other mycobacterial infections; *Pneumocystis carinii* pneumonia; chronic cryptosporidiosis; toxoplasmosis of the central nervous system (CNS); esophageal or lower respiratory tract candidiasis; disseminated cryptococcosis; pulmonary, gastrointestinal, CNS, or ocular cytomegalovirus infection; disseminated herpes simplex infection; and (cancers) Kaposi's sarcoma, primary B-cell lymphoma, and non-Hodgkin's lymphoma
— clinical findings of common infections are often atypical (e.g., increased frequency of extrapulmonary tuberculosis)

DIAGNOSIS

— serologic tests for HIV antibodies (ELISA, IFA, Western blot)
— isolation of virus

INFECTIOUS AGENT

— human immunodeficiency virus, types 1 and 2 (retroviruses)
— types 1 and 2 are serologically and geographically distinct but have similar epidemiologic and pathologic characteristics
— humans are reservoirs

MODE OF TRANSMISSION

— sexual exposure to an infected person
— exposure to the blood or blood products (transfusions and needle sharing) or tissues (transplantation) of an infected person
— transmitted from mother to fetus
— routine social or community contact with HIV-infected persons carries no risk of transmission

DISTRIBUTION

— worldwide
— more than 200,000 reported cases of AIDS in the United States as of January 1992; approximately 1 million additional persons asymptomatically infected with HIV
— worldwide, 8 to 10 million persons infected with HIV-1 by June 1990
— HIV-2 is currently endemic only in West Africa, although cases have appeared in Europe, South America, North America, and other parts of Africa
— cases were initially clustered among male homosexuals, intravenous drug users, prostitutes, and transfusion recipients
— distribution patterns have changed in the past 10 years and continue to change (fewer cases of transfusion-induced HIV disease, more cases of infection acquired from heterosexual sex, more cases of transplacental transmission)

INCUBATION PERIOD AND COMMUNICABILITY

— days to months until virus is detectable in the blood
— months to years before appearance of clinical HIV disease (about half of HIV-infected persons will have developed AIDS 10 years after infection in the absence of specific antiviral treatment)
— period of communicability is unknown but is presumed to begin early after onset of HIV infection and to extend through life

TREATMENT

— early recognition and treatment of treatable infections and neoplasms (often chronic suppressive/maintenance therapy is recommended because of high infection relapse rates)
— there are currently three Food and Drug Administration (FDA)-

approved anti-HIV agents: zidovudine (AZT), dideoxyinosine (also known as VIDEX or ddI), and dideoxycytodine (also known as HIVID or ddC; approved for use only in combination with AZT); these agents do not cure HIV disease but have been shown to slow its progression

PREVENTION AND CONTROL

— screening of blood (and other tissue) donors
— avoidance of sexual intercourse (vaginal, anal, oral) with persons known or suspected to be infected with HIV
— use of latex condoms and spermicide to reduce the risk of sexual transmission (there is no risk of HIV transmission in a long-term, mutually monogamous, heterosexual relationship between two partners known not to be infected with HIV)
— caution by health care workers in handling, using, and disposing of needles and other sharp instruments, and wearing of latex gloves when coming into contact with bodily fluids of any patient

FACTORS FACILITATING EMERGENCE

— urbanization
— changes in lifestyles/mores
— increased intravenous drug abuse
— international travel
— medical technology (transfusions)

Human Papillomavirus (HPV)

DISEASE(S) AND SYMPTOMS

— a variety of skin and mucous membrane lesions, from the common wart to laryngeal warts (in infants infected by their mothers during birth) to venereal warts (most often seen in the moist areas in and around the genitalia and anus)
— HPV has been strongly implicated in the etiology of cervical cancer (especially HPV types 16 and 18)

DIAGNOSIS

— usually based on lesion appearance
— in some cases, excision and histological examination are necessary

INFECTIOUS AGENT

— human papillomavirus (there are at least 60 types identified)

MODE OF TRANSMISSION

— usually by direct contact
— also by autoinoculation (e.g. by a shaving razor) and by contact with contaminated floors
— genital warts are sexually transmitted
— virus can be transmitted from mother to infant during birth

DISTRIBUTION

— worldwide

INCUBATION PERIOD AND COMMUNICABILITY

— 1 to 20 months; average is 2 to 3 months
— period of communicability is unknown but is probably at least as long as visible lesions persist

TREATMENT

— freezing of warts with liquid nitrogen
— application of salicylic acid or podophyllin to remove warts
— interferon has been shown to be effective in the treatment of genital warts
— surgical removal or laser therapy is required for laryngeal and cervical warts

PREVENTION AND CONTROL

— avoidance of direct contact with lesions
— use of a condom during sexual intercourse

FACTORS FACILITATING EMERGENCE

— possibly increases in sexual activity

Human Parvovirus B19

DISEASE(S) AND SYMPTOMS

Erythema infectiosum
— classic infection in childhood is characterized by erythema of cheeks (slapped cheek appearance) and rash on extremities
— adults have more severe illness, with fever and arthritis that can last for months or years
— may cause aplastic crisis in patients with chronic hemolytic anemias

DIAGNOSIS

— made on clinical grounds, can be confirmed by testing for antibodies

INFECTIOUS AGENT

— human parvovirus B19, a single-stranded DNA virus

MODE OF TRANSMISSION

— most commonly, contact with infectious respiratory secretions
— also transmitted transplacentally and via blood and blood products

DISTRIBUTION

— worldwide; common in children

INCUBATION PERIOD AND COMMUNICABILITY

— 4 to 20 days to development of rash
— probably not communicable after onset of rash; immunosuppressed persons with chronic infection may be communicable up to years after onset

TREATMENT

— supportive only

PREVENTION AND CONTROL

— isolation not practical in community at large
— hospitalized patients with transient aplastic crisis should be isolated
— hand washing after patient contact

FACTORS FACILITATING EMERGENCE

— a pervasive virus that has only recently drawn increased attention
— as a hematogenous infection, it may increase in importance in immunosuppressed persons and as a threat to the blood supply

Human T-Cell Leukemia Virus (HTLV), Types 1 and 2

DISEASE(S) AND SYMPTOMS

Adult T-cell leukemia/lymphoma (ATLL); chronic progressive myelopathy; tropical spastic paraparesis (TSP)
— lymphadenopathy, hepatomegaly, splenomegaly, lymphomatous meningitis
— cutaneous lesions (generalized erythroderma, papules, nodules, plaques, and maculopapular rashes)
— fever and abdominal symptoms may occur
— arthritis is frequently reported
— disease ranges from subacute to rapidly lethal (median survival for ATLL is 8 months)

DIAGNOSIS

- isolation of the virus from the blood
- detection of antibodies

INFECTIOUS AGENT

- human T-cell leukemia virus
- type 1 has been implicated in the causation of leukemia and lymphoma by serologic, virologic, and epidemiologic evidence
- type 2 was initially isolated from two cases of hairy cell leukemia (causality has not yet been established)

MODE OF TRANSMISSION

- person-to-person transmission by blood (transfusions and shared needles) and by sexual contact
- transplacental transmission is possible

DISTRIBUTION

- virus is present on all continents
- cases of HTLV-1 infection have clustered in the Caribbean, southwestern Japan, parts of Central and South America, Africa, Italy, and the southern United States
- HTLV-2 is commonly found in intravenous drug abusers

INCUBATION PERIOD AND COMMUNICABILITY

- incubation period is several years and may be as long as 20 years
- communicability is unknown

TREATMENT

- response of ATLL to conventional chemotherapeutic regimens has been poor
- corticosteroids are helpful in some cases

PREVENTION AND CONTROL

- avoidance of sexual or blood contact with an infected person
- screening of donated blood for the virus (types 1 and 2)

FACTORS FACILITATING EMERGENCE

- medical technology (transfusion)
- possibly increased intravenous drug abuse

Influenza A Virus

DISEASE(S) AND SYMPTOMS

Drift influenza; pandemic influenza
— sudden onset of fever, myalgias, cough, headache, and profound fatigue
— nasal discharge, sore throat, and hoarseness are common
— fever lasts from 1 to 5 days; respiratory symptoms and malaise may persist another 7 to 14 days
— severe cases involve complications such as pneumonia
— infection can be fatal, especially in the elderly and in those debilitated by chronic cardiac, pulmonary, renal, or metabolic disease, as well as in the immunosuppressed
— pandemic influenza is typically more severe, since populations have no immunity to pandemic strains

DIAGNOSIS

— recognition is commonly by epidemiological characteristics
— isolation of virus from respiratory tract
— detection of viral antigen in respiratory secretions

INFECTIOUS AGENT

— influenza A virus, an RNA virus that undergoes frequent mutations
— virus isolates are described by character of hemagglutinin (H) and neuraminidase antigens; type A includes 3 subtypes (H1N1, H2N2, and H3N2)
— emergence of completely new subtypes (antigenic shift) occurs at irregular intervals and typically results in pandemic influenza
— minor antigenic changes (antigenic drift) are responsible for annual epidemics and regional outbreaks

MODE OF TRANSMISSION

— airborne spread among crowded populations in enclosed spaces
— transmission also occurs by direct contact with mucus of an infected person (influenza virus can persist for hours in dried mucus)
— transmission from animal to human has been demonstrated rarely

DISTRIBUTION

— worldwide
— in temperate regions, influenza outbreaks occur during colder months
— in tropical regions, influenza occurs year round

INCUBATION PERIOD AND COMMUNICABILITY

— 1 to 2 days
— period of communicability is probably 3 to 5 days from clinical onset

TREATMENT

— amantadine and rimantadine, if given early, shorten clinical illness in acute influenza A

PREVENTION AND CONTROL

— immunization (vaccine is less effective in the elderly, in the immunosuppressed, and in people who have chronic renal failure)
— prophylactic amantadine is recommended for selected individuals (e.g., those at high risk of complications from immunization)

FACTORS FACILITATING EMERGENCE

— antigenic drift leads to small changes in the virus
— significant mutations in the virus (antigenic shift) may result from animal-human virus reassortment

Japanese Encephalitis Virus

DISEASE(S) AND SYMPTOMS

Japanese encephalitis virus disease
— clinical features range from inapparent to fatal
— mild infections involve fever, headache, and myalgias
— severe disease involves high fever, nausea, vomiting, and altered consciousness
— hyperthermia, seizures, paralysis, and coma can occur
— convalescence is prolonged; up to 80 percent of survivors experience neurologic sequelae
— with optimal care, case fatality rate is 10 percent (as high as 40 percent in young children and in persons over 65 years of age)

DIAGNOSIS

— isolation of the virus from cerebrospinal fluid or blood
— isolation of viral antibodies from the blood and cerebral spinal fluid

INFECTIOUS AGENT

— Japanese encephalitis virus
— pigs are important amplification hosts for the virus

MODE OF TRANSMISSION

- bite of an infective mosquito
- transplacental transmission has been documented
- not directly transmitted from person to person

DISTRIBUTION

- widely distributed in eastern and southern Asia, the far eastern Commonwealth of Independent States, and the Pacific islands

INCUBATION PERIOD

- 6 to 8 days

TREATMENT

- supportive only

PREVENTION AND CONTROL

- mosquito control
- an inactivated vaccine is widely used in Japan (95 percent efficacy in clinical trials)
- a live, attenuated vaccine has been used in China

FACTORS FACILITATING EMERGENCE

- changes in agricultural practices facilitating mosquito breeding

Lassa Virus

DISEASE(S) AND SYMPTOMS

Lassa fever
- gradual onset of fever, malaise, headache, dizziness, and sore throat
- nausea, vomiting, and diarrhea are common
- in severe cases, hypotension, shock, and seizures may result
- acute illness lasts 7 to 31 days, with an average of 12 days

DIAGNOSIS

- isolation of virus from blood, urine, or throat washings
- serological tests (ELISA or IFA)

INFECTIOUS AGENT

- Lassa virus, an arenavirus named after a town in Nigeria

MODE OF TRANSMISSION
- contact with excreta of infected rodents deposited on surfaces such as beds and floors, or in food
- transmission also occurs via contact with blood, secretions, or excretions of an infected person
- transplacental transmission can occur

DISTRIBUTION
- widely distributed over West Africa, especially Nigeria, Sierra Leone, and Liberia

INCUBATION PERIOD AND COMMUNICABILITY
- 8 to 14 days
- person-to-person transmission may occur during the acute febrile phase when virus is present in the throat

TREATMENT
- antiviral agents: ribavirin
- mechanical ventilation and renal dialysis may be required

PREVENTION AND CONTROL
- avoidance of contact with rats and infected persons
- strict isolation of infected persons

FACTORS FACILITATING EMERGENCE
- unknown

Measles Virus

DISEASE(S) AND SYMPTOMS

Measles
- fever, conjunctivitis, coryza, cough, and Koplic spots on the buccal mucosa
- red blotchy rash beginning on forehead and neck, later spreading to trunk and limbs

DIAGNOSIS
- usually made on clinical and epidemiological grounds

INFECTIOUS AGENT
- measles virus

MODE OF TRANSMISSION

— airborne transmission by droplet spread
— direct contact with the nasal or throat secretions of infected persons

DISTRIBUTION

— worldwide
— incidence in a population determined largely by levels of immunization

INCUBATION PERIOD AND COMMUNICABILITY

— 10 to 14 days
— infective virus is present from the 5th day of incubation through 4 days after onset of rash
— measles is one of the most highly communicable infectious diseases (measles virus can survive in droplet nuclei for more than 2 hours)

TREATMENT

— none

PREVENTION AND CONTROL

— immunization with live measles vaccine
— children should be kept out of school at least four days after the onset of rash

FACTORS FACILITATING EMERGENCE

— deterioration of public health infrastructure supporting immunization

Norwalk and Norwalk-like Agents

DISEASE(S) AND SYMPTOMS

Gastroenteritis, epidemic diarrhea
— vomiting, diarrhea, headache, and low-grade fever lasting 2 to 3 days
— disease often occurs in outbreaks involving people of all age groups

DIAGNOSIS

— identification of the agent in the stool by electron microscopy and/or immunologic assay (RIA and ELISA)

INFECTIOUS AGENTS

— Norwalk agent (virus-like), Snow Mountain agent, Hawaii agent, and other Norwalk-like agents

MODE OF TRANSMISSION

— most likely fecal-oral transmission
— respiratory transmission may occur via aerosolized vomitus
— alleged vehicles of transmission include drinking water, swimming water, and uncooked foods (shellfish and salads)

DISTRIBUTION

— worldwide
— in developing countries, disease is more common in children; in the United States, disease typically occurs in older children and adults

INCUBATION PERIOD AND COMMUNICABILITY

— typical incubation period is 1 to 2 days
— disease is communicable up to 2 days after diarrhea stops

TREATMENT

— supportive only (e.g., oral fluid replacement)

PREVENTION AND CONTROL

— effective preventive measures are undetermined
— possibly avoidance of alleged vehicles of transmission

FACTORS FACILITATING EMERGENCE

— increased recognition

Rabies Virus

DISEASE(S) AND SYMPTOMS

Rabies
— primarily a disease of animals; all warm-blooded mammals are susceptible
— acute encephalomyelitis
— fever, malaise, myalgia, vomiting, agitation or hydrophobia upon attempt to swallow
— initial symptoms followed by hyperventilation, aphasia, paralysis, seizures
— cardiac arrhythmias and coma can follow

DIAGNOSIS

— isolation and identification of rabies virus from saliva, cerebrospinal fluid, urine, brain, or other tissue

INFECTIOUS AGENT

— rabies virus
— dogs are most common reservoir host; in some areas, vampire bats, mongooses, wolves, foxes, raccoons, and other wild and domestic animals are important reservoir hosts; also, newly emerging in felines in the eastern United States

MODE OF TRANSMISSION

— a bite (that breaks the skin) from an infected animal; bites around head, face, or hands carry highest risk of infection
— mucous membrane exposure to saliva of an infected animal

DISTRIBUTION

— worldwide; causes an estimated 30,000 human deaths per year, mostly in developing countries

INCUBATION PERIOD AND COMMUNICABILITY

— 1 to 2 months
— period of communicability for animals includes week before clinical signs and throughout the course of the disease

TREATMENT

— immediate and thorough cleansing of bite wound
— administration of rabies immune globulin (RIG) around wound and intramuscularly to prevent infection, and vaccine intramuscularly to prevent infection
— the only treatment for disease is supportive; more than 99% of patients with symptomatic infection die

PREVENTION AND CONTROL

— pre-exposure vaccination is recommended for persons whose occupations or travel will place them at risk for exposure to rabid animals
— vaccination of dogs and cats
— isolation and destruction of infected animals

FACTORS FACILITATING EMERGENCE

— changing movements of reservoir host species
— absence or failure of rabies control programs

Rift Valley Fever Virus

DISEASE(S) AND SYMPTOMS

Rift Valley fever
— abrupt onset of fever, severe headache, myalgias, and arthralgias
— complications include jaundice and hemorrhagic complications
— encephalitis and retinitis may occur
— some survivors are left with neurologic sequelae and permanent visual damage
— (in animals: enzootic hepatitis)

DIAGNOSIS

— virus isolation from the blood
— demonstration of virus antibodies in the cerebrospinal fluid or acute serum

INFECTIOUS AGENT

— Rift Valley fever virus

MODE OF TRANSMISSION

— bite of an infective mosquito
— contact with infected animals or their tissues
— possible transmission via unpasteurized milk
— not directly transmitted from person to person

DISTRIBUTION

— widespread in Africa; initially described in Rift Valley in Kenya

INCUBATION PERIOD

— 3 to 5 days

TREATMENT

— supportive only

PREVENTION AND CONTROL

— an inactivated vaccine is available for persons at high risk of infection (veterinarians, laboratory personnel) in endemic areas
— a candidate live, attenuated vaccine is under development
— immunization of animals
— mosquito control

FACTORS FACILITATING EMERGENCE

— importation of infected mosquitoes and/or animals
— creation of mosquito habitats through dam building and irrigation

Ross River Virus

DISEASE(S) AND SYMPTOMS

Ross River fever
— a self-limited disease characterized by arthritis (especially in the wrist, knee, ankle, and small joints of the extremities), which lasts from days to months
— a maculopapular rash on the trunk and limbs commonly follows the onset of arthritis; rash resolves within 7 to 10 days
— fever is frequently present, lasting 6 to 7 days
— in 25 percent of cases, rheumatic symptoms continue one year or longer

DIAGNOSIS
— isolation of virus from serum
— detection of virus antibodies in serum

INFECTIOUS AGENT
— Ross River virus

MODE OF TRANSMISSION
— bite of an infective mosquito
— transplacental transmission may occur
— not directly transmitted from person to person
— virus reservoir is probably the kangaroo

DISTRIBUTION
— Australia, Tasmania, Papua New Guinea, Indonesia, and several South Pacific islands

INCUBATION PERIOD
— 3 to 11 days

TREATMENT
— supportive only

PREVENTION AND CONTROL
— mosquito control

FACTORS FACILITATING EMERGENCE
— importation of infected mosquitoes and/or travel by infected people
— creation of mosquito habitats through dam building and irrigation

Rotavirus

DISEASE(S) AND SYMPTOMS

Rotaviral enteritis
— varies from asymptomatic to severe and sometimes fatal
gastroenteritis; group A viruses predominate in infants and young
children, group B in older children and adults
— watery diarrhea, vomiting, low-grade fever, and dehydration
— illness typically lasts 3 to 10 days

DIAGNOSIS
— identification of the virus in the stool by immunologic assay
(ELISA), electron microscopy, or isolation in cell culture

INFECTIOUS AGENT
— one of three groups (A, B, or C) of rotavirus (A is the most common
cause of illness in humans)

MODE OF TRANSMISSION
— primarily fecal-oral
— fecal-respiratory transmission may also occur

DISTRIBUTION
— worldwide

INCUBATION PERIOD AND COMMUNICABILITY
— incubation period is 1 to 2 days
— virus shedding occurs throughout duration of illness and continues
for several days following the disappearance of symptoms

TREATMENT
— supportive only (e.g., oral fluid replacement)

PREVENTION AND CONTROL
— effective preventive measures are uncertain
— avoid exposure of infants to persons with acute gastroenteritis
— passive immunization by oral immunoglobulin has been effective
in protecting low-birth-weight newborns
— a number of oral vaccines are in various stages of
development

FACTORS FACILITATING EMERGENCE
— increased recognition

Venezuelan Equine Encephalitis (VEE) Virus

Disease(s) and Symptoms

Venezuelan equine encephalitis
— sudden onset of fever, chills, severe headache, nausea, and vomiting
— pharyngitis and facial erythema may be present
— central nervous system manifestations (stupor, coma, seizures, and spastic paralysis) can accompany severe cases
— most infections are fairly mild; symptoms last 3 to 5 days
— in patients with encephalitis, illness typically lasts 3 to 7 days

DIAGNOSIS

— isolation of the virus or of viral antibodies in the blood
— sometimes based on epidemiological grounds (in areas that have experienced a recent equine epizootic)

INFECTIOUS AGENT

— Venezuelan equine encephalomyelitis virus
— virus is maintained in rodents
— transmission cycle involves horses, which serve as the major source of virus to infect mosquitoes

MODE OF TRANSMISSION

— bite of an infective mosquito
— transmission also occurs transplacentally and in laboratories via inhalation
— not directly transmitted from person to person
— no evidence of aerosol transmission from horses to humans

DISTRIBUTION

— disease is enzootic and epizootic in tropical South America, Central America, the Caribbean, southern North America, and Mexico

INCUBATION PERIOD

— 2 to 5 days

TREATMENT

— supportive only

PREVENTION AND CONTROL

— mosquito control
— a live, attenuated vaccine is available for laboratory workers and other adults at high risk of infection

— a killed, attenuated vaccine exists for cases in which the live vaccine
is ineffective
— control of infection in horses by vaccination

FACTORS FACILITATING EMERGENCE

— introduction into new regions via infected mosquitoes and horses

Yellow Fever Virus

DISEASE(S) AND SYMPTOMS

Yellow fever
— clinical features range from inapparent to fatal
— typical attacks are characterized by abrupt onset, fever, chills,
headache, muscle pain, nausea, and vomiting
— as disease progresses, jaundice, hemorrhagic complications, and
renal failure may occur
— pulse may be slow despite high fever
— the case fatality rate among indigenous populations of endemic
regions is less than 5 percent; this rate may exceed 50 percent
among nonindigenous groups and in epidemics
— recovery is slow but complete in survivors

DIAGNOSIS

— isolation of virus from the blood
— demonstration of viral antigen in the blood or liver tissue by ELISA

INFECTIOUS AGENT

— Yellow fever virus

MODE OF TRANSMISSION

— bite of an infective mosquito
— not directly transmitted from person to person

DISTRIBUTION

— disease is endemic in tropical South and Central America and in
Africa
— potential for outbreaks exists in other areas where vector mosquito is
found (including the United States)

INCUBATION PERIOD

— range is 3 to 14 days; usually 1 to 6 days

— blood of patients is infective for mosquitoes 3 to 5 days after onset of illness

TREATMENT

— supportive only

PREVENTION AND CONTROL

— a live viral vaccine prepared from chick embryos is safe and highly effective (more than 95 percent of those vaccinated will have immune response within 7 to 10 days; immunity lasts at least 10 years)
— mosquito control

FACTORS FACILITATING EMERGENCE

— lack of effective mosquito control
— lack of widespread vaccination
— urbanization in the tropics
— increased air travel

EMERGENT PROTOZOANS, HELMINTHS, AND FUNGI

Anisakis

DISEASE(S) AND SYMPTOMS

Anisakiasis, herring worm disease, cod worm disease
— severe epigastric pain, nausea, vomiting, fever
— obstruction, ulceration, and bleeding in the gastrointestinal tract are possible

DIAGNOSIS

— recognition of the 2 to 3 cm. larva invading the oropharynx
— visualization of larvae through gastroscopic examination

INFECTIOUS AGENT

— larval nematodes of the Anisakidae family, common parasites of marine mammals and fish

MODE OF TRANSMISSION

— ingestion of larvae in raw or undercooked fish, squid, or octopus (larvae are colorless, tightly coiled, and not easily seen in fish flesh)
— not transmitted directly from person to person

DISTRIBUTION

— most cases are reported from Japan
— cases are also sporadically reported from North and South America, Europe, Asia, and the South Pacific
— infected fish can potentially be shipped to any region of the world

INCUBATION PERIOD

— 1 to 12 hours for gastric attachment; 7 to 14 days for intestinal attachment

TREATMENT

— endoscopic removal of larva
— surgery may be necessary to remove obstruction

PREVENTION AND CONTROL

— heating marine fish to 140°F for 10 minutes or freezing at –4°F for at least five days kills the larvae

FACTORS FACILITATING EMERGENCE

— increasing popularity of raw fish dishes in the United States and elsewhere

Babesia

DISEASE(S) AND SYMPTOMS

Babesiosis
— fever, fatigue, chills, and hemolytic anemia lasting from several days to a few months

DIAGNOSIS

— blood smear contains red blood cells with visible parasites

INFECTIOUS AGENT

— *Babesia microti* and other *Babesia* species (protozoan parasites)
— nymphal *Ixodes* ticks (carried by deer mice) are vectors; adult ticks live on deer

MODE OF TRANSMISSION

— bite of a nymphal *Ixodes* tick
— not directly transmitted from person to person
— occasional transmission by blood transfusion has been reported

DISTRIBUTION

- widespread in areas where ticks are present
- majority of cases are from northeastern United States
- also reported from France and other European countries

INCUBATION PERIOD

- variable; 1 week to 12 months reported

TREATMENT

- a combination of antiparasitic agents (clindamycin and quinine) has been effective in most patients
- exchange blood transfusion may be required in patients with very high-grade parasitemia

PREVENTION AND CONTROL

- avoidance of tick exposure in endemic areas (protective clothing, tick repellant)
- control of rodents around human habitations

FACTORS FACILITATING EMERGENCE

- reforestation and subsequent increase in deer population
- housing development in wooded areas

Candida

DISEASE(S) AND SYMPTOMS

Candidiasis
- fungal infections usually confined to the superficial layers of skin or mucous membranes: oral thrush, intertrigo, vulvovaginitis, paronychia, or onychomycosis
- ulcers may be formed in the esophagus, gastrointestinal tract, or bladder
- dissemination in the blood may produce lesions in other organs (kidney, spleen, liver, lung, endocardium, eye, or brain)

DIAGNOSIS

- microscopic demonstration of yeast cells in infected tissue or body fluid
- fungal culture

INFECTIOUS AGENT

— species of the fungus, *Candida*

MODE OF TRANSMISSION

— contact with secretions or excretions of mouth, skin, or vagina of infected persons, or with the feces of infected persons
— passage from mother to infant during childbirth
— endogenous spread
— disseminated candidiasis can originate from indwelling urinary catheters and percutaneous intravenous catheters

DISTRIBUTION

— worldwide
— the fungus (*C. albicans*) is often part of the normal human flora

INCUBATION PERIOD AND COMMUNICABILITY

— incubation period is variable
— infection is presumably communicable while lesions are present

TREATMENT

— topical antifungal agents: imidazole, nystatin
— oral clotrimazole troches or nystatin suspension is effective for treatment of oral thrush
— oral ketoconazole is effective for treatment of infected skin and mucous membranes of the mouth, esophagus, and vagina

PREVENTION AND CONTROL

— detection and treatment of infection early to prevent systemic spread
— detection and treatment of vaginal candidiasis during third trimester of pregnancy to prevent neonatal thrush
— amelioration of underlying causes of infection (e.g., removal of indwelling venous catheters)

FACTORS FACILITATING EMERGENCE

— immunosuppression
— medical management (catheters)
— antibiotic use

Cryptococcus

DISEASE(S) AND SYMPTOMS

Cryptococcosis
— a fungal infection, usually presenting as a subacute or chronic meningitis
— skin may show acneiform lesions, ulcers, or subcutaneous tumor-like masses
— infection of lungs, kidneys, prostate, bone, and liver may occur
— untreated cryptococcal meningitis terminates fatally within several months

DIAGNOSIS

— visualization of fungus on microscopic examination of cerebrospinal fluid
— tests for antigen in serum and cerebrospinal fluid

INFECTIOUS AGENT

— *Cryptococcus* species, typically *C. neoformans*, a fungus
— fungus grows saprophytically in external environment (can be isolated from the soil in many parts of the world)
— fungus can consistently be isolated from old pigeon nests and pigeon droppings

MODE OF TRANSMISSION

— presumably by inhalation
— waterborne transmission can also occur
— not transmitted directly from person to person or between animals and people

DISTRIBUTION

— worldwide
— infection occurs mainly in adults
— disseminated or central nervous system cryptococcosis is often a sentinel infection for HIV-infected persons
— infection also occurs in dogs, cats, horses, cows, monkeys, and other animals

INCUBATION PERIOD

— unknown

TREATMENT

— antifungal agents: amphotericin B is effective in many cases
— very difficult to cure in persons with HIV disease

PREVENTION AND CONTROL

— careful removal (preceded by chemical decontamination and wetting
with water or oil to prevent aerosolization) of large accumulations of
pigeon droppings

FACTORS FACILITATING EMERGENCE

— immunosuppression

Cryptosporidium

DISEASE(S) AND SYMPTOMS

Cryptosporidiosis
— a parasitic infection of the epithelial cells of the gastrointestinal,
biliary, and respiratory tracts of man, as well as other vertebrates
(birds, fish, reptiles, rodents, cats, dogs, cattle, and sheep)
— symptoms of infection include watery diarrhea, nausea, vomiting,
malaise, myalgias, and, in about half of cases, fever
— symptoms usually come and go, but subside in fewer than 30 days in
most healthy, immunocompetent persons
— immunocompromised persons may not be able to clear the parasite,
with disease becoming prolonged and fulminant and contributing to
death

DIAGNOSIS

— identification of oocysts in fecal smears
— identification of parasites in intestinal biopsies

INFECTIOUS AGENT

— *Cryptosporidium*, a protozoan parasite

MODE OF TRANSMISSION

— fecal-oral spread from contaminated fingers, food, and water
— occasional transmission by aerosolized organisms has been reported

DISTRIBUTION

— worldwide; organism has been found wherever sought

INCUBATION PERIOD AND COMMUNICABILITY

— probably 1 to 12 days
— oocysts, the infectious stage of the parasite, appear in the stool from the onset of symptoms to several weeks after symptoms resolve
— outside the body, oocysts can remain infective for 2 to 6 months in a moist environment

TREATMENT

— fluid and electrolyte replacement; nutritional support
— effective, specific therapy has not yet been identified

PREVENTION AND CONTROL

— careful handling of animal excreta
— hand washing by those in contact with calves and other animals with diarrhea
— effective water treatment

FACTORS FACILITATING EMERGENCE

— development near watershed areas
— immunosuppression

Giardia lamblia

DISEASE(S) AND SYMPTOMS

Giardiasis
— infection of the upper small intestine
— frequent diarrhea, bloating, abdominal cramps, fatigue, low-grade fever, malaise, and weight loss
— symptoms typically subside after 2 to 3 weeks, but chronic or relapsing diarrhea may occur

DIAGNOSIS

— identification of cysts or trophozoites in feces or of trophozoites in biopsy material from the small intestine

INFECTIOUS AGENT

— Giardia lamblia, a protozoan parasite

MODE OF TRANSMISSION

— ingestion of cysts in fecally contaminated food or water

— direct person-to-person spread via hand-to-mouth transfer of cysts from an infected individual (especially in day care centers and chronic care institutions)

DISTRIBUTION

— worldwide; causes both sporadic outbreaks and epidemics

INCUBATION PERIOD AND COMMUNICABILITY

— incubation period ranges from 3 days to 6 weeks; usually 1 to 3 weeks
— infected persons can be a source of infection for as long as they carry the organism

TREATMENT

— antiparasitic agents: quinacrine, metronidazole, furazolidine

PREVENTION AND CONTROL

— avoidance of drinking untreated surface water
— disposal of feces in a sanitary manner

FACTORS FACILITATING EMERGENCE

— infection in the animal population (beavers and dogs)
— capability of the organism to survive in water supply systems that use superficial water
— immunosuppression
— international travel

Microsporidia

DISEASE(S) AND SYMPTOMS

Microsporidiosis
— chronic gastroenteritis, diarrhea, and wasting in patients with HIV disease
— conjunctivitis, scleritis, diffuse punctate keratopathy, and corneal ulceration have also been reported, primarily in patients with HIV disease
— other findings include fever, hepatitis, muscle weakness, and neurologic changes

DIAGNOSIS

— requires electron microscopy of biopsy specimen

INFECTIOUS AGENT

— protozoan parasites from the phylum Microspora (phylum consists of about 80 genera, of which at least four cause human disease: *Encephalitozoon*, *Enterocytozoon*, *Nosema*, and *Pleistophora*)
— microsporidia typically infect animals and have only recently been recognized as human pathogens

MODE OF TRANSMISSION

— unknown; probably by ingestion of contaminated food or water
— spores of some species survive up to 4 months in the environment

DISTRIBUTION

— worldwide
— human infections have been reported from Africa, North and South America, Asia, and Europe
— the majority of reported patients have been immunosuppressed

INCUBATION PERIOD AND COMMUNICABILITY

— unknown

TREATMENT

— no clearly effective therapy is available
— some patients have improved with antiparasitic drugs pyrimethamine and metronidazole

PREVENTION AND CONTROL

— unknown at this time

FACTORS FACILITATING EMERGENCE

— immunosuppression
— parasite is newly recognized

Plasmodium

DISEASE(S) AND SYMPTOMS

Malaria
— fever, headache, nausea, vomiting, diarrhea, myalgias, and malaise
— in 30 to 40 percent of acute cases, the spleen is enlarged and liver may be tender
— respiratory and renal failure, shock, acute encephalopathy, pulmo-

nary and cerebral edema, coma, and death may result from severe cases (especially *P. falciparum* infections)
— duration of an untreated primary attack ranges from 1 week to 1 month or longer; relapses of febrile illness can occur at irregular intervals for up to 2 to 5 years
— chronically infected persons develop hyperreactive malarial splenomegaly or nephrotic syndrome
— case fatality rates among untreated children and nonimmune adults exceed 10 percent

DIAGNOSIS

— identification of characteristic intraerythrocytic parasites on a blood smear

INFECTIOUS AGENT

— *Plasmodium falciparum*, *P. vivax*, *P. ovale*, and *P. malariae*
— protozoan parasites with an asexual cycle in humans and sexual cycle in mosquitoes

MODE OF TRANSMISSION

— bite of an infective mosquito
— not directly transmitted from person to person
— transmission by transfusion and transplacental transmission account for a small percentage of infections

DISTRIBUTION

— indigenous malaria persists in about 100 tropical and subtropical countries
— disease occurs in Africa, Asia, Mexico, Central and South America, the Caribbean, the South Pacific Islands, and in parts of the Commonwealth of Independent States
— worldwide, an estimated 200 to 300 million infections occur annually, with 2 to 3 million deaths (most are from *P. falciparum*)
— chloroquine-resistant *P. falciparum* strains have been reported from endemic areas in Africa, Asia, and the Americas; continued spread of resistance is expected

INCUBATION PERIOD

— 10 to 30 days, depending on virus strain
— transmission by transfusion can occur as long as asexual forms of the parasite remain in the circulating blood (for *P. malariae*, this can be more than 40 years)

Treatment

- — chloroquine is drug of choice unless resistant *P. falciparum* is suspected
- — quinine plus tetracycline, pyrimethamine and sulfadiazine/ clindamycin, or mefloquine should be used for resistant *P. falciparum* strains
- — resistance of *P. falciparum* malaria to all antimalarials has been reported; in these cases, combination therapy and repeated courses of treatment may be necessary

Prevention and Control

- — mosquito control
- — chemoprophylactic regimens (be sure to obtain updated information)

Factors Facilitating Emergence

- — urbanization
- — changing parasite biology
- — environmental changes
- — drug resistance
- — air travel

Pneumocystis carinii

Disease(s) and Symptoms

Pneumocystis carinii pneumonia
- — progressive dyspnea, tachypnea, and cyanosis
- — pneumonia is often fatal in malnourished, chronically ill, and premature infants, as well as in adults who are immunocompromised

Diagnosis

- — demonstration of the organism in material from bronchial brushings, open lung biopsy, and lung aspirates
- — no satisfactory culture method or serologic test is in routine use at present

Infectious Agent

- — *Pneumocystis carinii*, a protozoan parasite (with genetic similarities to a fungus)

MODE OF TRANSMISSION

— unknown in man (airborne transmission has been reported in rats)
— subclinical infection may be common

DISTRIBUTION

— worldwide
— the disease affects 60 percent of patients with human immunodeficiency virus (HIV) disease

INCUBATION PERIOD AND COMMUNICABILITY

— unknown; symptoms typically appear 1 to 2 months after onset of immunosuppression
— period of communicability is unknown

TREATMENT

— cotrimoxazole is first choice drug; pentamidine is also used

PREVENTION AND CONTROL

— prophylaxis with cotrimoxazole in immunocompromised patients

FACTORS FACILITATING EMERGENCE

— immunosuppression

Strongyloides stercoralis

DISEASE(S) AND SYMPTOMS

Strongyloidiasis
— transient rash at site of parasite penetration into the skin
— coughing and wheezing may develop when parasite passes through lungs
— abdominal symptoms occur when adult female parasite invades intestinal mucosa
— abdominal pain, diarrhea, nausea can be chronic and relapsing
— in the immunocompromised host, infection may become disseminated, resulting in wasting, pulmonary involvement, and death

DIAGNOSIS

— identification of larvae in stool specimens or duodenal aspirates

INFECTIOUS AGENT

- *Strongyloides stercoralis*, a nematode
- larvae penetrate skin, enter blood vessels, travel to lungs, migrate up respiratory tree to the pharynx, where they enter the gastrointestinal tract (where the female lays eggs)

MODE OF TRANSMISSION

- penetration of skin or mucous membrane by infective larvae (usually from fecally contaminated soil)
- free-living form of the parasite can be maintained in the environment (soil) for years
- transmission also occurs via oral-anal sexual activities

DISTRIBUTION

- worldwide; most common in tropical and subtropical areas

INCUBATION PERIOD AND COMMUNICABILITY

- larvae can be found in stool 2 to 3 weeks after exposure
- infection is potentially communicable as long as living worms remain in the intestine

TREATMENT

- antiparasitic agents: thiabendazole, albendazole, ivermectin

PREVENTION AND CONTROL

- disposal of feces in a sanitary manner
- avoidance of skin-soil contact in endemic areas

FACTORS FACILITATING EMERGENCE

- international travel
- immunosuppression

Toxoplasma gondii

DISEASE(S) AND SYMPTOMS

Toxoplasmosis
- a systemic protozoan disease, frequently present as an acute mononucleosis-like disease (malaise, myalgias, fever)
- immunocompromised persons tend to have severe primary infection with pneumonitis, myocarditis, meningoencephalitis, hepatitis, chorioretinitis, or some combination of these

— congenital toxoplasmosis causes chorioretinitis, fever, jaundice, rash, and brain damage

DIAGNOSIS

— based on clinical signs, as well as on demonstration of the organism in body tissues or fluids

INFECTIOUS AGENT

— *Toxoplasma gondii*, a protozoan parasite
— cats and other felines are reservoirs
— intermediate hosts are sheep, goats, rodents, swine, cattle, chicken, and birds

MODE OF TRANSMISSION

— ingestion of oocysts (on fingers or in food contaminated with cat feces) or cysts in raw or undercooked meat
— transplacental transmission
— transmission through blood transfusion and tissue transplantations has been reported
— not directly transmitted from person to person (except in utero)

DISTRIBUTION

— worldwide
— prevalence of seropositivity is higher in warm, humid climates and is influenced by presence of cats and by eating habits

INCUBATION PERIOD

— 1 to 3 weeks

TREATMENT

— antiparasitic agents (pyrimethamine plus sulfadiazine) for persons with severe disease
— no treatment is needed for most healthy, immunocompetent hosts

PREVENTION AND CONTROL

— thorough cooking of meats
— daily disposal of cat feces and disinfection of litter pans (pregnant women should avoid contact with litter pans)
— thorough hand washing after handling of raw meat
— prophylactic treatment for patients with HIV disease

FACTORS FACILITATING EMERGENCE

— immunosuppression
— increase in cats as pets

C

Global Resources for
Infectious Disease Surveillance

U.S. and U.S. Affiliated

U.S. Department of Defense

ARMY
1. Walter Reed Army Institute of Research (WRAIR)
2. Armed Forces Institute of Pathology (AFIP)
3. U.S. Army Medical Research Institute of Infectious Diseases (USAMRIID)
4. U.S. Army Medical Research Units (USAMRU):
   - Brasilia, Brazil
   - Nairobi, Kenya
   - Seoul, Korea
   - Bangkok, Thailand
5. Armed Forces Medical Intelligence Center (AFMIC)
6. Armed Forces Epidemiology Board (AFEB)
7. Global Epidemiology Working Group (GEWG)

NAVY
1. Navy Medical Research and Development Command (NMRDC)
2. Navy Medical Research Units (NAMRU):
   - Indonesia
   - Philippines
   - Egypt
   - Peru

Public Health Service

NATIONAL INSTITUTES OF HEALTH (NIH)

1. Fogarty International Center
2. National Institute of Allergy and Infectious Diseases (NIAID)
   * International Collaborations in AIDS Research (ICAR)
       Mexico (Harvard University)
       Senegal (Harvard University)
       Malawi (Johns Hopkins University)
       Uganda (Case Western Reserve University)
       Zaire (Tufts University)
       Brazil (Cornell University)
   * International Collaborations in Infectious Disease
       Research (ICIDR)
       Brazil (Salvador) (Cornell University)
       Brazil (Forteleza) (University of Virginia)
       Brazil (Belo Horizonte) (Vanderbilt University)
       Brazil (Osvaldo Cruz Institute) (Harvard University)
       Venezuela (Albert Einstein College)
       Sudan (Brigham Young University)
       Israel (Columbia University)
   * Tropical Medicine Research Centers (TMRC)
       Colombia
       Brazil
       Philippines
   * Intramural
       Malaria Research and Training Center, Mali
       Ain Shams University, Egypt (research on vectors of
       disease)
   * International Tropical Medicine Research Network (not
       yet operational)

CENTERS FOR DISEASE CONTROL (CDC)

1. National Center for Infectious Diseases (NCID)
2. National Center for Prevention Services (NCPS)
3. Medical Entomology Unit, Guatemala
4. Epidemic Intelligence Service   (EIS)
   * Egypt
   * Puerto Rico
   * Sierra Leone
5. Field Epidemiology Training Projects (FETP)

- Thailand
- Indonesia
- Mexico
- Taiwan
- Saudi Arabia

International

World Health Organization, Geneva, Switzerland

1. Special Programme for Research and Training in Tropical
   Diseases (TDR)
2. Special Programme for Control of Diarrheal Diseases
3. International Centre for Diarrheal Disease Research,
   Bangladesh (ICDDR,B)
4. WHO Collaborating Centres: the WHO sponsors collaborations
   between laboratories around the world on many research topics,
   including such infectious disease subspecialties as:
   - Acquired immunodeficiency syndrome
   - AIDS research (Projet SIDA)
   - Arbovirus reference and research
   - Enteric phage typing
   - Epidemiology of leptospirosis
   - Epidemiology training
   - Evaluation and testing of new insecticides
   - Host and parasite studies on malaria
   - Immunization activities
   - *Klebsiella*
   - *Mycobacterium leprae*
   - Mycotic diseases
   - Plague
   - Reference and research in enteroviruses
   - Reference and research in *Escherichia*
   - Reference and research in rabies
   - Reference and research in *Shigella*
   - Reference and research in syphilis serology
   - Reference and research on viral hepatitis
   - Research, training, and eradication of dracunculiasis
   - Rickettsial reference and research
   - *Salmonella*
   - Smallpox and other poxvirus infections
   - *Staphylococcus* phage typing
   - Surveillance, epidemiology, and control of influenza

- Trepanomatoses
- Virus reference and research (respiratory virus diseases other than influenza)
- Virus reference and research (special pathogens)

5. Pan American Health Organization (PAHO)—network of surveillance labs:

- Osvaldo Cruz Foundation (FIOCRUZ), Rio de Janeiro, Brazil
- Carlos Malbran Institute, Buenos Aires, Argentina
- National Institute of Health, Bogota, Colombia
- National Hygiene Institute "Rafael Rangel", Caracas, Venezuela
- Central American Nutrition Institute (INCAP), Guatemala, Guatemala
- Caribbean Epidemiology Center (CAREC), Port of Spain, Trinidad
- Evandro Chagas Institute, Belem, Brazil
- National Health Institute, Santiago, Chile
- National Institute for Diagnosis and Epidemiological Reference (INDRE), Mexico City, Mexico

Pasteur Institutes
- Algiers, Algeria
- Brabant, Belgium
- Bangui, Central African Republic
- Paris, France
- Cayenne, French Guiana
- Noumea, New Caledonia
- Tehran, Iran
- Antananarivo, Madagascar
- Casablanca, Morocco
- Tangier, Morocco
- Dakar, Senegal
- Novi Sad, Yugoslavia

Consultative Group on International Agriculture Research (CGIAR)

The International Clinical Epidemiology Network (INCLEN)

National Epidemiology Boards (NEB)

Community Epidemiology and Health Management Network (CEN)

D

Committee and Staff Biographies

COMMITTEE

JOSHUA LEDERBERG (Co-chair), Ph.D., is University Professor and Sackler Foundation Scholar at Rockefeller University, New York. After receiving his Ph.D. at Yale, he served as professor of genetics at the University of Wisconsin, then at Stanford University, before coming to Rockefeller in 1978. His lifelong research, for which he received the Nobel Prize in 1958, has been in the genetic structure and function of microorganisms. Dr. Lederberg has also been actively involved in artificial intelligence research (in the computer sciences) and in the National Aeronautics and Space Administration experimental programs seeking life on Mars. He has been a consultant for the biotechnology industry (especially Cetus and Affymax Corporations) as well as for government and the international community. (For example, he has long had a keen interest in international health and has served for six years on the World Health Organization's Advisory Health Research Council.) Dr. Lederberg received the National Medal of Science in 1989, at which time his consultative role was specifically cited. He has been a member of the National Academy of Sciences since 1957, and a charter member of the Institute of Medicine; he has also served as chairman of the President's Cancer Panel and now chairs the Congress's Technology Assessment Advisory Council. From 1978 to 1990, Dr. Lederberg served as president of Rockefeller University. As University Professor, he continues his research activities there in the field of transcriptional specificities of bacterial mutagenesis.

ROBERT E. SHOPE (Co-chair), M.D., is professor of epidemiology at the Yale University School of Medicine. Internationally known for his ex-

265

pertise in discovering and identifying newly emerged microbes, he was a member of the teams that found and characterized Lassa virus, the rabies-related viruses, Lyme disease, and, most recently, the virus that causes Venezuelan hemorrhagic fever. The Yale Arbovirus research unit, which he directs, is the World Health Organization Centre for Arbovirus Research and Reference. This center is responsible for supplying diagnostic reference reagents internationally. Dr. Shope is past president of the American Society of Tropical Medicine and Hygiene and a fellow of the American Academy of Microbiology.

BARRY R. BLOOM, Ph.D., is an investigator of the Howard Hughes Medical Institute and Weinstock Professor of Microbiology and Immunology at the Albert Einstein College of Medicine in New York. He received his B.A. degree and an honorary Sc.D. degree from Amherst College, and his Ph.D. from Rockefeller University. He has served as a consultant to the White House on international health, as president of the American Association of Immunologists, and as president of the Federation of American Societies of Experimental Biology. Dr. Bloom is chairman of the Scientific and Technical Advisory Committee to the United Nations Development Program/World Bank/World Health Organization (WHO) Special Program for Vaccine Development. Dr. Bloom also serves on the Board on Science and Technology for International Development of the National Research Council and on the National Vaccine Advisory Board. He is a member of both the National Academy of Sciences and the Institute of Medicine.

ROBERT L. BUCHANAN, Ph.D., is research leader of the Microbial Food Safety Research Unit at the United States Department of Agriculture (USDA) Agricultural Research Service's Eastern Regional Research Center, where he conducts and coordinates research on controlling the transmission of human diseases in foods. He received his Ph.D. in food science from Rutgers University, which was followed by postdoctoral studies in mycotoxicology at the University of Georgia. Prior to joining USDA, he was an associate professor at Drexel University. Dr. Buchanan has served on the National Advisory Committee for Microbiological Criteria for Foods and the International Commission for Microbiological Specifications for Foods. He is a member of the American Academy of Microbiology.

JOHN R. DAVID, M.D. is professor and chairman of the Department of Tropical Public Health at Harvard School of Public Health and professor of medicine at Harvard Medical School. Dr. David received his M.D. from the University of Chicago and is board certified in internal medicine. His research focuses on cellular immunology, especially on the function of migration inhibitory factor (MIF), the first lymphokine, which he co-discovered; and on infectious diseases, primarily leishmaniasis, schistosomiasis, and tuberculosis. He is past president of the American Society of Tropical Medicine and Hygiene and a longtime consultant for the World Health Organization and the Special Program for Research and Training in Tropical Diseases of the World Bank/United Nations Development Fund/World Health Organization.

CIRO A. DE QUADROS, M.D., M.P.H., is the immunization advisor for the Pan American Health Organization (PAHO), the World Health Organization (WHO)'s Regional Office for the Americas. Dr. De Quadros received his M.D. and M.P.H. degrees is his native Brazil, where he began his career in epidemiology and public health. Before joining the WHO in 1970, he worked as a medical officer in health centers in the rural Northeast and Amazon regions of Brazil and taught epidemiology and public health in the National School of Public Health of the Osvaldo Cruz Foundation in Rio de Janeiro. Since 1970, Dr. De Quadros has been active in disease surveillance and control. He was the WHO's chief epidemiologist for the smallpox eradication program in Ethiopia from 1970 to 1977, when he transferred to PAHO in Washington, D.C., to head its Immunization Program. Dr. De Quadros is also adjunct associate professor in the Department of International Health of the Johns Hopkins School of Hygiene and Public Health and has published several papers on the control of vaccine-preventable diseases. He was the recipient of the 1988 Johns Hopkins School of Hygiene and Public Health Dean's Medal and the 1989 Child Survival Award, presented by the U.S. Committee for UNICEF and the Task Force for Child Survival.

PATRICIA N. FULTZ, Ph.D., is associate professor in the Department of Microbiology at the University of Alabama at Birmingham School of Medicine, and holds the title of scientist in the university's Center for AIDS Research and Comprehensive Cancer Center. Dr. Fultz received her Ph.D. from the University of Texas at Dallas and previously held positions as a visiting scientist at the Centers for Disease Control, where she was head of the AIDS Animal Model Studies, and as research associate professor at Emory University. She has served on numerous National Institutes of Health ad hoc research review groups and committees related to animal models for AIDS, as a consultant to the World Health Organization on this same subject, and as a consultant to French and German organizations involved in human immunodeficiency virus vaccine development. Currently, Dr. Fultz is a member of the NIH AIDS Related Research Review Group ARR-A and is on the editorial board of *AIDS Research and Human Retroviruses* and the *Journal of Medical Primatology*. Her primary research interests are in the pathogenesis of retroviral infections and vaccine development.

JOHN J. HOLLAND, Ph.D., is a professor in the Department of Biology and Institute for Molecular Biology at the University of California at San Diego. He received his Ph.D. at the University of California at Los Angeles and did postdoctoral work at the University of Minnesota. Dr. Holland has been a member of the faculties of the University of Minnesota, University of Washington, and University of California at Irvine prior to assuming his present position. He and his colleagues have investigated cellular, molecular, and biochemical aspects of infection by RNA viruses. Their present research interests center on the extreme genetic variability of RNA virus genomes, their heterogenous population structure, and their capacity for considerable biological adaptability and rapid evolution.

DEAN T. JAMISON, Ph.D., is staff director for the World Bank's *World Development Report*, 1993, in the Office of the Chief Economist of the World Bank. He is there on leave from the University of California at Los Angeles where he is a professor in the Department of Community Health Sciences and in the Department of Education. Professor Jamison's research interests lie in the economics of health and education. In particular, his current focus is on cost-effectiveness assessment of health interventions in developing countries; he is co-editing a major reference volume in this area, *Disease Control Priorities in Developing Countries* (forthcoming from Oxford University Press). Dr. Jamison serves as co-chair of the Institute of Medicine's Board on International Health and is a member of the Scientific and Technical Advisory Committee of the World Health Organization's Special Programme for Research and Training in Tropical Diseases.

EDWIN D. KILBOURNE, M.D., is Distinguished Service Professor at the Mount Sinai School of Medicine. He is a physician-virologist who has held professorships in medicine, public health, and microbiology. His special research interest is influenza in all its aspects, and he has made important contributions to our knowledge of influenza virus genetics, epidemiology, and vaccine development. Dr. Kilbourne is the author or co-author of books on influenza, preventive medicine and human ecology, and public health. He is a member of the National Academy of Sciences and is currently chairman of the board of directors of the Aaron Diamond AIDS Research Center of the City of New York.

ADEL A. F. MAHMOUD, M.D., Ph.D., is John H. Hord Professor and chairman of the Department of Medicine, Case Western Reserve University, and physician-in-chief of the University Hospitals of Cleveland. He received his M.D. from the University of Cairo and his Ph.D. from the University of London. Dr. Mahmoud's research focuses on the epidemiology and immunology of schistosomiasis and other major global helminthic infections, as well as the biology and function of eosinophils. He serves on the World Health Organization's Advisory Board Panel on Parasitic Diseases as well as the National Advisory Allergy and Infectious Diseases Council. Dr. Mahmoud is co-editor of *Tropical and Geographic Medicine*. He has been the recipient of many awards including the Bailey K. Ashford Medal of the American Society of Tropical Medicine and Hygiene and the Squibb Award of the Infectious Diseases Society of America. He currently serves as president of the International Society of Infectious Diseases.

GERALD L. MANDELL, M.D., is Owen R. Cheatham Professor of the Sciences, professor of medicine, and chief of infectious diseases at the University of Virginia. He received his M.D. from Cornell University Medical College. Dr. Mandell is co-editor of *Principles and Practice of Infectious Diseases*, as well as president-elect of the Infectious Diseases Society of America and former chairman of the American Board of Internal Medicine's Section on Infectious Diseases. His research, for which he holds a MERIT Award from the National Institutes of Health, has focused on the biology of phagocytic cells.

STEPHEN S. MORSE, Ph.D., is assistant professor at Rockefeller University in New York, where he has been on the faculty since 1985. Prior to that time, he was assistant professor of microbiology at Rutgers University. A virologist and immunologist, Dr. Morse received his Ph.D. from the University of Wisconsin-Madison and was a National Cancer Institute postdoctoral fellow in the Department of Microbiology and Immunology of the Medical College of Virginia. Dr. Morse chaired the organizing committee and was chair of the Conference on Emerging Viruses, sponsored by the National Institute of Allergy and Infectious Diseases and the Fogarty International Center of the National Institutes of Health (NIH), in conjunction with Rockefeller University, which was held in Washington in May 1989; he was also a member of the organizing committee of the NIH Conference on Emerging Microbes and Microbial Diseases, Washington, November 1991, and a consultant to the Congress's Office of Technology Assessment in 1989–1990. He is the editor of *Emerging Viruses* (Oxford University Press, 1992) and of the forthcoming *Evolutionary Biology of Viruses* (Raven Press). Dr. Morse is a councillor of the Microbiology Section, New York Academy of Sciences, and a corporation member of the Marine Biological Laboratory (Woods Hole); professional society memberships include the American Association of Immunologists, American Society for Microbiology, American Society for Virology, American Association of Pathologists, and Sigma Xi. His research has addressed viral effects on T lymphocyte development and function, using mouse thymic virus as a model. (This is a naturally occurring mouse herpesvirus that causes the deletion of $CD4^+$ cells in the developing thymus.)   He has also investigated methods for studying viral evolution.

JUNE E. OSBORN, M.D., is dean and professor of epidemiology at the University of Michigan School of Public Health and professor of pediatrics and communicable diseases in the Medical School.   She is trained as a virologist as well as a pediatric infectious disease specialist and has served in a number of advisory roles for the federal government, universities, and private foundations.   Dr. Osborn was elected to membership in the Institute of Medicine in 1986 and was a member of the steering committee for the National Academy of Sciences/Institute of Medicine study, *Confronting AIDS*. Currently, she is a member of the World Health Organization's Global Commission on AIDS and since 1989 has served as chair of the U.S. National Commission on AIDS.

WILLIAM C. REEVES, Ph.D., is professor emeritus of epidemiology in the School of Public Health at the University of California at Berkeley, where he has been a faculty member since 1946; he served as dean of the school from 1967 to 1971.   He received the doctorate in medical entomology and parasitology in 1943 and the M.P.H. in epidemiology in 1949 from the University of California at Berkeley.   He has served as a consultant to the surgeons general of the U.S. Army and the U.S. Public Health Service and to the National Institute of Allergy and Infectious Diseases, Centers for Disease Control, World Health Organization, and Pan American Health Organization.   He is past president of the American Society of Tropical Medicine and Hygiene and has been the recipient of many awards including the Walter Reed Medal from the above society, the John Snow Award from the American Public Health Association, and the Medal for Distinguished Civilian Service to the U.S. Army.   Dr. Reeve's research has focused on the epidemiology and control of vector-borne diseases.

PHILIP K. RUSSELL, M.D., is professor of international health at the Johns Hopkins School of Hygiene and Public Health.   He received his M.D. from the University of Rochester in 1958 and, following an internship, began a 31-year career in the U.S. Army Medical Department.   Dr. Russell served in various positions during his career with the Army, including director and commandant of the Walter Reed Army Institute of Research, assistant surgeon general for research and development, and commander of the U.S. Army Medical Research and Development Command.   He received several awards for his work, including the Distinguished Service Medal, before retiring as a major general in 1990.   Dr. Russell has served on numerous scientific committees and is presently a member of the Board of Scientific Counselors of the National Center for Infectious Diseases,

Centers for Disease Control, and chairman of the Management Committee of the Children's Vaccine Initiative Consultative Group. He is also scientific advisor to the National Vaccine Program and a consultant in infectious diseases to the surgeon general of the Army.

ALEXIS SHELOKOV, M.D., is director of medical affairs—and, until recently, director of vaccine research—at the Salk Institute, Government Services Division. Born and raised in China, he developed an early interest in epidemic infectious diseases; following graduation from Stanford University Medical School and a period of clinical training, he made a career commitment to study the etiology, pathogenesis, and epidemiology of epidemic infectious diseases, as a basis for their control and prevention. Dr. Shelokov served as virology laboratory chief at the National Institutes of Health and has held professorships in microbiology at the University of Texas and in epidemiology at Johns Hopkins University. He has been a member of a number of advisory committees for the federal government, universities, and private foundations, as well as for the Pan American Health Organization and World Health Organization. Dr. Shelokov is board certified in preventive medicine.

P. FREDERICK SPARLING, M.D., is J. Herbert Bate Professor and chairman of the Department of Medicine and professor of microbiology and immunology at the University of North Carolina School of Medicine in Chapel Hill. He was formerly Chairman of the Department of Microbiology and Immunology at the same institution. Dr. Sparling is an infectious disease physician and has published extensively in the area of sexually transmitted infections (STI) and bacterial pathogenesis, including particularly *Neisseria gonorrhoeae*, the cause of gonorrhea. In recent years his interests have also included the epidemiology, treatment, and prevention of STIs, and behaviors as risk factors for the acquisition of these infections. He now directs an STI Cooperative Research Center, one of five recently established in the United States. The focus of the center is the molecular basis of pathogenesis by multiple microorganisms that cause STIs and the epidemiological and behavioral factors that contribute to STIs in rural core transmitter populations. Dr. Sparling has been a member of numerous national organizations and has chaired a National Institutes of Health/National Institute of Allergy and Infectious Diseases) study section. Among his honors he lists receipt of the Joseph Smadel Award from the Infectious Diseases Society of America.

ANDREW SPIELMAN, Ph.D., is professor of tropical public health at the Harvard School of Public Health, where he explores the role of arthropods in human disease. His studies on Lyme disease have defined the manner in which ticks, deer, and rodents perpetuate this zoonosis, and developed a now-standard method for malaria diagnosis. He also received the Medal of Honor from the American Mosquito Control Association for establishing the biological basis for the first insect growth regulator. Dr. Spielman holds a Merit Award from the National Institutes of Health and has advised, among others, the United States Agency for International Development, Centers for Disease Control, National Institutes of Health, Pan American Health Organization, and Walter Reed Army Institute of Research.

STAFF

STANLEY C. OAKS, JR., Ph.D., is a study director in the Division of Health Sciences Policy at the Institute of Medicine (IOM). He received his Ph.D. in microbiology from the University of Maryland, College Park. Following a 20-year career in the U.S. Army Medical Department, where he was involved in clinical and research microbiology and vaccine product management, he joined the IOM's Division of International Health in 1990. The report of his previous IOM study, *Malaria: Obstacles and Opportunities*, was published in October 1991. Dr. Oaks is a fellow of the American Academy of Microbiology. His professional interests include clinical microbiology, rickettsial diseases, and tropical infectious diseases.

ELIZABETH E. MEYER is a research associate in the Division of Health Sciences Policy at the Institute of Medicine. She received a B.A. degree in biopsychology from Cornell University. Previously, Ms. Meyer served as research associate for the Institute of Medicine study, *Mapping the Brain and Its Functions*.

Glossary

acaricide   a pesticide that kills mites and ticks.

AIDS   acquired immunodeficiency syndrome, the end stage of HIV disease.

aminoglycoside   a class of antibiotic that acts by inhibiting microbial protein synthesis.

antibody   a protein produced by the immune system in response to the introduction of a substance (an antigen) recognized as foreign by the body's immune system. Antibody interacts with the other components of the immune system and can render the antigen harmless, although for various reasons this may not always occur.

antigen   a molecule capable of eliciting a specific antibody or T-cell response.

antigenic   having the properties of an antigen.

arbovirus   shortened form of arthropod-borne virus. Any of a group of viruses that are transmitted to man and animals by mosquitoes, ticks, and sand flies; they include such agents as yellow fever and eastern, western, and Venezuelan equine encephalitis viruses.

arenavirus   any of a group of viruses composed of pleomorphic virions of varying size, one large and one small segment of single-stranded RNA, and ribosomes within the virions that cause the virus to have a sandy appearance. Examples are Junin, Machupo, and Lassa fever viruses. Rodents are common reservoirs of the arenaviruses.

arthropod   as used in this report, refers to insects and ticks, many of which are medically important as vectors of infectious diseases.

arthropod-borne   capable of being transmitted by insect and tick (arthropod) vectors.

B lymphocyte one of two general categories of lymphocytes (white blood cells) involved in the humoral immune response. When help is provided by T lymphocytes, B lymphocytes produce antibodies against specific antigens.

bacillus rod-shaped bacteria.

bacteremia refers to the presence of bacteria in the blood.

beta-lactam an active portion of an antibiotic (e.g., a penicillin or cephalosporin) that is part of the chemical structure of the antibiotic and that can be neutralized by a beta-lactamase produced by certain microorganisms (e.g., some staphylococci).

beta-lactamase an enzyme that neutralizes the affect of an antibiotic containing beta-lactam.

BL-4 level of containment required for safe handling of the most contagious pathogenic microbes.

calicivirus a family of small viruses; includes vesicular exanthem and seal plague viruses.

carbapenem a class of antibiotic.

cellular immunity, cell-mediated immunity a type of immune response in which subpopulations of T-cells (helper T-cells and killer T-cells) cooperate to destroy cells in the body that bear foreign antigens, such as bacteria.

cephalosporin a class of antibiotic.

clonal of or pertaining to a group of genetically identical organisms derived from a single parent or a DNA population derived from a single DNA molecule by replication in a bacterial or eucaryotic host cell.

coagulase-negative refers to the inability of an organism, particularly staphylococci, to produce an enzyme that, in concert with a blood plasma cofactor, catalyzes the formation of fibrin from fibrinogen.

coding sequence the order of nucleotide bases in a nucleic acid that specifies the production of a particular product, such as a protein. A change in the coding sequence (e.g., as a result of a mutation) can result in a change in the product.

DDT 1,1,1-trichloro-2,2-bis(*p*-chlorophenyl)ethane or chlorophenothane, a pesticide.

deletion mutation a mutation that results from the deletion of one or more amino acids present in the genetic material of the organism undergoing the mutation.

disease as used in this report, refers to a situation in which infection has elicited signs and symptoms in the infected individual; the infection has become clinically apparent.

DNA   deoxyribonucleic acid, a carrier of genetic information (i.e., heredi-
tary characteristics) found chiefly in the nucleus of cells.

DNA virus   a virus that contains only DNA as its genetic material.

droplet nuclei   the very small particles of moisture expelled when a person coughs, sneezes, or speaks that may transfer infectious organisms to
another person who inhales the droplets.

ELISA   enzyme-linked immunosorbent assay. An immunological technique
used for the quantitation of antigen or antibody in a sample such as
blood plasma or serum. In the assay, enzyme-labeled antigen or antibody is bound to a solid surface (such as beads, tubes, or microplate
wells). After addition of the sample and a substrate, the presence of
the desired antigen, antibody, or antigen-antibody complex is indicated by a color change based on a reaction of the enzyme with the
substrate.

endemic   the condition in which a disease is present in a human community at all times.

endogenous   developing or originating from within the individual.

enzootic   refers to a disease (can be either low or high morbidity) that is
endemic in an animal community.

epidemic   the condition in which a disease spreads rapidly through a community in which that disease is normally not present or is present at a
low level.

epizootic   a disease of generally high morbidity that spreads rapidly through
an animal population.

escape mutant   refers to the formation of a mutation in a population of
microorganisms that allows the mutant organism to escape the immune
response directed against it.

etiologic agent   the organism that causes a disease.

etiology   the cause or origin of a disease.

fluoroquinolone   a class of antibiotic.

genetic adaptability   the ability of a microorganism to adapt to its environment, often allowing it to avoid detection or an immune response
generated against it.

genome   the complete genetic composition of an organism (e.g., human,
bacterium, protozoan, helminth, or fungus), contained in a chromosome
or set of chromosomes or in a DNA or RNA molecule (e.g., a virus).

gram-negative   refers to the inability of a microorganism to accept a certain stain. This inability is related to the cell wall composition of the
microorganism and has been useful in classifying bacteria.

gram-positive   refers to the ability of a microorganism to retain a certain stain. This ability is related to the cell wall composition of the microorganism and has been useful in classifying bacteria.

hemagglutinin a molecule, such as an antibody or lectin, that agglutinates red blood cells.

hemorrhagic fever a group of diverse, severe epidemic viral infections of worldwide distribution but occurring especially in tropical countries that are usually transmitted to humans by arthropod bites or contact with virus-infected rodents or monkeys and that share common clinicopathologic features (e.g., fever, hemorrhaging, shock, thrombocytopenia, neurological disturbances). Examples are Argentine, Bolivian, and Venezuelan hemorrhagic fevers; chikungunya; Rift Valley fever; and Ebola and Marburg virus diseases.

HIV disease the broad spectrum of opportunistic infections and diseases that occur in an individual infected with the human immunodeficiency virus.

humoral immunity antibody-mediated immunity; one of the mechanisms, using antibodies found in the blood and other body fluids, that the body uses to fight off infections.

hyperendemic the condition in which a disease is present in a community at all times and with a high incidence.

iatrogenic any adverse condition, such as an infection, in an individual occurring as the result of treatment by a physician.

immunocompromised a condition (caused, for example, by the administration of immunosuppressive drugs or irradiation, malnutrition, aging, or a condition such as cancer or HIV disease) in which an individual's immune system is unable to respond adequately to a foreign substance.

immunosuppression the retardation or cessation of an immune response as a result of, for example, anticancer drugs.

incidence as used in epidemiology, the number of new cases of a disease that occur in a defined population within a specified time period; the rate of occurrence.

infection implies that an agent, such as a virus or bacterium, has taken up residence in a host and is multiplying within that host—perhaps with no outward signs of disease. Thus, it is possible to be infected with an agent but not have the disease commonly associated with that agent (although disease may develop at a later time).

intramolecular recombination recombination that occurs within a single molecule, as opposed to between two molecules.

larvicide a material used to kill larval forms of pests and disease vectors.

lentivirus a subfamily of the retroviruses.

mechanical vector a vector, not essential to the life cycle of the agent, that transmits an agent without itself becoming infected.

microbial traffic the transfer of existing microbes to new host populations.

monoclonal antibody immunoglobulins derived from a single clone of plasma cells. Monoclonal antibodies constitute a pure population because they are produced by a single clone in vitro and are chemically and structurally identical.

mutation a transmissible change in the genetic material of an organism, usually in a single gene.

neuraminidase sialidase; an enzyme that catalyzes the hydrolysis of glucosidic linkages between a sialic acid residue and a hexose or hexosamine residue in glycoproteins, glycolipids, and proteoglycans. Neuraminidase is a major antigen of myxoviruses.

nonsense mutation a mutation in which one of the three terminator codons (used to signal the end of a polypeptide) in messenger RNA appears in the middle of a genetic message, causing premature termination of transcription, resulting in the production of generally nonfunctional polypeptides.

nosocomial infection hospital-acquired infection; an infection not present or incubating prior to admittance to the hospital.

opportunistic infection an infection caused by an organism that ordinarily does not cause disease but under circumstances such as impaired immunity, becomes pathogenic.

organoleptic capable of receiving a sense impression. Organoleptic inspections are based on sensory perceptions (e.g., fish smells fresh or spoiled).

pandemic an epidemic that occurs worldwide.

pathogen a microorganism that causes disease.

pathogenic capable of causing disease.

PCR see polymerase chain reaction.

plasmid an extrachromosomal, self-replicating structure found in bacterial cells that carries genes for a variety of functions not essential for cell growth. Plasmids consist of cyclic double-stranded DNA molecules that replicate independently of the chromosomes and can be transmitted from one cell to another by conjugation or transduction. Episomes are genetic elements that can replicate in either of two alternative states—independently in the cytoplasm or as an integrated portion of the bacterial chromosome.

point mutation a mutation resulting from a change in a single base pair in the DNA molecule, resulting from the substitution of one nucleotide for another.

polymerase chain reaction a laboratory method of amplifying low levels of specific microbial DNA or RNA sequences.

polymorphic appearing in different forms.

prevalence as used in epidemiology, the total number of cases of a disease in existence at a specific time and within a well-defined area; the percentage of a population affected by a particular disease at a given time.

provirus the genome of a virus integrated into the chromosome of the host cell. It is transmitted to all daughter cells.

quasispecies a mixture of distinct but closely related viral genomes that exists in a virus-infected individual.

recombination the formation of new combinations of genes as a result of crossing over (sharing of genes) between structurally similar chromosomes, resulting in progeny with different gene combinations than in the parents.

reservoir any person, animal, arthropod, plant, soil, or substance (or combination of these) in which an infectious agent normally lives and multiplies, on which it depends primarily for survival, and in which it reproduces itself in such manner that it can be transmitted to a susceptible vector.

retrovirus any of a large family of RNA viruses that includes lentiviruses and oncoviruses, so called because they carry reverse transcriptase.

reverse transcriptase RNA-directed DNA polymerase; an enzyme, such as is found in the human immunodeficiency virus, that catalyzes the reaction that uses RNA as a template for double-stranded DNA synthesis.

RNA ribonucleic acid.

RNA virus a virus that contains RNA as its genetic material.

selective pressure pressure exerted on an organism by its environment that causes a change in the organism's ability to cope with that environment.

septicemia, septicemic systemic disease associated with the presence and persistence of microorganisms in the blood.

seroconversion the change of a serologic test result from negative to positive as a result of antibodies induced by the introduction of microorganisms into the host.

serological the use of immune serum in any of a number of tests (agglutination, precipitation, enzyme-linked immunosorbent assay, etc.) used to measure the response (antibody titer) to infectious disease; the use of serological reactions to detect antigen.

seronegative   negative result in a serological test; that is, the inability to detect the antibodies or antigens being tested for.

seropositive   positive result in a serological test.

serotype   the characterization of a microorganism based on the kinds and combinations of constituent antigens present in that organism; a taxonomic subdivision of bacteria based on the above.

slow virus   any virus causing a disease characterized by a very long preclinical course and a very gradual progression of symptoms.

strain   a subgrouping of organisms within a species, characterized by some particular quality.

syndrome   a set of symptoms that may occur concurrently.

tubercle bacillus   the bacterium that causes tuberculosis, *Mycobacterium tuberculosis.*

variolation   a procedure, not used today, in which material from the pustule of an individual infected with smallpox (variola virus) was scratched into the skin of an infected person to induce immunity to the disease.

vector   a carrier, especially an arthropod, that transfers an infective agent from one host (which can include itself) to another.

vector-borne   transmitted from one host to another by a vector.

virulence   the degree of pathogenicity of an organism as evidenced by the severity of resulting disease and the organism's ability to invade the host tissues.

zoonosis   a disease of animals transmissible to humans.

zoonotic pool   the population of animals infected with nonhuman microbes that present a potential threat of transmission to humans.

Acronyms and Abbreviations

AABB – American Association of Blood Banks
ACIP – Immunization Practices Advisory Committee
AFIP – Armed Forces Institute of Pathology
AIDS – acquired immunodeficiency syndrome
ARC – American Red Cross
ASM – American Society for Microbiology
ATLL – adult T-cell leukemia/lymphoma
AZT – azidothymidine
BCG – bacille Calmette-Guerin
BRDPI – Biomedical Research and Development Price Index
BSE – bovine spongiform encephalopathy
CDC – Centers for Disease Control
CEN – Community Epidemiology and Health Management Network
CERTC – Clinical Epidemiology Research and Training Center
CEU – Clinical Epidemiology Unit
CIN – cervical intraepithelial neoplasia
CMV – cytomegalovirus
CSF – cerebrospinal fluid
DBCP – 1,2-dibromo-3-chloropropane
DDT – 1,1,1-trichloro-2,2-bis(p-chlorophenyl)ethane; chlorophenothane
DHF/DSS – dengue hemorrhagic fever/dengue shock syndrome
DNA – deoxyribonucleic acid
DoD – Department of Defense
DOT – directly observed therapy
EIS – Epidemic Intelligence Service
EPA – Environmental Protection Agency

FCCSET – Federal Coordinating Council for Science, Engineering, and Technology

FDA – Food and Drug Administration

FETP – Field Epidemiology Training Program

FIFRA – Federal Insecticide, Fungicide, and Rodenticide Act

FWS – U.S. Fish and Wildlife Service

GMI – Gorgas Memorial Institute

GML – Gorgas Memorial Laboratory

HAM/TSP – HTLV-I-associated myelopathy/tropical spastic paraparesis

HBV – hepatitis B virus

HFRS – hemorrhagic fever with renal syndrome

HIV – human immunodeficiency virus

HPV – human papillomavirus

HSV – herpes simplex virus

HTLV – human T-cell leukemia virus, human T-lymphotropic virus

IADB – InterAmerican Development Bank

ICAR – International Collaboration in AIDS Research

ICDDR, B – International Center for Diarrheal Disease Research, Bangladesh

ICIDR – International Collaboration in Infectious Disease Research

ICMRT – International Centers for Medical Research and Training

ICTDR – International Centers for Tropical Disease Research

IHPP – International Health Policy Program

INCIDR – Intramural NIAID Center for International Disease Research

INCLEN – International Clinical Epidemiology Network

IOM – Institute of Medicine

MAP – modified atmosphere packaging

MARU – Middle America Research Unit

MDRTB – multidrug-resistant tuberculosis

MIC – minimum inhibitory concentration

MMR – measles-mumps-rubella (vaccine)

MRSA – methicillin-resistant *Staphylococcus aureus*

NAMRU – U.S. Navy Medical Research Unit

NCID – National Center for Infectious Diseases

NCVDG – National Cooperative Vaccine Development Group

NEB – National Epidemiology Boards

NETSS – National Electronic Telecommunications System for Surveillance

NHSC – National Health Service Corps

NIAID – National Institute of Allergy and Infectious Diseases

NIH – National Institutes of Health

NNDSS – National Notifiable Disease Surveillance System

NNISS – National Nosocomial Infections Surveillance System

PAHO – Pan American Health Organization

PCR – polymerase chain reaction

PHS – U.S. Public Health Service
RFP – request for proposal
RNA – ribonucleic acid
SIV – simian immunodeficiency virus
STD – sexually transmitted disease
TB – tuberculosis
TDR – WHO Special Programme for Research and Training in Tropical
   Diseases
TDRU – Tropical Disease Research Unit
TMRC – Tropical Medicine Research Center
USAID – U.S. Agency for International Development
USAMRIID – U.S. Army Medical Research Institute of Infectious Diseases
USDA – U.S. Department of Agriculture
UTI – urinary tract infection
VDP – WHO Vaccine Development Programme
VRDB – Vaccine Research and Development Branch
WHO – World Health Organization
YARU – Yale Arbovirus Research Unit

Index

B

Babesiosis, 76, 248-249
Bacillus microbial control agents,
    102
Bacteria, 53, 63
    genetic changes, 89-92
    listing of, 36-37, 199-217
    passim
    virulence factors, 89-90, 91
    see also specific types
Behavioral factors, 1, 14, 48, 67,
    167-168
    see also Diet; Drug abuse; Land
    use factors; Sexual behavior;
    Travel
Beta-lactam antibiotics, 94
Bilge water, 81, 107
Biological control agents, 165
Biorational pesticides, 165
Biotechnology, 20
    attenuated organisms, 153-154
Birds, 30
Black Death, 17
Blood contamination, 59, 60, 78*n*
Body lice, 112
Borrelia burgdorferi, 28, 72, 76,
    200-202
Botulism, 66
Bovine spongiform encephalopathy
    (BSE), 64-65, 217-218
Brazilian purpuric fever, 90-92,
    208
Bubonic plague, 17, 22

C

Caliciviruses, 46-47
California, vector control in, 162
California serogroup viruses, 218-
    219
Campylobacter jejuni, 202-203
Candida, 249-250
Catheterization, 59

Cell lines, and virus infection, 82,
    84
Cellulitis, 199-200
Centers for Disease Control
    (CDC), 9, 11, 130, 131, 147-
    148, 164
    Division of Vector-Borne
        Infectious Diseases, 162
    Epidemic Intelligence Service
        (EIS), 9, 148
    Field Epidemiology Training
        Program (FETP), 9, 148
    Foreign Quarantine Division, 23
    Hospital Infections Program, 4,
        58, 121
    Immunization Practices
        Advisory Committee (ACIP),
        153
    National Center for Infectious
        Diseases (NCID), 9, 147
    National Nosocomial Infections
        Surveillance System
        (NNISS), 4, 58, 121-122
    National Notifiable Diseases
        Surveillance System
        (NNDSS), 3, 118-120
    overseas labs, 126, 262-263
    quarantine stations, 22-23
    surveillance activities, 5, 118-
        123, 131, 138-139
    vaccine purchase, 153-138
Cervical cancer, 105-106
Ceviche, 69, 107
Chickens, 19
Chikungunya virus, 44, 219-220
Children, vaccination of, 138, 155
China
    influenza monitoring, 130
    schistosomiasis outbreak, 112
Chlamydia spp., 36, 105, 203-205
Chloroquine, 29, 100-101
Cholera, 68, 107-108, 139, 215-
    216